# MEDICAL
# ENCYCLOPEDIA
# OF MOSES
# MAIMONIDES

# MEDICAL ENCYCLOPEDIA OF MOSES MAIMONIDES

## FRED ROSNER

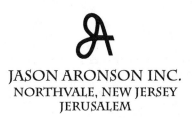

JASON ARONSON INC.
NORTHVALE, NEW JERSEY
JERUSALEM

This book was set in 11 pt. Galliard by Alpha Graphics in Pittsfield, NH.

**Library of Congress Cataloging-in-Publication Data**
Rosner, Fred.
    Medical encyclopedia of Moses Maimonides / by Fred Rosner.
        p.   cm.
    Includes index.
    ISBN 0-7657-5997-7 (alk. paper)
    1. Maimonides, Moses, 1135-1204—Contributions in medicine.
2. Medicine in rabbinical literature.   3. Medicine, Medieval.
I. Title.
R135.5.R665   1998
610'.9'02—dc21

97-41034
CIP

Manufactured in the United States of America. Jason Aronson Inc. offers books and cassettes. For information and catalog write to Jason Aronson Inc., 230 Livingston Street, Northvale, NJ 07647.

"Blessings rest on a man's home only on account
of his wife" (Baba Metzia 59a)


TO SARANNE


given to me as "a precious gift" (Yebamot 63b)
in honor of our fortieth year of marriage

# CONTENTS

# Contents

# Contents

# Contents

# Contents

# Contents

# PREFACE

My interest in Moses Maimonides was markedly enhanced during my post doctoral training in internal medicine and hematology at Maimonides Medical Center in Brooklyn, New York. That is when I began a ten year collaboration with the late Professor Suessman Muntner of Jerusalem, Israel, in the translation into English of the ten authentic medical treatises of Maimonides, which he had edited and published in Hebrew. In 1969, our translation of *Maimonides' Treatises on Hemorrhoids and Responsa* appeared (Lippincott) followed by *The Medical Aphorisms of Moses Maimonides* (Yeshiva University, Vol. 1, 1970, Vol. 2, 1971; reprinted by Bloch in 1973).

In 1974, I published *Sex Ethics in the Writings of Maimonides* (Bloch; reprinted by Jason Aronson in 1994), followed by *Maimonides' Glossary of Drug Names* in 1979 (American Philosophical Society) and *Medicine in the Mishneh Torah of Maimonides* in 1984 (Ktav; reprinted by Jason Aronson in 1997). Over the next decade, the Maimonides Research Institute in Haifa, Israel, published all ten authentic Maimonidean medical writings in seven volumes. These are *Maimonides' Treatises on Poisons, Hemorrhoids and Cohabitation* (1984); his *Commentary on the Aphorisms of Hippocrates* (1987); *The Medical Aphorisms of Moses Maimonides* (1989); his *Three Treatises on Health* (1990); his *Extracts from Galen: The Art of Cure* (1992); his *Treatise on Asthma* (1993); and his *Glossary of Drug Names* (1995). Professor Kottek and I edited the Proceedings of a Conference on *Moses Maimonides: Physician, Scientist and Philosopher* (Jason Aronson, 1993) and I recently published *The Medical Legacy of Moses Maimonides* (Ktav, 1998).

My interest in Maimonides is not limited to his medical writings. In 1975, I published an English translation of Maimonides' *Introduction to His Mishnah Commentary* (Feldheim; reprinted by Jason Aronson in 1995) followed by his *Mishnah Commentary on Tractate Sanhedrin* (Sepher-Hermon, 1981). I also translated and annotated *Maimonides' Treatise on Resurrection* (Ktav, 1982; reprinted by Jason Aronson in 1997). Finally, I published *The Existence and Unity of God, Three Trea-*

*tises Attributed to Moses Maimonides* (Jason Aronson, 1990) and *Six Treatises Attributed to Maimonides* (Jason Aronson, 1991). The latter two books represent edited and annotated translations of several spurious works falsely attributed to Maimonides, including the famous "Physician's Prayer," which was probably authored by Marcus Herz in Germany in 1783. Western readers now have access to the medical and non-medical writings of the great medieval Sage, Moses Maimonides. The present *Medical Encyclopedia of Moses Maimonides* allows the English reader to quickly access Maimonides' views on many medical topics and provides source material and references for the interested reader who wishes to obtain more detail on a specific subject.

I am greatly indebted to Professor Jacob Dienstag for suggesting the idea of an Encyclopedia of Maimonides and to Professor Samuel Kottek for writing the Foreword. Both men have been a source of encouragement and scholarship for me over the years. I consult with them frequently on Maimonidean-related matters. I thank the publisher Mr. Arthur Kurzweil and his dedicated staff of professionals at Jason Aronson, Inc., for the high quality and attractive format of the *Encyclopedia*. I am also thankful to my secretary, Mrs. Mary Sozomenu, for secretarial assistance.

Fred Rosner, M.D.

# FOREWORD

In October 1990, only a few weeks before the Gulf War, we organized in Jerusalem a conference on the topic "Moses Maimonides, Physician, Scientist and Philosopher." In the brief introductory remarks he provided for the book of Proceedings of the conference, which Professor Rosner and I edited together, my late mentor Professor Joshua Leibowitz remarked: "In medicine, as in other spheres of human civilization, we can find inspiration and guidance in a physician of the past, broadminded, striving for accomplishment, scholar and humanist." This physician, this scholar, this humanist, was, of course, Moses ben Maimon, alias Maimonides.

In addition to a long series of works devoted to Biblical and Talmudic Medicine, to Medical Ethics, to Medicine and Jewish Law, Fred Rosner has dedicated most of his amazing activity to the translation and edition of Maimonides' medical works. Between 1984 and 1995, the ten medical works of Maimonides appeared in English, handsomely published by the Maimonides Research Institute (Haifa, Israel). These translations are not heavy critical editions aimed at specialists of medieval and/or Jewish-Arabic medical literature. They are easy to read, though provided with explanatory notes and occasional bibliographical details. Fred Rosner has also gathered medical and paramedical data from Maimonides' *Mishneh Torah* (1984). This book was translated into French in 1992. Rosner has moreover offered a translation of the Introduction to the *Commentary on the Mishnah* (1975, reprinted 1996) and an edition of the *Treatise on Resurrection* (1982, reprinted 1997). He has even edited several spurious works that had been attributed to Maimonides (1991). Few living scholars, if any, can claim to have such a wide and comprehensive familiarity with Maimonides' medical works.

It was therefore quite logical, while taking into consideration the wide interest that Maimonides arouses among physicians and laypeople,

Jewish as well as Gentile, that Fred Rosner would undertake the project that gave birth to the present volume. This *Medical Encyclopedia of Moses Maimonides* will be a convenient tool for those who wish to conduct research on medical and para-medical topics through Maimonides' works. After an introduction on the life and works of Maimonides, Rosner provides some 450 entries of different length on items that include diseases, materia medica, hygiene, medical ethics and halakhah, and names of scholars and translators related to Maimonidean scholarship.

Such a compilation forcibly implies a choice—Rosner's choice: one who possesses the broadest knowledge is obviously the most able to choose key-words. This Encyclopedia of Maimonides' statements of medical and para-medical interest is a testimony of Rosner's outstanding contribution to this topic on which he has been toiling for more than thirty years.

Samuel S. Kottek, M.D.
The Harry Friedenwald Chair of History of Medicine
The Hebrew University-Hadassah Medical School

# MOSES MAIMONIDES
# THE PHYSICIAN

Moses, son of Maimon (acronym RaMBaM in Hebrew, Abu Imram Musa Ibn Maimun in Arabic, and Maimonides in Greek) was born in Cordova, Spain, on March 30, 1138, corresponding to Passover eve of the Hebrew year 4898. His mother died in childbirth, and consequently his father *dayan* (judge) Maimon raised him. Persecution by the Almohades, a fanatical group from North Africa, forced the Maimon family to flee Cordova in the year 1148. The family wandered through southern Spain and northern Africa for the next ten years and finally settled in Fez, Morocco.

Little is known of Maimonides' early life and medical education. There are no sources indicating that Maimonides had any formal medical education. In his *Medical Aphorisms*, he mentions "the elders before whom I have read"; this is a rare allusion to some semiprivate study of medicine. A few times he mentions the son of Ibn Zuhr, from whom he heard teachings of the latter's illustrious father

(the great physician Abu Merwan Ibn Zuhr), whom Maimonides held in great esteem.

Maimonides must have been an avid reader, since his medical writings show a profound knowledge of ancient Greek authors in Arabic translations and Moslem medical works. Hippocrates, Galen, and Aristotle were some of his Greek medical inspirations, and Rhazes of Persia, al-Farabi, and Ibn Zuhr, the Spanish-Arabic physician, are Moslem authors frequently quoted by Maimonides.

The Maimon family left Morocco in 1165, traveled to Palestine, landing in Acco, and from there went to Egypt, where they settled in Fostat (old Cairo). Maimonides turned to medicine as a livelihood after the death of his father in 1166 and the death of his brother in a shipwreck shortly thereafter. Maimonides was left with his brother's wife and child to support, and, after a year's illness following his brother's death, entered into the practice of medicine. He was appointed Court Physician to Vizier

*1*

al-Fadhil, Regent of Egypt during the absence of the Sultan, Saladin the Great, who was fighting in the Crusades in Palestine. It was at this time that Richard the Lion-Hearted, also fighting in the Crusades, is reported to have invited Maimonides to become his personal physician, an offer that Maimonides declined. His reputation as a physician grew in Egypt and neighboring countries, and his fame as theologian and philosopher became worldwide.

In 1193, Saladin died and his eldest son, al-Afdal Nur ad Din Ali, a playboy, succeeded him. As a result, Maimonides' medical duties became even heavier, as described in the famous letter he wrote to his friend, disciple, and translator, Rabbi Samuel Ibn Tibbon, in the year 1199:

I live in Fostat and the Sultan resides in Cairo; these two places are two Sabbath limits [marked-off areas around a town within which it is permitted to move on the Sabbath; approximately 1.5 miles] distant from each other. My duties to the Sultan are very heavy. I am obliged to visit him every day, early in the morning, and when he or any of his children or concubines are indisposed, I cannot leave Cairo but must stay during most of the day in the palace. It also frequently happens that one or two of the officers fall sick and I must attend to their healing. Hence, as a rule, every day, early in the morning, I go to Cairo and, even if nothing unusual happens there, I do not return to Fostat until the afternoon. Then I am famished but I find the antechambers filled with people, both Jews and gentiles, nobles and common people, judges and policemen, friends and enemies—a mixed multitude who await the time of my return.

I dismount from my animal, wash my hands, go forth to my patients, and entreat them to bear with me while I partake of some light refreshment, the only meal I eat in twenty-four hours. Then I go to attend to my patients and write prescriptions and directions for their ailments. Patients go in and out until nightfall, and sometimes, even as the Torah is my faith, until two hours and more into the night. I converse with them and prescribe for them even while lying down from sheer fatigue. When night falls, I am so exhausted that I can hardly speak.

In consequence of this, no Israelite can converse with me or befriend me [on religious or community matters] except on the Sabbath. On that day, the whole congregation, or at least the majority, comes to me after the morning service, when I instruct them as to their proceedings during the whole week. We study together a little until noon, when they depart. Some of them return and read with me after the afternoon services until evening prayer. In this manner, I spend the days. I have here related to you only a part of what you would see if you were to visit me.

Maimonides was also the spiritual leader of the Jewish community of

Egypt. At age 30, in the year 1168, shortly after settling in Fostat, he completed his first major work, the *Commentary on the Mishnah*. In 1178, ten years later, his magnum opus, the *Mishneh Torah*, was finished. This monumental work, a fourteen-book compilation of all biblical and talmudic law, remains a classic to this day. In 1190, Maimonides' great philosophical masterpiece, the *Guide for the Perplexed*, was completed.

Maimonides died on December 13, 1204 (20 Tebet, 4965), and was allegedly buried in Tiberias. Legend relates that Maimonides' body was placed upon a donkey and the animal set loose. The donkey wandered and wandered and finally stopped in Tiberias. That is the site where the great Maimonides was buried.

Maimonides was a prolific writer. We have already noted his famous trilogy, the *Commentary on the Mishnah*, the *Mishneh Torah*, and the *Guide for the Perplexed*. Each of these works alone would have indelibly recorded Maimonides' name for posterity. However, in addition, he also wrote a *Book on Logic* (*Maamar ha-Higayon*), a *Book of Commandments* (*Sefer ha-Mitzvot*), an *Epistle to Yemen* (*Iggeret Teman*), a *Letter of Apostasy* (*Iggeret Hashamad*), a *Treatise on Resurrection* (*Maamar Tahiyat ha-Metim*), commentaries on several tractates of the Talmud, and over six hundred responsa. Several additional works, including the

so-called *Prayer of Maimonides*,[1] are attributed to him but are, in fact, spurious, the prayer having been written in 1783.

Besides all the books we have just enumerated, Maimonides also wrote ten medical works.[2] The first is called *Extracts from Galen*, or *The Art of Cure*. Galen's extensive medical writings required two volumes just to catalogue and index them all. Maimonides, therefore, extracted what he considered the most important of Galen's pronouncements and compiled them verbatim in a small work intended primarily for the use of medical students. This work, like all of Maimonides' medical books, was originally written in Arabic. At least two Arabic manuscripts exist today, one in Hebrew and one in Arabic letters. This work, until recently, had not been published in any language, but brief excerpts therefrom in both English and Hebrew appeared in a Hebrew periodical.[3] A complete English translation by Uri Barzel appeared in 1992.[4]

The second of Maimonides' medical writings is the *Commentary on the Aphorisms of Hippocrates*. The famous aphorisms of Hippocrates were translated from the Greek into Arabic by Hunain Ibn Ishaq in the ninth century. Two incomplete Arabic manuscripts exist. Maimonides wrote his commentary on this translation. A good medieval translation into Hebrew was made by Moses ben Samuel

Ibn Tibbon. In this work, Maimonides occasionally criticizes both Hippocrates and Galen when their views differ from his own. For example, in Chapter 5, Hippocrates is quoted as having said, "A boy is born from the right ovary, a girl from the left," in response to which Maimonides remarks: "A man should be either prophet or genius to know this." The introduction to this work was edited in the original Arabic, with two Hebrew and one German translation, by Steinschneider in 1894.[5] The entire work was published by Hasida in 1935[6] and again in a definitive edition by Muntner in 1961.[7] Bar Sela and Hoff published Maimonides' interpretation of the first aphorism of Hippocrates.[8] This is the famous aphorism that has been called the motto or credo of the art of medicine: "Life is short, and the art long, the occasion fleeting, experience fallacious, and judgment difficult. The physician not only must be prepared to do what is right himself, but also must make the patient, the attendants, and the externals cooperate." I have published Maimonides' *Introduction* to this work[9] as well as the entire work[10] in English.

The third, and most voluminous, of Maimonides' medical works is the *Medical Aphorisms of Moses* (*Pirkei Moshe*). This book is composed of fifteen hundred aphorisms based mainly on Greco-Latin medical writers. There are twenty-five chapters,

each dealing with a different area of medicine, including anatomy; physiology; pathology; symptomatology and diagnosis; etiology of disease and therapeutics; fevers; bloodletting; laxatives and emetics; surgery; gynecology; hygiene; exercise; bathing; diet; drugs; and medical curiosities. A complete Arabic original manuscript exists in the Gotha library in Germany. A Hebrew translation was made in the thirteenth century and published in Lemburg, Poland, in 1834 and again in Vilna in 1888.[11] The definitive Hebrew edition is that of Muntner, dated 1959.[12] Maimonides' *Aphorisms*[13] was also translated into Latin in the thirteenth century and appeared as an incunabulum in Bologna in 1489 and again in Venice in 1497, followed by several printed Latin editions.[14] Only small fragments of this work appeared in a western language[15] until the complete English version prepared by Muntner and me was published in two volumes[16] and reprinted.[17] I published a revised and improved translation in 1989.[18]

A few excerpts from this most important work will demonstrate the flavor of Maimonidean medical thinking. Maimonides speaks of cerebrovascular disease: "One can prognosticate regarding a stroke, called apoplexy. If the attack is severe, he will certainly die but if it is minor, then cure is possible, though difficult. . . . The worst situation that can occur following a stroke is the complete irreversible suppression of respiration."

Maimonides explains that diabetes mellitus was seldom seen in cold Europe, whereas it was frequently encountered in warm Africa. He also reports this disease to be associated with the drinking of suave water of the River Nile (Maimonides lived in Fostat, or old Cairo). There follows the English translation of this most important aphorism, no. 69, from the eighth chapter.

> Moses says: I, too, have not seen it in the West [Spain, where Maimonides was born, or Morocco, where he fled from the persecution of the Almohades] nor did any one of my teachers under whom I studied mention that they had seen it [diabetes]. However, here in Egypt, in the course of approximately ten years, I have seen more than twenty people who suffered from this illness. This brings one to the conclusion that this illness occurs mostly in warm countries. Perhaps the waters of the Nile, because of their suaveness, may play a role in this.

An accurate description of obstructive emphysema is provided during a lengthy discussion of respiratory disease: ". . . reason [for respiratory embarrassment] is narrowing of the organs of respiration, then the breast is seen to greatly expand. This expansion produces rapid and cut off [respirations]."

Clubbing of the fingers associated with pulmonary disease, already described by Hippocrates, is beautifully depicted: "With an illness affecting the lungs called *hasal*, namely phthisis, there develops rounding of the nail as a rainbow." The signs and symptoms that occur in pneumonia are remarkably accurately described: "The basic symptoms which occur in pneumonia and which are never lacking are as follows: acute fever, sticking [pleuritic] pain in the side, short rapid breaths, serrated pulse and cough, mostly [associated] with sputum." Hepatitis is just as beautifully described: "The signs of liver inflammation are eight in number as follows: high fever, thirst, complete anorexia, a tongue which is initially red and then turns black, biliary vomitus, initially yellow egg yolk in color which later turns dark green, pain on the right side which ascends up to the clavicle. . . . Occasionally a mild cough may occur and a sensation of heaviness which is first felt on the right side and then spreads widely." Thus, the *Medical Aphorisms of Moses*.[19]

The fourth of Maimonides' medical writings is his *Treatise on Hemorrhoids*. This work was written, as Maimonides says in the introduction, for a nobleman—probably a member of the Sultan's family. There are seven chapters dealing with normal digestion, foods harmful to patients with hemorrhoids, beneficial foods, and general and local therapeutic measures such as sitz baths, oils, and fumigations. Maimonides disapproves of bloodletting or surgery for hemorrhoids except in severe cases. Maimonides' whole approach to the problem seems to bespeak a modern medical trend. The *Treatise on Hemorrhoids* was first published by Kroner in 1911 in Arabic, Hebrew, and German.[20] A general description of the work in English, by Bragman, appeared in 1927.[21] The definitive Hebrew edition is that of Muntner, dated 1965,[22] and an English translation of the entire work was published by me and Muntner in 1969.[23] An improved, more fully annotated English translation was recently published.[24] In the introduction to this work, Maimonides describes the reason for writing it:

> There was a youth, [descended] from knowledgeable, intelligent and comprehending forebears, from a prominent and renowned family, distinguished and charitable and of great means, in whom the affliction of hemorrhoids occurred at the mouth of the rectum, that interested me in his problem and placed the task [of healing them] upon me. These irritated him on some occasions and he treated them in the customary therapeutic manner until the pain subsided and the protruding hemorrhoids became reduced and returned to the interior of the body so that his [bodily] functions returned to normal. Because this [illness] recurred so many times, he considered having them extirpated in order to uproot this malady from its source so that it not return again. I informed him of the danger inherent

in this, in that it is not clear if these hemorrhoids are of the variety which should be excised or not, since there are people in whom they have once been [surgically] extirpated and in whom other hemorrhoids develop. This is because the causes which gave rise to the original ones remained and, therefore, new ones develop.

Here Maimonides provides an insight into the etiology of disease in general, in that he regards operative excision of hemorrhoids with skepticism, because surgery does not remove the underlying causes that produced the hemorrhoids in the first place.

The fifth work is Maimonides' *Treatise on Sexual Intercourse*, written for the nephew of Saladin, the Sultan al-Muzaffar Omar Ibn Nur ad-Din. The Sultan indulged heavily in sexual activities and asked Maimonides, his physician, to help him to increase his sexual potential. The work consists mainly of recipes of foods and drugs that are either aphrodisiac or antiaphrodisiac in their actions. Maimonides advises moderation in sexual intercourse and describes the physiology of sexual temperaments. There are two versions to this book, a short authentic and a longer spurious version. Both were first edited and published by Kroner in 1906 in Hebrew and German.[25] Ten years later, Kroner published the true short version from the original Arabic manuscript in Granada.[26] An Italian edition appeared in 1906,[27] and English[28] and Spanish[29] translations were published in 1961. The definitive Hebrew edition of both authentic[30] and spurious[31] versions of Maimonides' books on sex is that of Muntner, dated 1965. A new English translation of the true work, by me, was published[32] and reprinted.[33] Sex and health in the writings of Maimonides are also discussed by Harvey.[34]

The sixth medical book of Moses Maimonides is his *Treatise on Asthma*. The patient for whom this book was written suffered from violent headaches that prevented him from wearing a turban. The patient's symptoms began with a common cold, especially in the rainy season, forcing him to gasp for air until phlegm was expelled. The patient asked whether a change of climate would be beneficial. Maimonides, in thirteen chapters, explains the rules of diet and climate in general and those rules specifically suited for asthmatics. He outlines the recipes of food and drugs and describes the various climates of the Middle East. He states that the dry Egyptian climate is efficacious for sufferers from this disease, and warns against the use of very powerful remedies. The first critical edition of this work appeared in Hebrew in 1940, edited by Muntner.[35] Additional manuscripts became available after World War II, and a corrected, improved, and revised second Hebrew edition appeared in 1963.[36] Only three hundred copies of this edition were printed, and thus a third edition was published by Muntner in 1965.[37] An English version of Maimonides' book on asthma was published in 1963,[38] and a French translation in 1965.[39] I have commented extensively on this work elsewhere,[40] and published a revised and improved English translation in 1994.[41]

The last chapter of this work deals with concise admonitions and aphorisms that Maimonides considered "useful to any man desirous of preserving his health and administering to the sick." The chapter begins as follows: "The first thing to consider . . . is the provision of fresh air, clean water, and a healthy diet." Fresh air is described in some detail: "City air is stagnant, turbid and thick, the natural result of its big buildings, narrow streets, the refuse of its inhabitants . . . one should at least choose for a residence a wide-open suite . . . living quarters are best located on an upper floor . . . and ample sunshine. . . . Toilets should be located as far as possible from living rooms. The air should be kept dry at all times by sweet scents, fumigation and drying agents. The concern for clean air is the foremost rule in preserving the health of one's body and soul." Those who consider air pollution control to be of recent origin would do well to take note of Maimonides' prophetic statements of eight hundred years ago.

The seventh medical work of Maimonides is his *Treatise on Poisons and Their Antidotes*. It is one of the most interesting and popular works because it is very scientific and modern in its approach and was used as a textbook of toxicology throughout the Middle Ages. The book was written at the request of Maimonides' noble protector, the Grand Vizier and Supreme Judge al-Fadhil, who asked Maimonides to write a treatise on poisons for the layman's guidance before the arrival of a physician. In the introduction, Maimonides praises al-Fadhil and his feats in war and peace. He mentions al-Fadhil's orders to import from distant lands ingredients lacking in Egypt but necessary for the preparation of two antidotes against poisonings, the "great theriac" and the "electuary of Mithridates."

The first section of the book deals with snake and dog bites and with scorpion, bee, wasp, and spider stings. The first chapter concerns the conduct of the victim in general. Thus Maimonides states as follows:

> When someone is bitten, immediate care should be taken to tie the spot above the wound as fast as possible to prevent the poison from spreading throughout the body; in the meantime, another person should make cuts with a lancet directly above the wound, suck vigorously with his mouth and spit out. Before doing that, it is advisable to disinfect the mouth with olive oil, or with spirit in oil. . . .

> Care should be taken that the sucking person has no wound in his mouth, or rotten teeth . . . should there be no man available to do the sucking, cupping-glasses should be applied, with or without fire; the heated ones have a much better effect because they combine the advantages of sucking and cauterizing at the same time. . . . Then apply the great theriac. . . . Apply to the wound some medicine which should draw the poison out of the body.

In his book on poisons, Maimonides also describes the long incubation period for rabies (up to forty days). Numerous Arabic, Hebrew, and Latin manuscripts are extant.[42] A German translation was published in 1873 by Steinschneider.[43] A French translation appeared in 1865 by Rabbinowicz and was reprinted in 1935.[44] An English translation of Steinschneider's German version is that of Bragman in 1926.[45] The definitive Hebrew edition of Muntner appeared in 1942,[46] and Muntner's English version was published in 1966.[47] I commented on this work[48] and published a fully annotated new English translation with commentary and bibliography.[49]

The eighth book is the *Regimen of Health* (*Regimen Sanitatis*), which Maimonides wrote in 1198 during the first year of the reign of Sultan al-Malik al-Afdal, eldest son of Saladin the Great. The Sultan was a frivolous, pleasure-seeking man of thirty, subject to fits of melancholy or depression owing to his excessive indulgences in wine and women and his warlike adventures against his own relatives and in the Crusades. He complained to his physician of constipation, dejection, bad thoughts, and indigestion. Maimonides answered his royal patient in four chapters. The first chapter is a brief abstract on diet taken mostly from Hippocrates and Galen. The second chapter deals with advice on hygiene, diet, and drugs in the absence of a physician. The third, extremely important, chapter contains Maimonides' concept of "a healthy mind in a healthy body," one of the earliest descriptions of psychosomatic medicine. He indicates that the physical well-being of a person is dependent on his mental well-being and vice versa. The final chapter summarizes his prescriptions relating to climate, domicile, occupation, bathing, sex, wine-drinking, diet, and respiratory infections.

The whole treatise on the *Regimen of Health* is short and concise, but to the point. This is the reason for its great success and popularity throughout the years. It is extant in numerous manuscripts. A Hebrew translation from the original Arabic was made by Moses ben Samuel Ibn Tibbon in 1244, and this version was reprinted several times in the nineteenth century (Prague, 1838; Jerusalem, 1885; Warsaw, 1886). Two Latin translations were made in the thirteenth century. Several fifteenth-century incunabula and sixteenth-century editions of these Latin versions exist. One of the first Hebrew editions is that of Bloch in 1838.[50] An annotated German translation by Winternitz was published in 1843,[51] and Russian[52] and Spanish[53] translations appeared in 1930 and 1961, respectively. The Arabic text with German and Hebrew translations was published by Kroner in 1925,[54] although he had already published the all-important Chapter 3 dealing with psychosomatic medicine eleven years earlier, in 1914.[55]

English translations of Chapter 3 have been published by Bragman,[56] Savitz,[57] and Butterworth[58] and that of the first two chapters published by Skoss.[59] The definitive Hebrew version is that of Muntner, dated 1957,[60] although the Maimonidean bibliographer Dienstag[61] cites several additional Hebrew editions. Three English translations of the entire work were published: in 1958 by Gordon;[62] in 1964 by Bar Sela, Hoff, and Faris;[63] and in 1990 by me.[64] Another German translation by Muntner appeared in 1966.[65] These numerous editions in many languages attest to the importance and popularity of Maimonides' *Regimen of Health.*

The ninth medical writing of Maimonides is the *Discourse on the Explanation of Fits.* This work has been called Maimonides' swan song, as it was thought to be the last of his medical works, having been written in the year 1200, four years before his death.

It was written for the Sultan al-Malik al-Afdal, and is sometimes considered to represent Chapter 5 of the *Regimen of Health*. The Sultan persisted in his overindulgences and wrote to Maimonides, who was ill himself, asking advice about his health. Maimonides confirms most of the prescriptions of the Sultan's other physicians regarding wine, laxatives, bathing, exercise, and the like, and, near the end, gives a detailed hour-by-hour regimen for the daily life of the Sultan. The original Arabic was edited and published with Hebrew and German translations by Kroner in 1928.[66] English editions by Bar Sela, Hoff, and Faris in 1964[67] and by myself and Muntner in 1969,[68] another German version by Muntner in 1966,[69] and another Hebrew edition by Muntner in 1969[70] are available. The best edition is that by Leibowitz and Marcus, titled *On the Causes of Symptoms*,[71] in which the text is presented in four languages (Arabic, Hebrew, Latin, and English) and accompanied by a running commentary, explanatory essays, and a comprehensive catalog of drugs. The most recent English version was published in 1990.[72]

The final authentic medical book of Maimonides is the *Glossary of Drug Names*. This work was discovered by Max Meyerhof, an ophthalmologist in Egypt, in the Aya Sofia library in Istanbul, Turkey, as Arabic manuscript no. 3711.[73] Dr. Meyerhof edited the original Arabic and provided a French translation with a detailed commentary, which he published in 1940 in Cairo.[74] A Hebrew edition by Muntner appeared in 1969,[75] and my English translations were published in 1979[76] and 1996.[77] The work is essentially a pharmacopoeia and consists of 405 short paragraphs containing names of drugs in Arabic, Greek, Syrian, Persian, Berber, and Spanish.

In summary, Maimonides' medical writings are varied, comprising extracts from Greek medicine, a series of monographs on health in general and several diseases in particular, and a more recently discovered pharmacopoeia demonstrating his extensive knowledge of Arabic medical literature and his familiarity with several languages. Some people believe that Maimonides' medical writings are not as original as his theological and philosophical works.[78] However, his medical works demonstrate the lucidity, conciseness, and formidable powers of systematization and organization so characteristic of all his writings. The *Book of Poisons*, the *Regimen of Health*, and the *Medical Aphorisms of Maimonides* became classics in their fields in medieval times.

Maimonides prescribes a healthy diet and lifestyle, considering them to be of such importance that he includes these rules, together with others of ethical content, in his legal *Code of Jewish Law*, the *Mishneh Torah*.[79] To Maimonides, however, bodily perfection is not the ultimate goal. Rather, together with material means and ethical values, it permits the attainment of perfection in knowledge. "Learned and experienced, strict and scrupulous, open-minded though critical, considering ethics and psychology not less crucial than diet and drugs, Maimonides was no doubt, at least in the eyes of his fellow men, an accomplished physician."[80] I conclude by citing a paragraph from my first paper on Maimonides:[81]

Maimonides died on December 13, 1204 [20 Tebet, 4965] and was buried in Tiberias, Palestine. The Christian, Moslem and Jewish worlds mourned him. His literary ability was incredible and his knowledge was encyclopedic. He mastered nearly everything known in the fields of theology, mathematics, law, philosophy, astronomy, ethics, and, of course, medicine. As a physician, he treated disease by the scientific [as opposed to empiric or popular] method, not by guesswork, superstition, or rule of thumb. His attitude towards the practice of medicine came from his deep religious background, which made the preservation of health and life a divine commandment. His inspiration lives on through the years and his position as one of the medical giants of history is indelibly recorded. He was physician to Sultans and Princes, and as Sir William Osler said, "He was Prince of Physicians." The heritage of his great medical writings is being more and more appreciated. To the Jewish people he symbolized the highest spiritual and intellectual achievement of man on this earth; as so aptly stated, "From Moses to Moses there never arose a man like Moses," and none has since.

---

1. F. Rosner, "The Physician's Prayer Attributed to Maimonides," *Bull. Hist. Med.*, 41 (1967):440–454.

2. F. Rosner, "Maimonides, the Physician: A Bibliography," *Bull. Hist. Med.*, 43 (1969):221–235; "Maimonides the Physician: A Bibliography," *Clio Medica*, 15 (1980):75–79.

3. U. Barzel, "The Art of Cure: A Non-Published Medical Book by Maimonides," *Harofe Haivri*, 2 (1955):82–83 (Heb.) and 165–177 (Eng.).

4. U.S. Barzel, *The Art of Cure. Extracts from Galen* (Haifa: Maimonides Research Institute, 1992).

5. M. Steinschneider, "Die Vorrede des Maimonides zu seinem Commentar über die Aphorismen des Hippokrates," *Ztschr. d. deutsch. Morgenland. Gesellsch.*, 48 (1894):218–234.

6. M.Z. Hasida (Bocian), *Perush le-Pirké Abukrat shel Ha-Rambam. Hassegullah* (Jerusalem) 1934–1945, 1–30 (stencil) (Heb.).

7. S. Muntner, *Moshe ben Maimon*, Commentary on the Aphorisms of Hippocrates, *Perush le-Pirké Abukrat* (Jerusalem: Mosad Harav Kook, 1961).

8. A. Bar Sela and H.E. Hoff, "Maimonides' Interpretation of the First Aphorism of Hippocrates," *Bull. Hist. Med.*, 37 (1968):347–354.

9. F. Rosner, "The Introduction of Maimonides to His 'Commentary on the Aphorisms of Hippocrates,'" *Clio Medica*, 11 (1976):59–64.

10. F. Rosner, *Moses Maimonides' Commentary on the Aphorisms of Hippocrates* (Haifa: Maimonides Research Institute, 1987).

11. Z. Magid, ed. *Medical Aphorisms of Maimonides* (*Pirkei Moshe*) (Vilna: L. Matz, 1888) (1st ed., Lemberg, 1834) (Heb.).

12. S. Muntner, *Moshe ben Maimon* (*Medical*) *Aphorisms of Moses in Twenty-Five Treatises* (*Pirké Moshe bi-Refuah*) (Jerusalem: Mosad Harav Kook, 1959) (Heb.: Eng. summary).

13. J.O. Leibowitz, "Maimonides' Aphorisms," *Koroth* 1 (1955):213–219 (Heb.); I–III (Eng. summary).

14. J.O. Leibowitz, "The Latin Translations of Maimonides' Aphorisms," *Koroth*, 6 (1973):273–281 (Heb.); XCIII–XCIV (Eng. summary).

15. W. Steinberg and S. Muntner, "Maimonides' Views on Gynecology and Obstetrics," *Am. J. Obst. Gynec.*, 91 (1965): 443–448; F. Rosner and S. Muntner, "Moses Maimonides' Aphorisms Regarding Analysis of Urine," *Ann. Int. Med.*, 71 (1969):217–220; "The Surgical Aphorisms of Moses Maimonides," *Amer. J. Surg.*, 119 (1970): 718–725; F. Rosner, "Moses Maimonides and Diseases of the Chest," *Chest*, 60 (1971):68–72.

16. F. Rosner and S. Muntner, Studies in Judaica, *The Medical Aphorisms of Moses Maimonides* (New York: Yeshiva University Press, 1970), vol. 1, p. 267; ibid. (Yeshiva University Press, 1971), vol. 2, p. 244.

17. F. Rosner and S. Muntner, Studies in Judaica, *The Medical Aphorisms of Moses Maimonides*, vol. 1 and vol. 2 (New York: Bloch, for Yeshiva University Press, 1973), pp. 264 and 244.

18. F. Rosner, *The Medical Aphorisms of Moses Maimonides* (Haifa: Maimonides Research Institute, 1989).

19. F. Rosner, "The Medical Aphorisms of Moses Maimonides," in J.O. Leibowitz, *Memorial Volume in Honor of S. Muntner* (Israel Inst. Hist. Med. Jerusalem, 1983), pp. 6–30.

20. H. Kroner, "Die Haemorrhoiden in der Medizin des XII und XIII Jahrhunderts," *Janus*, 16 (1911):441–46 and 644–718.

21. L.J. Bragman, "Maimonides' Treatise on Hemorrhoids," *New York State Med. J.*, 27 (1927):598–601.

22. S. Muntner, *Moshe ben Maimon: On Hemorrhoids* (*Birefuot Hatechorim*) (Jerusalem: Mosad Harav Kook, 1965) (Heb.).

23. F. Rosner and S. Muntner, *The Medical Writings of Moses Maimonides. Treatise on Hemorrhoids and Maimonides' Answers to Queries* (Philadelphia: Lippincott, 1969).

24. F. Rosner, *Moses Maimonides' Treatises on Poisons, Hemorrhoids, and Coitus* (Haifa: Maimonides Research Institute, 1984).

25. H. Kroner, *Ein Beitrag zur Geschichte der Medizin des XII Jahrhunderts an der Hand Zweier Medizinischer Abhandlungen des Maimonides auf Grund von 6 unedierten Handschriften* (Oberdorf-Bopfingen: Itzowsky, 1906).

26. H. Kroner, "Eine Medizinische Maimonides Handschrift aus Granada. Ein Beitrag zur Stilistik des Maimonides und Charakteristik der Hebräischen Ueberzetzungsliteratur," *Janus*, 21 (1916):203–247.

27. U. DeMartini, *Maimonides, Segreto dei segretti* (Rome: Istituto di storia della Medicina dell'Universita de Roma, 1960).

28. M. Gorlin, *Maimonides "On Sexual Intercourse"* (*Fi'l-Jima*) (Brooklyn, NY: Rambash, 1961).

29. E. Chelminski, "Notas introductorias al 'Guia sobre el contacto sexual' de Maimonides," *Anales de ars Medici* (Mexico) 5(4) (1961):240–248.

30. S. Muntner, *Moshe ben Maimon on the Increase of Physical Vigor* (*Maamar al hizuk koah ha-gavrah*) (Jerusalem: Mosad Harav Kook, 1965), pp. 35–65 (Heb.).

31. S. Muntner, "Pseudo-Maimonides on Sexual Life," in *Sexual Life, Collection of Medieval Treatises* (*Maamar al razei ha-chajim ha-miniyim*) (Jerusalem: Genizah, 1965).

32. F. Rosner, *Sex Ethics in the Writings of Moses Maimonides* (New York: Bloch, 1974).

33. F. Rosner, *Moses Maimonides' Treatises on Poisons, Hemorrhoids, and Coitus.*

34. W.Z. Harvey, "Sex and Health in Maimonides," in F. Rosner and S.S. Kottek, eds., *Moses Maimonides. Physician, Scientist and Philosopher* (Northvale, NJ: Jason Aronson, 1993) pp. 33–39 and 239–240.

35. S. Muntner, *Moshe ben Maimon* (*Maimonides*). *Sefer ha-Katzeret* (*The Book on Asthma*) (Jerusalem: Rubin Mass, 1940).

36. S. Muntner, *Rabbi Moses ben Maimon. Sefer ha-Katzeret or Sefer ha-Misadim* (*The Book on Asthma*) (Jerusalem: Genizah, 1963).

37. S. Muntner, *Moshe ben Maimon on Asthma* (*Sefer ha-Katzeret*) (Jerusalem: Mosad Harav Kook, 1965), pp. 67–119 (Heb.).

38. S. Muntner, *The Medical Writings of Moses Maimonides. Treatise on Asthma* (Philadelphia: Lippincott, 1963).

39. S. Muntner and I. Simon, "Le Traité de L'Asthme de Maïmonide (1135–1304) Traduit Pour la Première Fois en Français d'Après le Texte Hébreu," *Rév d'Hist. Méd. Héb.*, 16 (1963):171–186; 17 (1964):5–13, 83–97, 127–139, 187–196; 18 (1965):5–15.

40. F. Rosner, "Moses Maimonides' Treatise on Asthma," *Thorax*, 36 (1981): 245–251; *J. Asthma*, 21 (1984):119–129.

41. F. Rosner, *Moses Maimonides' Treatise on Asthma* (Haifa: Maimonides Research Institute, 1994).

42. F. Rosner, "Moses Maimonides' Treatise on Poisons," *J.A.M.A.*, 205 (1968):914–916.

43. M. Steinschneider, "Gifte und ihre Heilung," *Virchows Arch. F. Path. Anat.*, 57 (1873):62–120.

44. I.M. Rabbinowicz, *Traité des Poisons* (Paris: Lipschutz, 1935; 1st ed., 1865).

45. L.J. Bragman, "Maimonides' Treatise on Poisons," *Med. J. and Rec.*, 124 (1926):103–107.

46. S. Muntner, *Moshe ben Maimon* (*Maimonides*), *Samei ha-mavet ve-ha-refuot kenegdam* (*Poisons and Their Antidotes, or "The Treatise to the Honored One"*) (Jerusalem: Rubin Mass, 1942).

47. S. Muntner, *The Medical Writings of Moses Maimonides*, vol. 2: *Treatise on Poisons and Their Antidotes* (Philadelphia: Lippincott, 1966).

48. F. Rosner, "Moses Maimonides' Treatise on Poisons," *N.Y. State J. Med.*, 80 (1980):1627–1630.

49. F. Rosner, *Moses Maimonides' Treatises on Poisons, Hemorrhoids, and Coitus.*

50. S. Bloch, "Michtav ha-Rav Rabenu Moshe ben Maimon Be'ad ha-Sultan," *Kerem Hemed*, 3 (1838): 31–39.

51. D. Winternitz, *Das Diatetische Sendschreiben des Maimonides* (*Rambam*) *an den Sultan Saladin* (Vienna: Braumueller and Seidel, 1843).

52. I.K. Shmukler, *Pismo Moiseh Maimonida K Egipefskomu Sultanu. Gugienicheskie Sovetia Perevod S Drev-*

neevreiskogo Doctora I.K. Shmuklera (Kiev). Otdelnii Ottisk Iz, "Vrach Dela" #14–15 and 16. Charkov. "Nauchnaja Misl." Uchr. NKZ. UKSSR (1930).

53. E. Chelminsky, "La Preservacion de la Juventud" de Maimonides, Version Castellana, *Anales de Ars Medici* (Mexico), 5 (1961):303–344.

54. H. Kroner, "*Fi tadbir as sihhat*, Gesundheitsanleitung des Maimonides fur den Sultan al-Malik al-Afdhal," *Janus*, 27 (1923):101–116, 286–330, 28 (1924):61–74, 143–152, 199–217, 408–419, 455–472; 29 (1925):235– 58.

55. H. Kroner, *Die Seelenhygiene des Maimonides, Auszug aus der 3, Kapital des diatetischen Sendschreibens des Maimonides an den Sultan al Malik Alafdahl* (ca. 1198) (Frankfurt A.M.: J. Kauffmann, 1914).

56. L.J. Bragman, "Maimonides on Physical Hygiene," *Ann. Med. Hist.*, 7 (1925):140–143.

57. H. Savitz, "Maimonides' Hygiene of the Soul," *Ann. Med. Hist.*, 4 (1932):80–86.

58. C.E. Butterworth, "On the Management of Health," in R.L. Weiss and C.E. Butterworth, eds., *Ethical Writings of Maimonides* (New York: New York University Press, 1975), pp. 105–111.

59. S.L. Skoss, "The Treatises of Maimonides on Health Care," in *Portrait of a Jewish Scholar; Essays and Addresses* (New York: Bloch, 1957), pp. 99–116.

60. S. Muntner, *Moshe ben Maimon, Hanhagat ha-Briyut, Regimen Sanitatis, Letters on the Hygiene of the Body and of the Soul* (Jerusalem: Mosad Harav Kook, 1956).

61. J.I. Dienstag, "Translators and Editors of Maimonides' Medical Works: A Bio-Bibliographical Survey," in J.O. Leibowitz, ed., *Memorial Volume in Honor of S. Muntner* (Jerusalem: Israel Inst. His. Med., 1983), pp. 95–135.

62. H.L. Gordon, *Moses ben Maimon, The Preservation of Youth, Essays on Health (Fi Tadbir As-Sihha)* (New York: Philos. Lib., 1958).

63. A. Bar Sela, H.E. Hoff, and E. Faris, *Moses Maimonides' Two Treatises on the Regimen of Health* (Philadelphia: Am. Philos. Soc. [Trans. n.s. vol. 54, p. 4], 1964).

64. F. Rosner, *Moses Maimonides' Three Treatises on Health* (Haifa: Maimonides Research Institute, 1990).

65. S. Muntner, *Regimen Sanitatis oder Dietetik fur die Seele und den Korper mit Anhang der Medizinischen Responsen und Ethik des Maimonides* (Basel: S. Karger, 1966).

66. H. Kroner, "Der Medizinische Schwanengesang des Maimonides," *Janus*, 32 (1928):12–116.

67. A. Bar Sela, H.E. Hoff, and E. Faris, *Moses Maimonides' Two Treatises on the Regimen of Health.*

68. F. Rosner and S. Muntner, *Treatise on Hemorrhoids and Maimonides' Answers to Queries.*

69. S. Muntner, *Regimen Sanitatis.*

70. S. Muntner, *Moshe ben Maimon, Biyur Sheimot Ha-Refuot (Lexicography of Drugs*, and *Medical Responses)* (Jerusalem: Mosad Harav Kook, 1969).

71. J.O. Leibowitz and S. Marcus, *Moses Maimonides on the Causes of Symptoms* (Berkeley, CA: University of California Press, 1974).

72. F. Rosner, *Moses Maimonides' Three Treatises on Health.*

73. M. Meyerhof, "Sur Un Glossaire de Matière Médicale Arabe Composé par Maïmonide," *Bull. Inst. Egypte*, 17 (1935):223–235; "Sur Un Ouvrage Médicale Inconnu de Maïmonide," *Mélanges Maspéro*, 3 (1935–1940):1–7.

74. J. Meyerhof, *Un Glossaire de Matière Médicale, Composé par Maïmonide* (*Sarh Asma' al'Uqqar*), vol. 41 (Cairo: Mem. Inst. Egypte, 1940).

75. S. Muntner, *Moshe ben Maimon. Hanhagut Habriyut.*

76. F. Rosner, *Moses Maimonides' Glossary of Drug Names* (Philadelphia: American Philosophical Society, 1979).

77. F. Rosner, *Moses Maimonides' Glossary of Drug Names* (Haifa: Maimonides Research Institute, 1996).

78. E. Lieber, "The Medical Works of Maimonides: A Reappraisal," in F. Rosner and S.S. Kottek, eds., *Moses Maimonides. Physician, Scientist and Philosopher*, pp. 13–24 and 235–237.

79. M. Maimonides, *Mishneh Torah, Hilchot Deot*, Chapter 4.

80. S.S. Kottek, "Maimonides on the Perfect Physician," in F. Rosner and S.S. Kottek, eds., *Moses Maimonides. Physician, Scientist and Philosopher*, pp. 25–32 and 237–239.

81. F. Rosner, "Moses Maimonides (1135-1204)," *Annals of Internal Medicine*, 62 (1965):373–375.

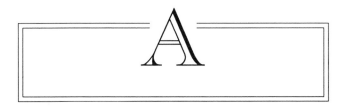

**ABDOMEN**—In his *Medical Aphorisms*,[1] Maimonides quotes Galen, who said that the eating of things that have begun to putrefy leads to worm formation in the abdomen (Chapter 6:21). Three types of abdominal worms are described: One resides in the perianal region (oxyuris?); another resembles gourd seeds and is found in the large intestine (taenia?); and the third resembles snakes (ascaris?) and is found in the small intestine. Worms develop in the abdomen from bad, irritating humor (ibid., 9:93). Worms and other abnormalities give rise to abdominal pain (ibid., 6:42 and 23:93). Paracentesis with the removal of abdominal fluid is described (ibid., 15:7). Abdominal injuries and the suturing of abdominal wounds are also discussed (ibid., 15:37).

In his *Commentary on the Aphorisms of Hippocrates*,[2] Maimonides points out that pressure on the abdomen assists in the expulsion of the placenta after childbirth (Chapter 5:49). Abdominal pain is discussed (ibid., 6:7) as well as ascites, which is treated by the elimination of the excess abdominal fluid (ibid. 6:14) by paracentesis (ibid., 6:28) or by diuretics (ibid., 15:36), or through the stools. The ancients thought that ascites or hydrops could be cured by elimination of the fluid in the stools, rather than through the urine. The Talmud is of the same opinion: "Much stool is a sign of much hydrops" (*Shabbat* 33a, *Bechorot* 44b). Otherwise, the patient's abdomen becomes filled with water and the patient dies (Chapter 7:55). A variety of abdominal ailments and their treatment are discussed in the *Extracts from Galen*.[3]

Elsewhere, Maimonides advocates the consumption of lean meat. Meat from an animal's abdomen is "fat and is all bad: It satiates but it corrupts digestion, suppresses the appetite and give rise to white humor."[4] In his legal code (*Mishneh Torah, Shabbat* 21:28), Maimonides rules that the abdomen may be anointed and massaged on the Sabbath, provided that both actions are performed simultaneously, so as to constitute a departure from the normal weekday procedure. [*See also* STOMACH and INTESTINES]

---

1. F. Rosner, *The Medical Aphorisms of Moses Maimonides* (Haifa: Maimonides Research Institute, 1989).

2. F. Rosner, *Maimonides' Commentary on the Aphorisms of Hippocrates* (Haifa: Maimonides Research Institute, 1987).

3. U.S. Barzel, *Maimonides' Art of Cure. Extracts from Galen* (Haifa: Maimonides Research Institute, 1992).

4. F. Rosner, *Moses Maimonides' Three Treatises on Health* (Haifa: Maimonides Research Institute, 1990), p. 27.

**ABORTION**—In his *Medical Aphorisms*,[1] Maimonides cites the physiological cause for abortion according to the medieval concept of disease being caused by a disequilibrium of the four body humors (Chapter 16: 22). He also states that a woman may abort because of exertional activity or because of steambathing "because a bath softens the body and the nerves" (ibid.,16:30). A woman may also miscarry following the excessive anointing of her head with oil because this produces and evokes coughing, the uterus becomes shaken up, and it expels the fetus (ibid.).

An unborn fetus, in Jewish law, is not considered to be a complete human being until it is born and, hence, may be destroyed to save the mother's life.[2] Therefore, both in relation to an ox goring a pregnant woman and inducing a miscarriage and in relation to a human being who assaults a woman, even unintentionally, causing accidental abortion, Maimonides speaks only of compensation for injury and pain that must be paid to the woman for the premature loss of her fetus. The fetus is considered to be an appendage of the mother and belongs jointly to her and her husband, and thus damages must be paid for its premature death. However, the one responsible is not culpable for involuntary homicide, since the unborn fetus is not considered to be a person or a full human being.[3]

In several places in his *Mishneh Torah*, Maimonides reiterates that an unborn fetus technically is not a human being and hence may (or must) be destroyed to preserve the mother's life. Second, once birth begins, the baby is considered to be a human being and cannot be destroyed even to save the mother because one is not allowed to destroy one life to save another, the only exception being the case of a pursuer. Third, Maimonides permits abortion or an embryotomy to save the mother's life not only because the unborn fetus is not a human being, but also because it is equated with a pursuer, whereby the fetus is considered to be pursuing the mother and trying to kill her.

An abortion conveys ritual uncleanness, as does a placenta. Women were said to bury their abortions in the fields, although abortions were sometimes thrown into cisterns. Only an abortus forty days old or older conveys uncleanness, a recognition of the fact that an embryo begins to take form forty days after conception. A woman becomes ritually unclean not only after giving birth to a healthy child, but also if she delivers a dead infant or even a small fetus. A habitual aborter is discussed by Maimonides when he says that "if she miscarries three times in succession, the presumption is that she is prone to miscarry—perchance he is not destined to build a family by her" (*Eeshut* 15:12).

---

1. F. Rosner, *The Medical Aphorisms of Moses Maimonides* (Haifa: Maimonides Research Institute, 1989).
2. F. Rosner, *Modern Medicine and Jewish Ethics*, 2nd ed. (Hoboken, NJ, and New York: Ktav and Yeshiva University Press, 1991), pp. 133–167.
3. F. Rosner, *Medicine in the Mishneh Torah of Maimonides* (New York: Ktav, 1984), pp. 170–174.

*ABSCESS*—In ancient and medieval times, phlebotomy was used to treat swellings such as tumors and abscesses. Galen, Hippocrates, and even Maimonides subscribed to this view.[1] In his *Commentary on the Aphorisms of Hippocrates*,[2] Maimonides points out that brain abscesses are life-threatening (Chapter 1:12). Patients with intestinal abscesses cannot tolerate purgation (ibid., 1:24). Abscesses in

the throat (scrofula or tonsillitis?) occur mostly in children (ibid., 2:26). The word "abscess" is also used to describe swollen or enlarged lymph nodes (ibid., 4:55). Abscesses may cause itching (ibid., 5:23). An internal abscess that ruptures may have serious consequences (ibid., 7:8). Such an abscess should be treated with astringent medications (ibid., 7:37).

In his *Medical Aphorisms*,[3] Maimonides quotes Galen, who defined an abscess as a pus inflammation (Chapter 2:25). Such abscesses can occur in any organ (ibid., 3:48) including the brain (ibid., 3:83) and the kidneys (ibid., 9:95). Some abscesses resemble "groat bags" (ibid., 2:61). The most favorable abscess is one that is on the verge of expelling its pus (ibid., 6:68). The treatment of soft tissue abscesses is to apply wool soaked in warm oil on them (ibid., 9:118).

Sometimes, for abscesses of the hands and feet, it suffices to apply thereon a sponge soaked in cold water with a little vinegar or styptic wine. However, for abscesses of the liver, one should not apply anything cold on them; rather, one cooks asparagus in wine, makes a lukewarm compress therefrom, and applies it at the beginning of the abscess. The same benefit is derived from compresses of quince oil, myrtle oil, mastic oil, spike oil, or wormwood oil. None of these should be used cold, nor should any oily substance be used for abscesses of the eyes or mouth (ibid., 9:126).

---

1. U.S. Barzel, *Maimonides' Art of Cure. Extracts from Galen* (Haifa: Maimonides Research Institute, 1992), p. 29.

2. F. Rosner, *Maimonides' Commentary on the Aphorisms of Hippocrates* (Haifa: Maimonides Research Institute), 1987.

3. F. Rosner, *The Medical Aphorisms of Moses Maimonides* (Haifa: Maimonides Research Institute, 1989).

*AGING*—In his *Medical Aphorisms*,[1] Maimonides quotes Galen, who said that a healthy regimen for the elderly consists of oil massages in the morning followed by exercise such as walking, washing in comfortably warm water, drinking wine, and consuming warming and moistening foods (Chapter 17:27). The weak and frail elderly should be fed small but frequent meals (ibid., 17:29). Bread for the elderly should be toasted, and milk is good only for old people who can digest it without developing flatulence (ibid., 17:30). In the summer they should eat fresh figs, and in the winter dry figs (ibid., 17:31). They should be given parsley, honey, and wine as diuretics and oil or prunes cooked in honey before meals to soften their stools (ibid., 17:32). Cooked rather than fried or roasted meat is preferable for the elderly (ibid., 17:34). Old age is divided into three stages (ibid., 17:35); it cannot be repulsed

or hindered, but it can be delayed by carefulness with the diet, much bathing, adequate sleep, pleasant walks, and the avoidance of that which dries or cools (ibid., 17:36). Specific remedies for constipation are discussed (ibid., 17:38). Tremors in the elderly are due to weakness of the power that supports and moves the body (ibid., 7:36).

In his *Treatise on Asthma*,[2] Maimonides warns old people against eating large meals (Chapter 6:1). Rather, a person should eat only when hungry, and even then not to full satiation (ibid., 6:3). A little wine is especially good for the elderly (ibid., 7:1). Strong purgatives should not be used to treat constipation (ibid., 9:5). The regular use of enemas is said not only to cleanse the intestines and improve digestion, but also to delay aging (ibid., 9:8). Bloodletting, with the removal of large quantities of blood, is harmful to the elderly (ibid., 13:46).

In his *Commentary on the Aphorisms of Hippocrates*,[3] Maimonides explains that aged people tolerate fasting better than younger people because they have less natural body heat and therefore require less food (Section 1:12–14). Elderly people, in general, have fewer illnesses than young people and children because they control their diets better. However, their resistance to disease is weak, and when they become ill, healing is more difficult (ibid., 2:39). Old people are most comfortable during late summer and early autumn (ibid., 3:18). During old age, black bile prevails and causes confusion of the mind and sleeplessness (ibid., 3:30). Other illnesses of old age include shortness of breath, cough, urinary retention, pain in the joints, vertigo, apoplexy, dimness of vision, and dullness of hearing (ibid., 3:31).

The "potion of youth," or a concoction known as the Great Itrifal (a compounded myrobalan electuary containing many ingredients), delays aging and is detailed in Maimonides' *Regimen on Health*[4] (Chapter 3:10–11). [*See also* LONGEVITY]

1. F. Rosner, *The Medical Aphorisms of Moses Maimonides* (Haifa: Maimonides Research Institute, 1989).

2. F. Rosner, *Moses Maimonides' Treatise on Asthma* (Haifa: Maimonides Research Institute, 1994).

3. F. Rosner, *Maimonides' Commentary on the Aphorisms of Hippocrates* (Haifa: Maimonides Research Institute, 1987).

4. F. Rosner, *Moses Maimonides' Three Treatises on Health* (Haifa: Maimonides Research Institute, 1990).

*AIR*—The ancients thought that blood and air (pneuma) flow through arteries and veins. Galenic medicine distinguished between natural, vital (animalistic), and psychic pneumas. The ancient Jewish sages divided the pneumas into four categories. The Jewish book of mysticism known as the *Zohar* (*Ruth* 84a) quotes Rabbi Rachimai, who said that just as the body has four fundamental elements, a person has four powers, which are *nefesh*, *ruach* (pneuma), *nishmata*, and *nishmata yetera*. Elsewhere (*Genesis Rabbah* 14:10), we read: The soul has five names: *nefesh*, *ruach*, *neshama*, *yeduda*, and *chaya*. In his *Treatise on Health*,[1] Maimonides asserts that:

> It is first necessary to pay attention to the improvement of the air and then to the improvement of the water and after that to the improvement of the foods. This is so because what the physicians call pneumas are thin vapors found in the body of living beings. Their origin and their fundamental substance are derived from the air which is inhaled from without. The vapor which is found in the blood of the liver and in the vessels which emanate from it is called the Natural Spirit. The vapor which is found in the blood of the heart and the pulsating vessels is called the Vital Spirit and the vapor which is found in the chambers of the brain and which is disseminated therefrom through the hollowness of the nerves is called the Psychic Spirit. The source of all of them and most of their substance is derived from the air which is inhaled from without and, if this air is rancid or putrid or turbid, all the pneumas change and their characteristics become the opposite of what they should be.

The rabbis state (*Genesis Rabbah* 14:11) that one should praise the

Lord for every breath that a person breathes. Further, the main site of life is the nostrils (*Yoma* 85a), as it is written: "all in whose nostrils was the breath of life" (Genesis 7:22).

Concern for clean air is articulated by Maimonides in both his *Treatise on Health* and his *Treatise on Asthma*.[2] Even the talmudic sages were concerned about the cleanliness of the air. Thus, the streets of Jerusalem were cleaned every day (*Baba Metzia* 26a). Permanent threshing floors, tanneries, and cemeteries had to be distant from the cities (*Baba Batra* 25a). Garbage dumps and furnaces could not be situated in the city of Jerusalem (*Baba Kamma* 82b).

Finally, in his *Medical Aphorisms*,[3] Maimonides quotes Galen, who said that air occasionally collects beneath the skin (subcutaneous emphysema) and sometimes under the membranes that surround the bones (periostium), or sometimes beneath the membrane that covers one of the internal organs (gas gangrene or clostridial infection?). [*See also* AIR POLLUTION]

---

1. F. Rosner, *Moses Maimonides' Three Treatises on Health* (Haifa: Maimonides Research Institute, 1990), pp. 73–74.

2. F. Rosner, *Moses Maimonides' Treatise on Asthma* (Haifa: Maimonides Research Institute, 1994), pp. 107–109.

3. F. Rosner, *The Medical Aphorisms of Moses Maimonides* (Haifa: Maimonides Research Institute, 1989), p. 43.

**AIR POLLUTION**—In his *Treatise on Asthma*,[1] Maimonides states that clean air is one of six obligatory hygienic principles. Air should be kept fresh on hot days by spraying and sprinkling the floor with aromatic water or by using flowers, heat-abating leaves, and draft. Conversely, on cold, rainy days, the air should be fumigated with perfumes that warm the body. The last and most important chapter of Maimonides' *Treatise on Asthma* is concerned with concise admonitions and aphorisms, which he considered "useful to any man desirous of preserving his health [i.e., the patient] and administering to the sick [i.e., the physician]." The chapter begins as follows: "The first thing to consider . . . is the provision of fresh air, clean water and a healthy diet." Fresh air is then described in some detail:

> ". . . city air is stagnant, turbid and thick, the natural result of its big buildings, narrow streets, the refuse of its inhabitants . . . one should at least choose for a residence a wide-open site . . . living quarters are best located on an upper floor . . . and ample sunshine . . . toilets should be located as far as possible from living areas. The air should be kept dry at all times by sweet scents, fumigation and drying agents. The concern for clean air is the foremost rule in preserving the health of one's body and soul. . . ."

Maimonides appears to be describing air pollution, eight hundred years before it became recognized as an important problem in major industrial cities.

1. F. Rosner, *Moses Maimonides' Treatise on Asthma* (Haifa: Maimonides Research Institute, 1994).

*ALMONDS*—In his *Medical Aphorisms*, Maimonides quotes Galen, who said that almonds are among the most salutary of fruits and specifically strengthen the stomach and liver. He also cites Abu Merwan Ibn Zuhr, who said that almonds guard the exterior of the brain and protect the moistness of organs very well.[1] In his *Mishneh Torah* (*Deot* 4:11), Maimonides asserts that figs, grapes, and almonds are good whether fresh or dried. In his *Treatises on Health*, he says that dishes prepared with almonds, sugar, lemon juice, or wine are good in any season.[2]

In his *Treatise on Asthma*,[3] Maimonides endorses a remedy to clear the lungs of moisture, ease respiration, and eliminate the cough of asthma: Soak wheat bran overnight in hot water; filter it and add sugar and almond oil; place it on the fire until it resembles a julep, and drink when lukewarm. Also beneficial are almonds prepared with rose leaves, especially in the winter. Dried, sugar-coated almonds are said to aid the digestion, soften the stools, and facilitate the expulsion of wastes.

1. F. Rosner, *The Medical Aphorisms of Moses Maimonides* (Haifa: Maimonides Research Institute, 1989), pp. 306 and 349.
2. F. Rosner, *Moses Maimonides' Three Treatises on Health* (Haifa: Maimonides Research Institute, 1990), p. 144.
3. F. Rosner, *Moses Maimonides' Treatise on Asthma* (Haifa: Maimonides Research Institute, 1994).

*ALOE*—In his *Glossary of Drug Names*,[1] Maimonides defines aloe as the juice of the plant known as *sabir* or *al-muqr* in Arabic and *aloē* in Greek. It is a bitter plant employed as an emmenagogue and a gastric remedy. There are several varieties. The famous physician Abu Merwan Ibu Zuhr is cited by Maimonides as having said that the wood of aloe has the property of strengthening the stomach and benefiting it.[2] Aloe also eliminates bad mouth odors. In his *Regimen of Health*,[3] Maimonides recommends ligna aloe for cold illnesses. It is also an ingredient in the Great Itrifal electuary, which is a myrobalan-containing electuary. Aloe is also an ingredient in a barley distillate that is beneficial if imbibed shortly after bathing. In his *Extracts from Galen*,[4] Maimonides describes aloe as a medicine that "closes and glues," as a "dry medicine," as a "relaxing medicine," and as a stomach-strengthening medicine.

1. F. Rosner, *Moses Maimonides' Glossary of Drug Names* (Haifa: Maimonides Research Institute, 1996), no. 318.

2. F. Rosner, *The Medical Aphorisms of Moses Maimonides* (Haifa: Maimonides Research Institute, 1989), p. 349.

3. F. Rosner, *Moses Maimonides' Three Treatises on Health* (Haifa: Maimonides Research Institute, 1990).

4. U.S. Barzel, *Maimonides' The Art of Cure. Extracts from Galen* (Haifa: Maimonides Research Institute, 1992).

*AMPUTATION*—In his *Medical Aphorisms*,[1] Maimonides quotes Galen, who said that if a limb dies to the point of one's not sensing it when it is pricked or burned with fire, one should hasten to amputate it next to the demarcation site where there is healthy tissue before it becomes black (Chapter 15:10). Gangrene of a limb is obviously being described, with amputation as a life-saving measure. After amputation, the stump should be cauterized (ibid., 15:12). Amputation is again discussed later in this book (ibid., 15:60). Amputees are also described in the Talmud (*Baba Batra* 20a; *Yoma* 78b; *Yebamot* 102b; *Chagigah* 3a). [*See also* SURGERY]

1. F. Rosner, *The Medical Aphorisms of Moses Maimonides* (Haifa: Maimonides Research Institute, 1989), p. 349.

*AMULETS*—Contrary to considerable rabbinic opinion during the Middle Ages, which favored the use of amulets to ward off misfortune, sickness, or "evil spirits,"[1] Maimonides was strongly opposed to such practices.[2] He argues against the folly of amulet writers (*Mishneh Torah, Tefillin* 5:4) and condemns the use of religious objects, such as a Torah scroll, for the curing of illness (*Akum* 11:12). Maimonides rules that even though one may use second tithe oil for anointing, one may not pour it over a callus or a lichen eruption, or use it as an ingredient in an amulet, because second tithe is not meant to be used as a medicament (*Maaser Sheni* 3:16). He also states that a metal amulet is susceptible to ritual uncleanness like any other human adornment (*Kelim* 8:6), as is a piece of leather in which an amulet is wrapped (ibid., 7:11).

Elsewhere in his *Mishneh Torah*, Maimonides discusses the subject of amulets and preserving stones that were worn for medical purposes and thought to be efficacious (*Shabbat* 19:13–14). Perhaps amulets and the like were effective because of their placebo effect. The use of amulets in animals is also described by Maimonides (ibid., 20:13).

1. H.J. Zimmels, *Magicians, Theologians and Doctors: Rabbinical Responsa* (12th–19th centuries) (London: Goldston, 1952).

2. F. Rosner, *Medicine in the Mishneh Torah of Maimonides* (New York: Ktav, 1984), pp. 281–283.

*ANATOMY*—The first chapter of Maimonides' *Medical Aphorisms* is devoted exclusively to anatomy and physiology.[1] First is a description of nerves, tendons, ligaments, and blood vessels. Maimonides distinguishes sensory and motor nerves, and subdivides blood vessels into arteries, veins, and capillaries: "Arteries in the entire body communicate with veins and interchange some blood and air through these anastamoses which are so narrow as to be invisible to the eye." Arteries and veins are called "pulsating and nonpulsating" vessels, respectively. The circle of Willis is described, as is the lamina cribrosa: "The bone which protects the brain from the inside and the palate is hollow. Anatomists call it the sieve." Maimonides recognizes that "The spinal cord . . . is surrounded by the same two membranes that surround the brain." Morphological and physiological descriptions of many body structures and organs, such as the eyeball, the larynx, the spleen, the kidneys, the gallbladder, and others, are provided. Muscle action is described in its various phases, including voluntary contraction and passive relaxation.

In both his *Mishnah Commentary*[2] and his *Mishneh Torah*,[3] Maimonides enumerates the 248 and 251 members, respectively, in a man's and a woman's body. The Talmud has a similar list (*Bechorot* 45a). He also asserts that the chest is called "the key of the heart" because chest movement inflates the lung against the heart and, therefore, serves as a key in that it opens a passageway through which air can enter and exit. A Canaanite slave obtains his freedom if his master causes the loss of one of twenty-four of his limbs or organs, which Maimonides lists as the fingers of the hands and the feet, the earlobes, the tip of the nose, the tip of the breast in a woman or the tip of the membrum in a man. Physical blemishes that disqualify a priest from serving in the Temple are also listed and discussed in great detail in *Mishneh Torah*.

1. F. Rosner, *The Medical Aphorisms of Moses Maimonides* (Haifa: Maimonides Research Institute, 1989), pp. 6–25.

2. F. Rosner, "Medicine in Moses Maimonides' Commentary on the Mishnah," *Koroth* (Jerusalem) 9 (1988): 565–578.

3. F. Rosner, *Medicine in the Mishneh Torah of Maimonides* (New York: Ktav, 1984), pp. 123–134.

*ANENCEPHALY*—One chapter in Maimonides' *Mishneh Torah* deals with fetal development and embryology (*Issurei Biyah* 10:1ff). Various forms and shapes of abortuses render a woman ritually unclean (ibid., 5:13–15). Teratology and monster births are discussed in detail, including human abortuses resembling a domestic or wild animal, a bird, or a snake (ibid., 10:8–10). Esophageal atresia, anencephaly, spina bifida, and other congenital abnormalities are described by Maimonides as follows:

> If the fetus is born with an obstructed gullet, or if it lacks everything from the navel downwards and is, therefore, shapeless, or if its skull is shapeless, or if its face is covered over so that it is unrecognizable, or if it has two backs and two spines, or if the abortion consists of a head which has no recognizable articulation, or an arm without recognizable lines—a fetus of any of these kinds does not render the mother unclean through childbirth (ibid., 10:11).

*ANETH*—Maimonides recommends aneth (anethum graveolens) boiled in water and mixed with oil for someone who ingested a food containing deadly poison, to help him vomit.[1] Milk, butter, and honey should also be ingested and vomited. Then the specific antidote should be administered. In his *Regimen of Health*,[2] Maimonides prescribes a cassia fistula remedy containing seven kernels of aneth for patients with hard stools. Hectic fever is treated by feeding the patient barley groats and spelt wheat boiled in water with leek, aneth, salt, oil, and vinegar.[3] Aneth is also discussed in Maimonides' *Glossary of Drug Names*.[4]

1. F. Rosner, *Moses Maimonides' Treatises on Poisons, Hemorrhoids and Cohabitation* (Haifa: Maimonides Research Institute, 1984), p. 82.

2. F. Rosner, *Moses Maimonides' Three Treatises on Health* (Haifa: Maimonides Research Institute, 1990), p. 54.

3. U.S. Barzel, *Maimonides' The Art of Cure. Extracts from Galen* (Haifa: Maimonides Research Institute, 1992), pp. 175–176.

4. F. Rosner, *Moses Maimonides' Glossary of Drug Names* (Haifa: Maimonides Research Institute, 1996), nos. 279 and 363.

*ANGER*—In his *Mishneh Torah* (*Deot* 2:3), Maimonides asserts that anger is an extremely bad temperament, and that it is proper for man to distance himself from it to the opposite extreme. He should teach himself not to become angered even over something for which anger would be appropriate (see *Taanit* 4a). If he wishes to instill fear in his children and members of his household, or in the community—if he is the leader—and he wishes to be angry at them so that they revert to good, then he should show himself to be angry in front of them in order to chastise them; but his own mind should be at peace, just as with a man who simulates anger at a time when anger is called for, but who really is not angry (see *Shabbat* 105b). The sages of old stated: "He who becomes angry is as if he worships idols" (*Nedarim* 22a). They also stated that "He who becomes angry, if he is a wise man, his wisdom departs from him, and if he is a prophet, his prophecy leaves him" (*Pesachim* 66b). And the life of people of anger is no real life; therefore, they commanded one to remain far from anger until one does not become irritated even for things that arouse anger, and this is the good path (*Deot* 2:3).

In his *Medical Aphorisms*,[1] Maimonides quotes Galen, who said that emotional stress such as anxiety, happiness, or anger can lead to fainting and profuse perspiration (Chapter 7:3). Maimonides explains that such altered emotions cause the dissolution of life spirits (ibid., 7:12). Anger is also said to occur in people who have inadequate "warmth" in their heart (ibid., 8:31), perhaps an early reference to psychosomatic medicine.

_____

1. F. Rosner, *The Medical Aphorisms of Moses Maimonides* (Haifa: Maimonides Research Institute, 1989).


***ANIMAL EXPERIMENTATION—***
In the introduction to his *Mishnah Commentary*, Maimonides states that everything that was created in this world by Almighty God was created to serve humankind.[1] Animals may thus be used as beasts of burden and for food, providing that they are humanely slaughtered. Scientific experiments upon laboratory animals in the course of medical research that are designed to yield information that may lead to cure of disease are sanctioned by Jewish law as legitimate utilization of animals for the benefit of humankind. However, wherever possible, pain or discomfort should be eliminated or minimized by analgesia, anesthesia, or other means. Otherwise, the pain does not serve to satisfy a legitimate human need, and its infliction is prohibited. In addition, animal experimentation is permissible by Jewish law only if its purpose is to obtain practical benefits to humankind and not simply the satisfaction of intellectual curiosity.[2] Furthermore, if alternative means of obtaining the same information are available, such as tissue-culture studies, animal experimentation may be considered to fall under the category of unnecessary cruelty to animals, and therefore be prohibited. [*See also* CRUELTY TO ANIMALS]

_____

1. F. Rosner, *Maimonides' Introduction to his Commentary on the Mishnah* (Northvale, NJ: Jason Aronson, 1995).

2. F. Rosner, *Modern Medicine and Jewish Ethics*, 2nd ed. (Hoboken, NJ, and New York: Ktav and Yeshiva University Press, 1991), pp. 353–373.


***ANISE—***In his *Regimen of Health*,[1] Maimonides lists anise as one of many ingredients in the myrobalan electuary, known as the Great Itrifal, that improves the three digestions (as described by Galen and Hippocrates) and strengthens all the organs in general and the heart and stomach in particular. It also delays aging, liquefies white humor, prevents gases from ascending to the brain, strengthens the senses, helps coitus, and gladdens the spirit. Anise boiled in hot water is also an ingredient of syrups that soften the stool and excrete white bile or phlegm. Anise is also described by Maimonides in his *Glossary of Drug Names*,[2] where he describes it as the seed of the Roman fennel and that which the people of Maghrib know as sweet cumin.

1. F. Rosner, *Moses Maimonides' Three Treatises on Health* (Haifa: Maimonides Research Institute, 1990), pp. 57–58.

2. F. Rosner, *Moses Maimonides' Glossary of Drug Names* (Haifa: Maimonides Research Institute, 1996), no. 19.

*ANOREXIA*—The drinking of tepid water is said to produce body weakness and loss of appetite.[1] In his *Treatises on Health*, Maimonides says that satiety causes loss of appetite because the stomach is full and distended.[2] An emotional experience or psychological shock can produce anorexia or loss of appetite. In his *Mishneh Torah* (*Deot* 4:10), Maimonides advises that a person who wishes to be strong should not yield to his appetite by eating excessively or by consuming detrimental foods.

In his *Medical Aphorisms*,[3] Maimonides lists anorexia as one of the classic symptoms of liver inflammation (Chapter 6:55). He quotes Galen, who said that anorexia may occur at the beginning of bloody diarrhea (ibid., 6:90). As the illness progresses, the anorexia becomes more pronounced. Complete loss of appetite may represent a life-threatening situation (ibid., 6:94). Anorexia may also develop together with repulsion of food and nausea in patients with melancholy or splenic illness (ibid., 9:79). Capers are said to be an appetite stimulant because they liquefy the white bile and the phlegma in the stomach and excrete it in the stool (ibid., 21:37).

1. F. Rosner, *Moses Maimonides' Treatise on Asthma* (Haifa: Maimonides Research Institute, 1994), p. 72.

2. F. Rosner, *Moses Maimonides' Three Treatises on Health* (Haifa: Maimonides Research Institute, 1990).

3. F. Rosner, *The Medical Aphorisms of Moses Maimonides* (Haifa: Maimonides Research Institute, 1989).

*APHRODISIACS*—In his *Treatise on Sexual Intercourse*,[1] Maimonides describes aphrodisiac foods and medications. Such foods include lamb meat, pigeon meat, and all brains, especially the brains of chickens. Doves, other birds, and rooster testicles are extremely helpful in increasing sperm (Chapter 4). Also beneficial to increasing libido are bone marrow, chicken-egg yolks, the eggs of doves and partridges, and fresh milk as it issues from the nipples (ibid.). Aphrodisiac fruits include almonds, hazelnuts, grapes, pistachio and indican nuts, and black-pepper kernels. Also, honey and wine incite sexual desire (ibid.). Maimonides also describes various concoctions of foods and drugs that are either aphrodisiac or antiaphrodisiac in their effect.

In his *Medical Aphorisms*,[2] Maimonides reiterates the efficacy of fowl consumption to increase sexual potency (Chapter 20:69). Chicken eggs or testicles, especially if cooked with onion or turnip, are potent aphrodisiacs (20:71–72). There is some disagreement as to whether or not coconut is an aphrodisiac (20:86). Oophorectomy destroys a woman's libido (24:29).

Mandrakes (Gen. 29:35) and other aphrodisiacs are described in the Bible, the Talmud, and other ancient Jewish writings.[3] Maimonides does not enumerate mandrake as having aphrodisiac activity, but he lists this plant in his *Glossary of Drug Names*.[4]

---

1. F. Rosner, *Maimonides' Treatises on Poisons, Hemorrhoids and Cohabitation* (Haifa: Maimonides Research Institute, 1984), pp. 153–182.
2. F. Rosner, *The Medical Aphorisms of Moses Maimonides* (Haifa: Maimonides Research Institute, 1989).
3. F. Rosner, *Medicine in the Bible and the Talmud*, augmented edition (Hoboken, NJ, and New York: Ktav and Yeshiva University Press, 1995), 127–131.
4. F. Rosner, *Moses Maimonides' Glossary of Drug Names* (Haifa: Maimonides Research Institute, 1996).

*APOPLEXY*—In his *Medical Aphorisms*,[1] Maimonides quotes Galen, who said that one can prognosticate regarding a stroke called apoplexy. If it is severe, the patient will certainly die, but if it is minor, cure is possible, although difficult. The worst situation is the complete irreversible suppression of respiration (Chapter 6:1). A severe stroke causes death because apoplexy causes loss or marked derangement of important functions such as respiration, rational thinking, speech, the senses, and the pulse (ibid., 6:94). The cause of apoplexy is said to be the mobility of the "soul spirit" to move out of the head to the other organs because of either an abscess in the brain or the filling of the cerebral ventricles with phlegmatic humors (ibid., 23:61).

In his *Commentary on the Aphorisms of Hippocrates*,[2] Maimonides states that apoplexy usually occurs without fever (Section 2:19). He quotes Hippocrates, who, like Galen, said that if an attack of apoplexy is strong, the patient cannot recover. He then explains the cause of apoplexy and paralysis (ibid., 2:42). He disagrees with Hippocrates' claim that apoplexy and other illnesses occur in association with a lot of rain (ibid., 3:16). Hippocrates also said that apoplexy occurs in both the spring (ibid., 3:20) and the winter (ibid., 3:23), and that it is an affliction of old people (ibid., 3:31), to which Maimonides responds: "This is clear to one who is familiar with the constitution of old people" (ibid.). Later, he describes a "stertorous sound" or death rattle, which is a sign of imminent death in a speechless apoplexy patient (ibid., 3:51). He quotes Galen's and Hippocrates' assertion that illnesses of the black bile may lead to apoplexy or hemiplegia and are most apt to occur in a person between forty and sixty years of age (ibid., 6:56–57). Maimonides retorts by saying that the development of these two illnesses from the black bile is a rarity, and that they occur mostly as a result of the white humor, and from age sixty and up (ibid.).

1. F. Rosner, *The Medical Aphorisms of Moses Maimonides* (Haifa: Maimonides Research Institute, 1989).

2. F. Rosner, *Maimonides' Commentary on the Aphorisms of Hippocrates* (Haifa: Maimonides Research Institute, 1987).

*APPLES*—In one of his *Treatises on Health*,[1] Maimonides states that the consumption of apples and quinces after a meal is advisable for the maintenance of good health. Is this the source of the adage "An apple a day keeps the doctor away"? These and other fruits are astringent and bind the intestines, and therefore should be consumed immediately after the meal (*Mishneh Torah, Deot* 4:6). In his *Medical Aphorisms*,[2] Maimonides quotes Abu Merwan Ibu

Zuhr, who said that apples strengthen the brain and are salutary for the emaciated and enfeebled. However, apple flavoring gives rise to gases in the nerves and muscles (Chapter 20:74). The constipating action of apples or apple juice is also stated in Maimonides' *Extracts from Galen*,[3] where apples are said to be harmful to patients with tumors of the liver "because they close the mouth of the bile duct and cause it to shrink and prevent the bile from coming out." Apples are particularly harmful if the tumor is on the concave side of the liver. In his *Treatise on Asthma*,[4] he states that the Egyptians use apple juice as an ingredient in purgative medications.

1. F. Rosner, *Moses Maimonides' Three Treatises on Health* (Haifa: Maimonides Research Institute, 1990), p. 134.

2. F. Rosner, *The Medical Aphorisms of Moses Maimonides* (Haifa: Maimonides Research Institute, 1989).

3. U.S. Barzel, *Maimonides' The Art of Cure. Extracts from Galen* (Haifa: Maimonides Research Institute, 1992), pp. 105 and 158.

4. F. Rosner, *Moses Maimonides' Treatise on Asthma* (Haifa: Maimonides Research Institute, 1994), p. 129.

*APRICOTS*—In his *Causes of Symptoms*,[1] Maimonides allows the consumption of small amounts of apricots, pears, and quinces before meals to stimulate the appetite or after the meal as an astringent. He strongly objects, however, to the consumption of fresh fruits as foods because "they are rapidly transformed into harmful humors" (p. 135). He explains this objection further in the first chapter of his *Regimen of Health* and in his *Mishneh Torah* (*Deot* 4:11). Such opposition is understandable because of the rapid spoilage of soft fruit in a hot country such as Egypt. Apricots are also mentioned by Maimonides in his *Glossary of Drug Names* (drugs nos. 13 and 233).[2] [*See also* FRUITS]

---

1. F. Rosner, *Moses Maimonides' Three Treatises on Health* (Haifa: Maimonides Research Institute, 1990).

2. F. Rosner, *Moses Maimonides' Glossary of Drug Names* (Haifa: Maimonides Research Institute, 1996).

*ARISTOLOCHIA*—In his *Glossary of Drug Names*,[1] Maimonides describes the round and long forms of aristolochia, a plant whose root serves as an emmenagogue. In his *Treatise on Asthma*,[2] he advises oxymel syrup in seeds of aristolochia for stomach cleansing without vomiting. Aristolochia is also one of many ingredients in a commonly used purgative preparation that expels white humors and cleanses the head.

---

1. F. Rosner, *Moses Maimonides' Glossary of Drug Names* (Haifa: Maimonides Research Institute, 1996), no. 133.

2. F. Rosner, *Moses Maimonides' Treatises on Asthma* (Haifa: Maimonides Research Institute, 1994), pp. 82 and 104.

*ARMENGAUD BLASIUS*—Translator and physician to King James II of Aragon (1291–1327) and to Pope Clement V (1305– 1315), Armengaud made his translations from the Arabic or from the Hebrew, or at any rate with the help of Hebrew versions.[1] Among the works he translated is Maimonides' *Treatise on Asthma* (*Tractatus contra passionem asthematis*). This Latin translation, composed in 1302, was not printed. Latin translations of Maimonides' *Regimen of Health* and *Treatise on Poisons* are attributed to Armengaud, but are really the works of John of Capua.[2]

---

1. M. Steinschneider, *Hebraeische Uebersetzungen*, 1893 (facsimile reprint 1956), pp. 764, 767, 772, 778; ibid. *Die Europäischen Uebersetzungen aus dem Arabischen*, 1905 (facsimile reprint 1956), 33, no. 163 (2nd pagination).

2. A. Marx, *Jewish Quarterly Review*, new series 9 (1918):254–255.

*ARTERIES*—In his *Medical Aphorisms*,[1] Maimonides quotes Galen, who describes arteries and veins as pulsating and nonpulsating vessels that enter all body organs together and are deeply embedded therein.

Sometimes the veins and arteries are so close to each other that they adhere (Chapter 1:3). Arteries and veins come from the closest large blood vessels, except those that supply the breasts and the testicles. Here, the vessels arise from distal blood vessels to prolong the mixing of blood until the milk or semen, respectively, is thoroughly ripe (ibid., 1:4). All arteries have corresponding veins, with rare exceptions (ibid., 1:5). Large arteries, such as the hepatic and renal arteries and veins, the aorta, and the inferior vena cava are also described (ibid., 3:34). Maimonides discusses the carotid arteries in his *Mishnah Commentary* (*Chullin* 1:1), where he calls them "the pulsating vessels on the side of the neck." The expansion and contraction of arteries produces the pulse (*Aphorisms* 4:2). If the arteries fill with dark and viscous blood, disease will ensue (ibid., 7:24). Overfilled arteries may become visible to the naked eye (ibid., 8:57). Blood-borne infection and endocarditis seem to be described in the statement, "If putrefaction occurs in large arteries, a substance . . . reaches into the heart chambers and putrefies there" (ibid., 10:10). An excess of blood or abnormal blood in arteries should be treated with phlebotomy, followed by purgative medications to purify the humor in the blood (ibid., 12:39). Pulsating blood vessels may occur in tumors (ibid., 15:13), probably a reflection of their vascularity. Severance of an ar-

tery can result in fatal hemorrhage (ibid., 15:46). Although men and women differ in their reproductive organs, their arteries and veins throughout the body are of one kind—not only in number, but also in structure, function, and location (ibid., 16:10).

Elsewhere,[2] Maimonides describes wounds of blood vessels that tear and that leak blood. The blood flow can be treated by "blocking or stopping up the wound through which the blood leaks" by contracting the wound with a bandage or "by the clotting in it of fresh blood, or by things applied to it from the outside." He then details several such measures.

---

1. F. Rosner, *The Medical Aphorisms of Moses Maimonides* (Haifa: Maimonides Research Institute, 1989).

2. U.S. Barzel, *Maimonides' The Art of Cure. Extracts from Galen* (Haifa: Maimonides Research Institute, 1992), pp. 55–57.

*ARTHRITIS*—Maimonides quotes Hippocrates' statement that arthritis is one of the afflictions of old age. Arthritis is alleviated by pouring cold water over the affected joints, which, Maimonides explains, stops the pain-producing humor from going to them and also benumbs one's senses.[1] In his *Treatise on Asthma*, he writes that the cure for arthritis, podagra (gout), asthma, and other ailments "is not known or is difficult."[2] In his *Extracts from Galen*, Maimonides speaks of arthritis, sciatica, gout, and headaches as being due to excessive and faulty humors, and offers herbs and medications as treatments. He also discusses the formation of stones in the joints.[3]

In his *Medical Aphorisms*, Maimonides quotes Galen, who recommended a bland diet or bloodletting for patients suffering from arthritis.[4] Arthritis limited to the hip joint is called sciatica. If it occurs in the feet, it is called podagra. The abnormal humor, or chyme, is usually a raw or viscous one. Liquids within joints resemble mucin. Contractures may develop as a result of arthritis. Repeated several times is the therapeutic approach for gout and other forms of arthritis and joint pains: Eliminate the damaging chymes and prevent their reaccumulation. Local measures include both warmth and cold. [*See also* GOUT]

1. F. Rosner, *Maimonides' Commentary on the Aphorisms of Hippocrates* (Haifa: Maimonides Research Institute, 1987), pp. 88 and 137.

2. F. Rosner, *Moses Maimonides' Treatise on Asthma* (Haifa: Maimonides Research Institute, 1994), p. 47.

3. U.S. Barzel, *Maimonides' The Art of Cure. Extracts from Galen* (Haifa: Maimonides Research Institute, 1992), pp. 95 and 167.

4. F. Rosner, *The Medical Aphorisms of Moses Maimonides* (Haifa: Maimonides Research Institute, 1989).

**ASCITES**—In his *Medical Aphorisms*,[1] Maimonides quotes Galen's assertion that ascites (hydrops) is caused by an accumulation of humors in the abdomen and that it produces stretching and separation of vessels. The patient's pulse becomes hard, small, and accelerated, and certainly so if fever occurs (Chapter 4:41). Anasarca is caused by fluid accumulation within all solid body organs, and this produces a fluttering pulse (ibid.). The treatment for anasarca is to expel the white bile through laxatives and emetics followed by gargling to expel white bile from the head. Diuretics should also be used (ibid., 9:59). One should not hasten to puncture the abdomen to drain ascitic fluid unless it becomes unavoidable because the humors increase to such an extent that they weigh heavily on the patient and weaken him (ibid., 15:7). Diuretics are preferable (ibid., 15:36).

1. F. Rosner, *The Medical Aphorisms of Moses Maimonides* (Haifa: Maimonides Research Institute, 1989).

**ASPARAGUS**—In his *Glossary of Drug Names*,[1] Maimonides describes various species of asparagus to be medically used as diaphoretics. In his *Regimen of Health*,[2] he recommends asparagus roots as a healthful food. Asparagus seeds are one of many ingredients in the Great

Itrifal, an electuary that improves digestion and strengthens all body organs. In his *Treatise on Poisons*,[3] he prescribes asparagus root cooked in six ounces of wine as an antidote for the bite of a certain spider. In his *Medical Aphorisms*,[4] he asserts that asparagus increases semen and relieves a backache that is caused by white bile or by cold. Furthermore, if pregnant women eat a lot of asparagus hearts, their offspring will have improved characteristics and qualities. The Talmud (*Berachot* 51a, *Pesachim* 110b), and Maimonides in his *Mishnah Commentary* (*Nedarim* 6:10), state that asparagus is a beverage compounded from cabbage seed and other legumes that should be imbibed in the morning on an empty stomach.

---

1. F. Rosner, *Moses Maimonides' Glossary of Drug Names* (Haifa: Maimonides Research Institute, 1996), no. 111.
2. F. Rosner, *Moses Maimonides' Three Treatises on Health* (Haifa: Maimonides Research Institute, 1990), pp. 44 and 58.
3. F. Rosner, *Maimonides' Treatises on Poisons, Hemorrhoids and Cohabitation* (Haifa: Maimonides Research Institute, 1984), p. 63.
4. F. Rosner, *The Medical Aphorisms of Moses Maimonides* (Haifa: Maimonides Research Institute, 1989), pp. 307–308.

**ASTHENIA**—In his *Treatise on Asthma*,[1] Maimonides writes that the drinking of tepid water is a cause of bodily weakness, the diminution of one's constitution and the beginning of asthenia. Therefore, one should be extremely careful to avoid it. He also claims that excessive bloodletting can lead to fainting or severe, near-fatal asthenia. In his *Medical Aphorisms*,[2] Maimonides quotes Galen, who says that a faulty constitution of humors in organs can lead to weakness. Extreme weakness can produce mental confusion and forgetfulness.

---

1. F. Rosner, *Moses Maimonides' Treatise on Asthma* (Haifa: Maimonides Research Institute, 1994), pp. 72 and 126.
2. F. Rosner, *The Medical Aphorisms of Moses Maimonides* (Haifa: Maimonides Research Institute, 1989).

**ASTROLOGY**—The generally prevalent belief in astrology during the Middle Ages was fully shared by Jews, many of whom were convinced of the fundamental truth of the power of celestial bodies to influence human destiny. Moses Maimonides was one of the few who not only dared to raise his voice against this almost universally held belief, but even branded it as a superstition akin to idolatry.[1] He unequivocally prohibits anyone to influence his actions by astrology, as an offense punishable by disciplinary flogging. In his legal treatise on idolatry and heathen ordinances, he categorically rejects astrology and other superstitious practices and beliefs (*Mishneh Torah, Akum* 11:16).

In his famous *Letter to Yemen*, Maimonides denounces astrology as a fallacy and a delusion:

> I note that you are inclined to believe in astrology and in the influence of the past and future conjunctions of the planets upon human affairs. You should dismiss such notions from your thoughts. Cleanse your mind as one cleanses dirty clothes. Accomplished scholars, whether they are religious or not, refuse to believe in the truth of this science. Its postulates can be refuted by real proofs on rational grounds.

In his psychological and ethical treatise titled *The Eight Chapters* (*Shemonah Perakim*), Maimonides again sharply inveighs against astrology, denouncing it as a deception that is subversive to the faith and teachings of Judaism: "I have entered into this subject so that you may not believe the absurd ideas of astrologers, who falsely assert that the constellation at the time of one's birth determines whether one is to be virtuous or vicious."

In his *Letter on Astrology*, in answer to an inquiry from Jewish scholars of southern France, Maimonides exposes the foibles and fallacies of astrology.[2] Noteworthy in this letter is the oft-quoted comment that the Second Temple was destroyed and national independence forfeited because the Jews were occupied with astrology. Maimonides told his correspondents that he did not take the matter lightly, but had studied it thoroughly and came to the conclusion that astrology was an irrational illusion of fools who mistake vanity for wisdom and superstition for knowledge.

---

1. F. Rosner, "Moses Maimonides' Opposition to Astrology," *Journal of the American Medical Association*, 236 (1976):346.

2. A. Marx, "The Correspondence Between the Rabbis of Southern France and Maimonides About Astrology," *Hebrew Union College Annual* (1926): 311–358 and (1927):493–494.

**ASTRONOMY**—Maimonides' treatise on the sanctification of the New Moon is a masterpiece in astronomy. The treatise appears to be sharply divided into three sections: laws pertaining to the rite of sanctification and to the intercalation of months and years at the time of the Synedrium (*Mishneh Torah, Kiddush Hachodesh*, Chapters 1–5), the system of a continuous fixed calendar (Chapters 6–10), and an astronomical computation of the visibility of the new crescent (Chapters 11–19). Maimonides asserts that members of the ancient Jewish court had to be knowledgeable in astronomy and astronomical computations to determine in advance whether or not the new crescent would be visible at its proper time (ibid., 1:6, 2:4). In the second section of his treatise, he offers, with masterful lucidity and succinctness, a systematic exposition of calendaric regulation, including the lunar months and solar seasons, the mean conjunction of sun and moon, and the four seasons defined by the equinoxes and solstices. In the third section, he discusses the true position of the sun and moon on the eve of the thirtieth day of any month, calculates the moon's longitudinal and latitudinal positions, and computes the limits of visibility of the new crescent. Nonastronomical factors that may influence the visibility of the new crescent, such as weather conditions (ibid., 18:1), the transparency of the air (ibid., 18:2), and the topography of the site of observation (ibid., 18:4), are also discussed by Maimonides.

An analysis of this treatise, its date of composition, sources used by Maimonides, and his astronomical background and motivation in writing it are provided by Obermann in a lengthy introduction to the English translation of Maimonides' "Sanctification of the New Moon."[1]

In discussing scientific beliefs, in his treatise on oaths, Maimonides provides us with certain astronomical facts.

It is well known to wise men endowed with understanding and knowledge that the sun is one hundred and seventy times larger than the earth. If an ordinary person swears that the sun is larger than the earth, he is not liable to a flogging because of a false oath. For although the fact is as stated, this is not commonly known to any but the most eminent scholars, and no person is liable unless he swears about a thing well known to at least three ordinary persons, e.g., that a man is a man, or a stone a stone. Similarly , if he swears that the sun is smaller than the earth, even though this is not so, he is not liable to a flogging. For this subject is not familiar to all men, and it is, therefore, not like swearing that a man is a woman, as he is merely swearing about the way the sun appears to him, and he does indeed see it small. This holds good in all similar cases connected with calculations dealing with astronomical cycles, constellations, and geometrical measurements, and other scientific matters which are known only to some men (*Shebuot* 5:22).

Lengthy discussions by Maimonides on astronomy can also be found in his *Guide for the Perplexed* and in some of his letters.[2] The interested reader is referred to these sources for further detail.

---

1. J. Obermann, in *Sanctification of the New Moon*, trans. S. Gandz (New Haven, CT: Yale University Press, 1956).

2. L.D. Stitskin, *Letters of Maimonides* (New York: Yeshiva University Press, 1977).

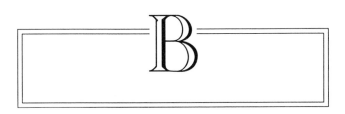

**BAR SELA, ARIEL**—A native Israeli physician, Bar Sela joined the faculty of the Baylor College of Medicine in 1959. Together with E. Hoff and Elias Faris, Bar Sela translated and edited in English *Moses Maimonides' Two Treatises on the Regimen of Health* (American Philosophical Society, 1964). Also with H.E. Hoff, Bar Sela authored an English translation of Maimonides' Interpretation of the First Aphorism of Hippocrates (*Bulletin of the History of Medicine*, 37 (1963):347–354).

**BARLEY**—In his *Medical Aphorisms*,[1] Maimonides quotes Galen, who said that barley gruel invigorates body strength and cleanses the respiratory passages of bad humors by dissolution and liquefaction (Chapter 8:25). Barley gruel's cleansing power can be increased by mixing some pepper therein (ibid., 21:8). Barley gruel also contains a cooling force for an inflamed eye (ibid., 21:9). Mixed with lentils, barley gruel is a most nutritious food (ibid.).

In his *Treatise on Asthma*,[2] Maimonides recommends small birds roasted or prepared with barley soup for patients with asthma. Also beneficial are certain fruits consumed with barley soup. Beets seasoned with barley gruel serve as an effective laxative. A dish made of barley with its peel is an effective emetic. Barley soup assists in expectoration in an asthmatic patient. In his *Extracts from Galen*[3] and in his *Treatises on Health*,[4] Maimonides discusses at length the virtues of barley, barley soup, and barley gruel for both healthy and sick people. Barley, barley beer, barley bread, barley flour, barley groats, and barley water are all discussed in the Talmud.[5]

---

1. F. Rosner, *The Medical Aphorisms of Moses Maimonides* (Haifa: Maimonides Research Institute, 1989).

2. F. Rosner, *Moses Maimonides' Treatise on Asthma* (Haifa: Maimonides Research Institute, 1994).

3. U.S. Barzel, *Maimonides' The Art of Cure. Extracts from Galen* (Haifa: Maimonides Research Institute, 1992).

4. F. Rosner, *Moses Maimonides' Three Treatises on Health* (Haifa: Maimonides Research Institute, 1990).

5. F. Rosner (translator), *Julius Preuss' Biblical and Talmudic Medicine* (Northvale, NJ: Jason Aronson, 1993).

*BARRENNESS*—In his *Mishnah Commentary*, Maimonides asserts that a barren woman cannot give birth because of the characteristics of her body. The tokens are that she does not have breasts like other women's breasts, she has no hair growing on her body like other women, her voice is deep so that one cannot distinguish between it and the voice of men, and the female pudenda do not project from her body as they do in other women (*Yebamot* 1:1).

In his *Mishneh Torah*, Maimonides describes the signs of barrenness in women (*Eeshut* 2:4–6) and men (ibid. 2:11–12). He distinguishes between a congenital or "sun-made" eunuch and acquired eunuchism secondary to illness, trauma, or surgery. He rules that if a eunuch performs a betrothal or if a barren woman is betrothed, the betrothal is completely valid (ibid., 4:10). Additional references to barrenness are found in *Mishneh Torah*[1] and are scattered throughout his medical writings.[2]

1. F. Rosner, *Medicine in the Mishneh Torah of Maimonides* (New York: Ktav, 1984), pp. 143–153.

2. F. Rosner, Moses Maimonides the Physician, in *Moses Maimonides: Physician, Scientist, and Philosopher* (F. Rosner and S.S. Kottek, eds.) (Northvale, NJ: Jason Aronson, 1993), pp. 3–12.

*BARZEL, URIEL S.*—A native Israeli physician, Barzel studied Arabic, Islamic culture, and philosophy. Since 1975, he has been Associate Professor of Medicine at the Albert Einstein College of Medicine of New York's Yeshiva University. Barzel published excerpts in Hebrew and English of *Maimonides' The Art of Cure. Extracts from Galen, Harofe Haivri, Hebrew Medical Journal*, 28 (1955):82–93 and 164–177) and later the entire work in English (Haifa: Maimonides Research Institute, 1992).

*BATHING*—In his *Mishneh Torah* (*Deot* 4:16–17), Maimonides recommends that healthy people should bathe every seven days, but not shortly after a meal or when hungry. The whole body should be washed with hot and then lukewarm water. Upon leaving the bath one should be careful not to catch a draft. It is good to sleep a little after a bath before eating. Excessive heat in a bathhouse may be harmful to one's health.

An entire chapter in Maimonides' *Medical Aphorisms*[1] is devoted to bathing based on the writings of Galen. Lengthy discussions of the indications and contraindications of bathing are also found in Maimonides' *Treatises on Health*,[2] *Treatise on Asthma*,[3] and *Extracts from Galen*.[4]

1. F. Rosner, *The Medical Aphorisms of Moses Maimonides* (Haifa: Maimonides Research Institute, 1989).

2. F. Rosner, *Moses Maimonides' Three Treatises on Health* (Haifa: Maimonides Research Institute, 1990).

3. F. Rosner, *Moses Maimonides' Treatise on Asthma* (Haifa: Maimonides Research Institute, 1994).

4. U.S. Barzel, *Maimonides' The Art of Cure. Extracts from Galen* (Haifa: Maimonides Research Institute, 1992).

*BEANS*—In his *Mishneh Torah* (*Deot* 4:9), Maimonides categorizes beans as a detrimental food that people should eat sparingly and only during the rainy (i.e., winter) season. In his *Treatise on Asthma*,[1] however, he recommends soup made from rue, beets, and chicken, cooked with beans, for asthmatic patients. He also describes a dish made of crushed beans (in Hebrew, *grissin shel pul*, a term frequently used in the Talmud, e.g., *Niddah* 9 and *Machshirin* 5) as an emetic. In his *Medical Aphorisms*,[2] he cites Abu Merwan Ibn Zuhr, who said that beans decrease the intellect. Beans, bean gruel, and bean soup are also discussed in the Talmud.[3]

------

1. F. Rosner, *Moses Maimonides' Treatise on Asthma* (Haifa: Maimonides Research Institute, 1994), pp. 58 and 62.

2. F. Rosner, *The Medical Aphorisms of Moses Maimonides* (Haifa: Maimonides Research Institute, 1989), p. 349.

3. F. Rosner (translator), *Julius Preuss' Biblical and Talmudic Medicine* (Northvale, NJ: Jason Aronson, 1993).

*BEETS*—In his *Treatise on Asthma*,[1] Maimonides describes beets as an ingredient of a laxative potion. Beet juice mixed with olive oil serves as an effective enema and preserves the health of people with hard, dry stools that are difficult to evacuate. In his *Medical Aphorisms*,[2] Maimonides quotes Galen, who said that radishes and beets are converted to blood in the body, but only a little and only after a very active preparatory process (Chapter 20:18). In his *Regimen of Health*,[3] Maimonides recommends beets as a healthy food, especially in the summer months. The medicinal and nutritive values of beets are also mentioned in the Talmud (*Berachot* 44b and *Sanhedrin* 64a, respectively). Beets are also efficacious against internal inflammation (*Gittin* 69b) and ward off the skin illness known as *raathan* (*Ketubot* 77b). The beet (*beta vulgaris*) is also described by Maimonides in his *Glossary of Drug Names*[4] as a species of carrot.

------

1. F. Rosner, *Moses Maimonides' Treatise on Asthma* (Haifa: Maimonides Research Institute, 1994), pp. 76–78.

2. F. Rosner, *The Medical Aphorisms of Moses Maimonides* (Haifa: Maimonides Research Institute, 1989), p. 296.

3. F. Rosner, *Moses Maimonides' Three Treatises on Health* (Haifa: Maimonides Research Institute, 1990), pp. 54 and 144.

4. F. Rosner, *Moses Maimonides' Glossary of Drug Names* (Haifa: Maimonides Research Institute, 1996), no. 361.

*BENVENISTE, SAMUEL*—A fourteenth-century Spanish physician and translator from Saragossa, Benveniste served as physician to Don Manuel, brother of King Pedro of Aragon. In about 1300, Benveniste translated Maimonides' *Treatise on Asthma* into Hebrew, probably from the Latin rather than the original Arabic. Benveniste's translation was edited with introduction and notes by Suessman Muntner.[1]

---

1. S. Muntner, *Moshe ben Maimon— Sefer Haketzeret (Maimonides' Book on Asthma)* (Jerusalem: Rubin Mass, 1940). Reprinted in 1963 by Geniza (Jerusalem) and in 1965 by Mossad Harav Kook (Jerusalem).

**BESTIALITY**—Bestiality is strongly condemned by Maimonides in his *Mishneh Torah*, where he states:

> If a man has a connection with an animal, or causes an animal to have connection with him, both are punishable by stoning, as it is said, "And thou shalt not lie with any beast" (Lev. 18:23), i.e., whether he is the active or passive participant in the act. Regardless of whether it is a domestic animal, a wild beast, or a fowl, in all these cases the penalty is death by stoning. Nor does Scripture differentiate between a fully grown animal and one not yet fully grown, seeing that it is said *any* beast, i.e., even a newly born beast. Whether he has connection in a natural manner or not, once he has initiated sexual contact with it, or has caused it to initiate contact with him, he is liable (*Issurei Biyah* 1:16).

An additional lengthy condemnation of bestiality is found in Maimonides' *Mishnah Commentary* (*Sanhedrin* 7:4).[1]

---

1. F. Rosner, *Maimonides' Commentary on the Mishnah, Tractate Sanhedrin* (New York: Sepher Hermon, 1981), pp. 86–94.

**BITES**—The first section of Maimonides' *Treatise on Poisons*[1] deals with the bites of snakes and mad dogs and the stings of scorpions, bees, wasps, and spiders. The recommended emergency care of the victim, including the application of a ligature proximal to the bite, incising the bite, and sucking out the poison, is as up-to-date as any modern textbook on toxicology or poisoning. Maimonides also describes simple and compounded remedies to draw out the poison when applied to the bite, and remedies to be taken internally. He details the preparation of the great theriacs or electuaries used by ancient and medieval physicians. Dietary measures for animal-bite victims are also discussed.

In his *Medical Aphorisms*,[2] Maimonides quotes Galen, who said that if a person is bitten by a scorpion and the poison descends into a nerve, an artery, or a vein, the bite produces extremely severe complications (Chapter 9:109). The poison must be emptied from the site of the bite by strong medications or suction cups, or by sucking out the poison with one's mouth (ibid., 9:119). Life-saving antidotes should be taken in maximal quantity, but without harming the patient's body (ibid., 21:49). For insect bites, one should drink the great theriac in diluted pure wine (ibid., 21:50). For crocodile bites, apply an ointment made from crocodiles to the wound, and it heals rapidly (ibid., 21:54).

In his *Extracts from Galen*,[3] Maimonides reiterates the treatment of an animal bite or sting: Alleviate the pain and remove the poison by medicines that pull strongly, by cupping glasses or hollow horns, by sucking out the poison with one's mouth, and by medicines that burn, like cauterization.

Finally, in his *Mishneh Torah* (*Shabbat* 10:25), Maimonides rules that because of possible danger to life, harmful reptiles, such as snakes and scorpions, may be captured on the Sabbath, even if their bite is not fatal, provided that the sole intention is to escape being bitten. For the same reason, wild beasts or reptiles whose bite is certain to be fatal may be killed on sight on the Sabbath (ibid., 11:4).

1. F. Rosner, *Moses Maimonides' Treatises on Poisons, Hemorrhoids and Cohabitation* (Haifa: Maimonides Research Institute, 1987), pp. 1–115.

2. F. Rosner, *The Medical Aphorisms of Moses Maimonides* (Haifa: Maimonides Research Institute, 1989).

3. U.S. Barzel, *Maimonides' The Art of Cure. Extracts from Galen* (Haifa: Maimonides Research Institute, 1992), p. 156.

**BLADDER**—In his *Medical Aphorisms*,[1] Maimonides quotes Galen, who said that the urinary bladder and the gallbladder receive (blood) vessels that nourish them and have tubes or ducts that remove superfluities or wastes from them (Chapter 1:63). The tubes or ducts referred to are obviously the urethra and the cystic duct, respectively. The urinary bladder is located near the uterus (ibid., 1:65). Excretion of wastes from a diseased urinary bladder may be difficult (ibid., 8:15). The bladder may be empty because the kidneys cease to function (ibid., 9:96). Polyuria and polydipsia are described as symptoms of diabetes in which the patient drinks large quantities of fluids and excretes them by way of the urinary bladder (ibid., 23:94). Galen incorrectly attributed this disease to an illness in the kidneys and bladder (ibid.).

Various medications and instruments (i.e., catheters) to treat different bladder disorders are discussed in Maimonides' *Extracts from Galen*.[2] A remedy to cleanse the bladder and excrete its contents consists of terebinth resin or radish juice.[3] [*See also* UROLOGY]

1. F. Rosner, *The Medical Aphorisms of Moses Maimonides* (Haifa: Maimonides Research Institute, 1989).

2. U.S. Barzel, *Maimonides' The Art of Cure. Extracts from Galen* (Haifa: Maimonides Research Institute, 1992).

3. F. Rosner, *Moses Maimonides' Treatise on Asthma* (Haifa: Maimonides Research Institute, 1994), p. 76.

**BLINDNESS**—In his *Mishneh Torah*, Maimonides rules that a blind person is considered to be legally in good health in terms of the validity of his buying, selling, and giving gifts (*Zechiyah Umatanah* 8:1). The blind, although they recognize voices and thus identify persons, are ineligible to testify in court by biblical law, as written: "He being a witness, whether he hath seen" (Lev. 5:1). Only one who can see may give evidence (*Edut.* 9:12). Someone blind in one eye, however, is eligible to serve as a witness (ibid.). Among the ten classes of people ineligible to give testimony in court, based primarily on biblical law, are blind people (ibid., 9:1). A person blind in one eye can also serve as a judge in civil, but not in capital, cases (*Sanhedrin* 11:11).

The Bible, the Talmud, and post-talmudic Hebrew writings contain a vast amount of literature pertaining to diseases of the eyes, including their etiology, blindness, diagnosis and treatment, and the position of the blind in Jewish law. The interested reader is referred to Preuss's classic book.[1]

1. F. Rosner (translator), *Julius Preuss' Biblical and Talmudic Medicine* (North-vale, NJ: Jason Aronson, 1994), pp. 259–284.

**BLOCH, SAMSON**—A native Polish author of Hebrew books, Bloch (1784–1845) is mainly known for his *Shebile Olam* (*Paths of the World*), a description of the geography and the nations of Asia and Africa. According to Wachstein,[1] Bloch is the editor of the earliest published Hebrew version of Maimonides' *Regimen of Health*, although his name is nowhere mentioned in the *Kerem Hemed* (1838, 3:31–39) in which it was published. The title in that periodical is *Michtav Harav Moshe ben Maimon be'ad ha Sultan* (*Letter of Moses Maimonides to the Sultan*).

1. B. Wachstein, *Die Hebraeische Publizistik in Wien*, 1:15–16, 267.

**BLOOD**—Maimonides subscribed to the medieval concept of the four body humors: blood (red bile), phlegm (white bile), melancholy (black bile), and choler (yellow bile). These humors correspond to the four qualities: hot, cold, dry, and wet. Disease was thought to be the result of an abnormal quality or quantity or mixture of humors. In his *Regimen of Health*, Maimonides warns against the consumption of certain fruits such as peaches, apricots, and raisins, which generate humors and cause the blood to boil (Chapters 1:12 and 3:6). Emotional experiences such as fright cause a person to become pale because the blood goes to the interior of the body (ibid., 3:10), apparently a description of peripheral vasoconstriction. The blood in the heart was thought to carry pneuma or vital spirit (ibid., 4:1), which is disseminated throughout the body by the arteries.

In another of his *Treatises on Health*,[1] Maimonides states that wine generates healthy blood similar to natural blood, which is hot and moist. Plethora represents an excess or overfilling of blood in the body and is treated by bloodletting. Such blood excess is also discussed by Maimonides in his *Extracts from Galen*,[2] where he states that it may be expelled by menstrual bleeding or other spontaneous bleeding that is sometimes difficult to stop. Overflow of blood due to rheum can be expelled by expectorating blood. He describes a boy who coughed up a large quantity of blood and who recovered after aggressive treatment. Other similar patients did not survive. The disease being treated is not identified, but may have been tuberculosis. In his *Treatise on Asthma*,[3] Maimonides reiterates the origin of the pneuma of the blood from the liver and its dissemination through the heart and great vessels to the entire body. Moderate drinking of cold water prevents putrefaction of blood in the vessels.

Finally, in his *Medical Aphorisms*,[4] Maimonides quotes Galen's assertion that very little and thin blood and pneuma flow in arteries, but thick pneuma flows in veins (Chapter 1:19). Blood is superior to all the humors (ibid., 2:1). Good blood is transformed into good nourishment for the body, whereas bad blood leads to decay and putrefaction (sepsis?) (ibid., 3:31). Completely cooked (i.e., metabolized) blood reaches the breasts (ibid., 3:38), where it is transformed into mother's milk (see the Talmud, *Bechorot* 6b and *Niddah* 9a). Blood not only nourishes organs, but maintains natural body heat (*Aphorisms* 3:46). Nasal bleeding or epistaxis is described (ibid., 6:17), as is hemoptysis (ibid., 9:37–38), hemorrhoidal bleeding (ibid., 6:81), and menstrual bleeding (ibid., 16:1–7). Remedies to stop hemorrhages are given (ibid., 15:47). Congested or coagulated blood (ibid., 6:91), thick blood (ibid., 7:24), and watery blood (ibid., 8:67) are characterized and their causes and effects described. Bloody diarrhea or black stools occur in liver disease (ibid., 6:82 and 89). Hematomas occur when blood flows outside the arteries under the skin (ibid., 24:13).

In his legal code (*Mishneh Torah*), Maimonides lists blood as one of the five liquids that render foodstuffs susceptible to ritual uncleanness (*Tumat Ochlin* 1:1). The consumption of blood is prohibited (ibid.,

6:1), which, as he explains in part in his *Guide for the Perplexed* (Section 3:48), is because blood is difficult to digest and constitutes a harmful nourishment.

---

1. F. Rosner, *Moses Maimonides' Three Treatises on Health* (Haifa: Maimonides Research Institute, 1990), pp. 131 and 137.
2. U.S. Barzel, *Maimonides' The Art of Cure. Extracts from Galen* (Haifa: Maimonides Research Institute, 1992).
3. F. Rosner, *Moses Maimonides' Treatise on Asthma* (Haifa: Maimonides Research Institute, 1994).
4. F. Rosner, *The Medical Aphorisms of Moses Maimonides* (Haifa: Maimonides Research Institute, 1989).

*BLOODLETTING*—The teachings of antiquity concerning the body humors and temperaments are rarely found in talmudic writings. However, the subject of bloodletting, or venesection, for plethora and as a hygienic or prophylactic measure is discussed in great detail in the Talmud.[1] The discussion includes the recommended amount, timing, and frequency of bloodletting, nourishment to be consumed before and after the procedure, instructions for its use, and bloodletting in animals.

Bloodletting was a commonly practiced procedure for the treatment of a variety of ailments and was sometimes hazardous. Maimonides rules that before bloodletting, the patient should recite a supplication to God for healing and that, after the treatment is over, he should say, "Blessed are Thou, Healer of the living" (*Mishneh Torah, Berachot* 10:12). Elsewhere in *Mishneh Torah* (*Deot* 4:1ff) and more extensively in *Medical Aphorisms*,[2] Maimonides discusses the subject of bloodletting. He asserts that one should not phlebotomize a youth below age fourteen or anyone over the age of seventy. One should not be guided by only the age of a particular patient, but "One should examine his facial appearance. This is because one finds many people who are only sixty years old who cannot tolerate phlebotomy at all, whereas others who are seventy years old can tolerate this well because their blood is plentiful and their strength is great." He further states that "the conditions and complications that militate against bloodletting . . . are as follows: convulsive disorders, severe insomnia, anginal type pain . . . someone who is extremely obese, or someone who is inordinately anxious, or a youngster or an elderly person or someone who is very fearful and cowardly, or someone who is not accustomed to giving blood . . . or someone plagued by diarrhea and colitis." The frequency, timing, and site of venesection, the quantity to be removed, and other facets of bloodletting are also discussed. During the procedure, "most important of all is to examine the status of the pulse. If one perceives that the pulse is changing either in its largeness [i.e., fullness] or evenness [i.e., rhythm], one should terminate the phlebotomy. It is obviously unnecessary for me to mention that venesection should cease immediately if a patient becomes faint."

Additional references to bloodletting are found throughout Maimonides' other medical writings.

----

1. F. Rosner, *Medicine in the Bible and the Talmud*, augmented edition (Hoboken, NJ: Ktav and Yeshiva University Press), 1995, pp. 150–161.

2. F. Rosner, *The Medical Aphorisms of Moses Maimonides* (Haifa: Maimonides Research Institute, 1989), pp. 213–223.

*BRAGMAN, LOUIS JOSEPH—* This New York State physician published several articles on Jewish medicine, including a general description of Maimonides' *Treatise on Hemorrhoids* (*New York State Journal of Medicine*, 27 (1927):598–601) and a free English translation of Maimonides' *Treatise on Poisons* (*Medical Journal and Record*, 124 (1926):103–107 and 169–171).

*BRAIN*—In his *Medical Aphorisms*,[1] Maimonides quotes Galen, who states that the brain is one of the unpaired organs of the body (Chapter 1:21). Many well-recognized anatomical structures of the brain are described, such as the anterior fontanelle in children (ibid., 1:41); the pia and dura mater, called the thin and the thick brain membrane (ibid., 1:42); the lamina cribrosa, called the sieve (ibid.); the circle of Willis, or the interweaving web of arteries (ibid., 1:43); and the spinal cord (ibid., 1:44). Headache-producing illnesses may originate in the arteries, veins, nerves, meninges, scalp, or brain substance itself (ibid., 6:59). Brain abscesses are of two varieties, cold and hot. Either can produce lethargy, insomnia, stupor, or confusion (ibid., 9:17–18). A variety of therapies are suggested (ibid., 9:18–20). Trauma to the brain itself because of a skull fracture is also described (ibid., 24:55).

In his *Commentary on the Aphorisms of Hippocrates*,[2] Maimonides quotes Hippocrates, who explains that phrenitis is a hot inflammation of the meninges (*birsam*, in Arabic), which produces melancholy that can be rectified if the illness-producing material moves in the opposite direction (Section 6:11). The word *birsam* is also mentioned in the Talmud (*Gittin* 69a), as is the term *kirsam* (*Chullin* 108b). If a person suffers a severe wound to the brain, he develops fever and vomiting owing to swelling of the brain (Section 6:50). Skull fractures and their consequences are again discussed (ibid., 7:24 and 50). Sneezing is said to occur if the brain is heated and the cerebral ventricles are moist, and the air therein descends and produces a noise (ibid., 7:51).

Melancholy is also discussed by Maimonides in his *Regimen of Health*[3] (Section 3:13), where he defines the psychic spirit as the vapor found in the cerebral ventricles (ibid., 4:1). The head should be washed only with hot water, because cold water dulls the brain and causes it to retain its superfluities (ibid., 4:11). To strengthen the brain, one should smell spices and blossoms (ibid., 4:13).

In his *Treatise on Asthma*,[4] Maimonides recommends aromatic herbs for asthmatics "to fortify the brain and dry out any humidity therein" (Chapter 11:1ff). He describes in detail an asthmatic woman for whom he prepared a remedy "to cleanse the lungs, strengthen the brain, and stop the catarrhs" (ibid., 12:5). Numerous references to the brain, including discussions of brain tumors, are found in Maimonides' *Extracts from Galen*.[5]

In his *Mishneh Torah*, Maimonides recognized the fatal outcome in an animal that has torn meninges (*Tumat Met* 6:1). He also describes the pia and dura mater, as well as the medulla oblongata, which he characterizes as "the beanlike structures which are the beginning of the nape of the neck" (ibid., 6:3).

1. F. Rosner, *The Medical Aphorisms of Moses Maimonides* (Haifa: Maimonides Research Institute, 1989).

2. F. Rosner, *Maimonides' Commentary on the Aphorisms of Hippocrates* (Haifa: Maimonides Research Institute, 1987).

3. F. Rosner, *Moses Maimonides' Three Treatises on Health* (Haifa: Maimonides Research Institute, 1990).

4. F. Rosner, *Moses Maimonides' Treatise on Asthma* (Haifa: Maimonides Research Institute, 1994).

5. U.S. Barzel, *Maimonides' The Art of Cure. Extracts from Galen* (Haifa: Maimonides Research Institute, 1992).

**BREAD**—In his *Medical Aphorisms*,[1] Maimonides quotes Galen, who said that the most valuable and most appropriate bread for someone who does not perform any physical exercise, or for the elderly, is bread that has been well baked in the oven and that contains a large quantity of sourdough. However, unleavened bread in all its forms is not appropriate for any type of individual (Chapter 10:16).

In his *Regimen on Health*, Maimonides recommends properly prepared wheat bread to maintain one's health. He then defines "properly prepared":

It should be made from fully ripened wheat after the superfluous moistures are dried out but which is not so old that it begins to spoil. The bread should not be made from refined flour; the flour should be passed through a sieve and its sourness should be perceptible, and one should add a proper amount of salt. But the bread should be made from coarse kernels, unpeeled and unpolished and its sourness should be noticeable. One should work it well while kneading and bake it in an oven. Know that everything that is made from wheat other than this bread is not a good food under any circumstances. Indeed, there are foods made from it which are extremely bad such as unleavened bread, boiled dough such as noodles and macaroni, flour boiled in *ditza* . . . , dough baked in a casserole, dough that is fried like a pancake covered with honey, and bread that is kneaded in olive oil or in any other oil. All these are bad foods for every man (Chapter 1:16).

The Talmud also praises the virtues of wheat bread (*Horayot* 13b). Maimonides also talks of the therapeutic value of thin bread in broth (ibid., 2:8). In one of his other *Treatises on Health*,[2] he reiterates the importance of bread as a healthful food in a regular diet. The flour should be sifted thoroughly until none of the bran remains. It should be breaded so well that its saltiness is evident and the fermentation clearly perceptible, and then baked in an earthen oven. Similar statements about bread, its preparation, and its efficacy are found in his *Treatise on Asthma*.[3] In his *Mishneh Torah* (*Deot* 4:10) he warns against eating large amounts of bread toasted in oil, or bread that was kneaded with oil, or fine meal that was completely sifted so that not a trace of bran remains (see *Pesachim* 2:7), unless they are needed as a medicine.

1. F. Rosner, *The Medical Aphorisms of Moses Maimonides* (Haifa: Maimonides Research Institute, 1989).

2. F. Rosner, *Moses Maimonides' Three Treatises on Health* (Haifa: Maimonides Research Institute, 1994), pp. 142–143.

3. F. Rosner, *Moses Maimonides' Treatise on Asthma* (Haifa: Maimonides Research Institute, 1994).

**BREASTS**—In his *Medical Aphorisms*,[1] Maimonides quotes Galen, who said that the breasts and the uterus were created to perform a single function (i.e., procreation) and, hence, share common arteries and veins (Chapter 3:40). Breast cancer is said to develop in women whose bodies are not cleansed by menstruation (ibid., 16:22). Women's milk to breastfeed their infants is described (ibid., 16:35). Maimonides is strongly critical of Galen's pronouncement that if a pubertal girl's right breast is larger than the left, she will have male offspring; and that if the left is larger, she will have female offspring (ibid., 24:18).

Maimonides quotes Hippocrates,[2] who said that if the breasts of a pregnant woman suddenly shrink in size, she will abort (Chapter 5:37). Maimonides comments on the interrelationship between the breasts and the uterus, and notes that the shriveling of the breasts indicates inadequate nutrition to both of these organs, which leads to abortion. He criticizes Hippocrates' assertion that if blood collects in a woman's breasts, it indicates madness (ibid., 5:40). To stop heavy menstrual bleeding, cupping glasses should be applied to the breasts (ibid., 5:50). Cupping glasses are also discussed in the Talmud (e.g., *Shabbat* 154b).

---

1. F. Rosner, *The Medical Aphorisms of Moses Maimonides* (Haifa: Maimonides Research Institute, 1989).
2. F. Rosner, *Maimonides' Commentary on the Aphorisms of Hippocrates* (Haifa: Maimonides Research Institute, 1987).

*BULIMIA*—In his legal code, the *Mishneh Torah* (*Shevitat Asor* 2:9), Maimonides rules that if someone is seized by ravenous hunger (bulimia), he may be fed on the Day of Atonement (Yom Kippur) until his eyes brighten. One may even feed him carrion or creeping animals (i.e., forbidden foods) immediately, and should not wait until permitted food becomes available. One need not go about searching for permitted food, but should immediately give him whatever comes to hand because of the danger to his life (*Maachalot Assurot* 14:16).

In his *Medical Aphorisms*,[1] Maimonides quotes Galen, who said that perverse craving for food occurs in women usually in the first trimester of pregnancy, and is due to superfluities in the folds of the stomach (Chapter 16:23). In fact, all disorders that develop in women with ravenous appetites or craving for unhealthy foods are due to disturbances at the mouth of the stomach (ibid., 16:24). Bulimia represents a cold, biting pain that develops at the mouth of the stomach and leads to syncope (ibid., 23:87). The therapy for this disorder includes astringent and warming medications (ibid., 23:87).

---

1. F. Rosner, *The Medical Aphorisms of Moses Maimonides* (Haifa: Maimonides Research Institute, 1989).

*BUTTER*—The biblical Hebrew term *chemah* probably refers either to butter, curd, buttermilk, or cream.[1] Quoting Galen, Maimonides says that the residue of milk that is churned and whose butter was removed is called buttermilk.[2] Butter and honey mixed together is an exceptionally valuable food for patients with expectoration that is due to pneumonia (*Aphorisms* 21:18). Furthermore, all types of butter, fresh or boiled, are good for all people.[3]

---

1. F. Rosner, "Milk and Cheese in Classic Jewish Sources," in *Medicine in the Bible and the Talmud*, augmented edition (Hoboken, NJ: Ktav and Yeshiva University Press, 1995), pp. 115–126.
2. F. Rosner, *The Medical Aphorisms of Moses Maimonides* (Haifa: Maimonides Research Institute, 1989), p. 376.
3. F. Rosner, *Moses Maimonides' Three Treatises on Health* (Haifa: Maimonides Research Institute, 1990), p. 27.

**BUTTERWORTH, CHARLES E.—** This American political scientist and philosopher had extensive training in Arabic studies and Islamic philosophy. He translated Chapter 3 of Maimonides' *Regimen of Health* into English and published it in *Ethical Writings of Maimonides*, R.L. Weiss and C.E. Butterworth, eds. (New York: New York University Press, 1975), pp. 105–111.

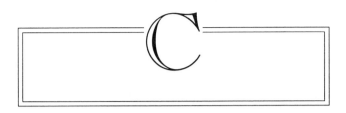

**CABBAGE**—In his *Medical Aphorisms*,[1] Maimonides quotes Abu Merwan Ibu Zuhr, who said that raw or cooked cabbage purifies the voice and removes hoarseness after shouting. In both his *Regimen of Health*[2] and *Mishneh Torah* (*Deot* 4:9), Maimonides lists cabbage as part of a group of vegetables that are bad for all people. The Talmud (*Shabbat* 38a) states that cabbage shrinks when it is cooked, but is thereby improved. Elsewhere (*Berachot* 44b), the Talmud asserts that cabbage is good for sustenance, and beets for healing. Cabbage also cures illness (ibid., 57b), especially if boiled (*Abodah Zarah* 29a). Maimonides also mentions cabbage in his *Glossary of Drug Names*.[3] [*See also* ASPARAGUS]

1. F. Rosner, *The Medical Aphorisms of Moses Maimonides* (Haifa: Maimonides Research Institute, 1989), p. 306.

2. F. Rosner, *Moses Maimonides' Three Treatises on Health* (Haifa: Maimonides Research Institute, 1990), p. 28.

3. F. Rosner, *Moses Maimonides' Glossary of Drug Names* (Haifa: Maimonides Research Institute, 1996), no. 184.

**CANCER**—In his *Extracts from Galen*,[1] Maimonides discusses several types of tumors that vary in color, size, location, consistency, and other features. He is obviously describing both cancers as well as abscesses or infections. The treatment for cancer is to first empty the active humor; then, one should prevent more humors from collecting in the blood vessels leading to the tumor. Black bile in a tumor signifies cancer. Scrofula (tuberculosis) is caused by the formation of a hard tumor in the soft tissues. Abscesses are hot tumors, often filled with red bile or blood. Surgery, cauterization, and various medications are treatments for cancer.

In his *Medical Aphorisms*,[2] Maimonides quotes Galen, who said that dissolving medications should be used to treat cancer (Chapter 9:120). In its early stages, cancer is curable by wide excisional surgery (ibid., 15:13) following purgation to eliminate the black biles (ibid., 15:18). The blood should be allowed to flow freely from the operative site. Then wound compresses should be applied (ibid.). Skin tumors are treated with dissolution, putrefaction, or surgical excision (ibid., 15:20). Breast cancer is said to occur in women whose bodies are not cleansed by menstruation (ibid., 16:22). Cancers always arise from black bile and may be solid or ulcerating (ibid., 23:46–48). Maimonides also quotes Hippocrates,[3] who said that a hidden (i.e., internal) cancer should not be treated because treatment may accelerate death. Some cancer patients survive for long periods without any specific therapy.

---

1. U.S. Barzel, *Maimonides' The Art of Cure. Extracts from Galen* (Haifa: Maimonides Research Institute, 1992), pp. 171–177.
2. F. Rosner, *The Medical Aphorisms of Moses Maimonides* (Haifa: Maimonides Research Institute, 1989).
3. F. Rosner, *Maimonides' Commentary on the Aphorisms of Hippocrates* (Haifa: Maimonides Research Institute, 1987), p. 175.

**CARDIOLOGY**—In his *Medical Aphorisms*,[1] Maimonides quotes Galen, who states that the right chamber of the heart was created for the benefit of the lung. If the lung dies, the right chamber of the heart also dies (Chapter 1:53). The liver is a right-sided organ, and the heart leans toward the left side. The heart attracts beneficial nourishment to itself and repulses that which is harmful (ibid., 3:32–33). Death always follows an extreme aggravation of a bad constitution of the heart (ibid., 3:97). If much cold humor comes to the heart during the height of a fever, the patient is near death. If the heart muscle itself becomes cool or heated, moist, or extremely weak, the cause is a bad constitution (ibid., 4:27). A bad combination of cardiac humors leads to palpitations of the heart (ibid., 6:49). Such sudden heart palpitations can occur in seemingly healthy people, in the young and the old (ibid., 9:113). All are helped by venesection and a light diet.

The exact diseases or conditions being described are not readily clear in modern terms. However, it is apparent that ancient and medieval physicians such as Galen, Maimonides, and others described the anatomy, physiology, and pathophysiology of the heart as understood in those days. Health was present if the four body humors (white bile, or phlegm; red bile, or blood; black bile; and yellow bile) were qualitatively and quantitatively normal. Disequilibrium of these humors leads to illness.

Maimonides ridicules Galen's statement that the benefit of testicles in living beings is greater than that of the heart. If a man's heart is excised, says Maimonides, can he remain alive and live a good life? Can he engage in sexual intercourse and show his male sexual potential? Obviously not! Maimonides agrees with Aristotle's thesis that the heart sends powers to each of the other organs, such as the brain and liver, so that these organs perform their special functions.

In his other medical treatises,[2] Maimonides speaks of extremely bad gases, especially melancholic vapors that enter the heart and the brain and corrupt their humors. He describes pain in the heart resulting in syncope and severe heartache following venesection for indigestion. He lists a variety of recipes to strengthen the heart and restore its normal rhythm. A special concoction is detailed for palpitations of the heart. Maimonides also speaks of sickness in the heart, dryness of the heart, and heart disturbances. He states that hectic fever, of necessity, affects the heart adversely.

---

1. F. Rosner, *The Medical Aphorisms of Moses Maimonides* (Haifa: Maimonides Research Institute, 1989).

2. F. Rosner, *The Medical Legacy of Moses Maimonides* (Hoboken, NJ: Ktav, 1998).

*CASTRATION*—Castration or the mutilation of the procreative organs is forbidden in man and animal (*Mishneh Torah, Issurei Biyah* 16:10). A priest (*kohen*) with maimed or crushed genitalia cannot serve in the Temple, nor may he eat of the heave offering (*Terumot* 7:13). Maimonides defines such individuals (*Issurei Biyah* 16:3–8), giving precise descriptions of a variety of anatomical genital abnormalities, including hypospadias,

anorchidia, and fistulas. He rules that these invalidities apply only to acquired traumatic conditions, but not in cases where a man was born with crushed or maimed genitals or without testicles, or if he contracted a disease that made these organs nonfunctional. These conditions are due to an act of heaven and do not disqualify a priest (ibid., 16:9). A similar discussion is found in Maimonides' *Mishnah Commentary* (*Yebamot* 8:12).

In his *Guide for the Perplexed* (3:49), Maimonides states that we must not injure in any way the organs of generation in living beings (Leviticus 22:24). This lesson is based on the principle of "righteous statutes and judgments" (Deuteronomy 4:8).

The induction of sterility without surgical or traumatic wounding or removal of the genitalia can also be effected by medical means, such as the consumption of a "potion of herbs" used to treat gonorrhea. As a side effect, this potion causes sterility. Maimonides rules that it is forbidden to give men or animals an oral contraceptive potion to render them sterile (*Issurei Biyah* 16:12). Sterilization—indeed, even direct castration—is permitted to obviate danger to life. [*See also* CONTRACEPTION and DANGER TO LIFE]

*CATAPLASMS*—In his *Medical Aphorisms*,[1] Maimonides quotes Galen, who said that cataplasms or poultices help to warm the body

(Chapter 8:2). Warm cataplasms in the winter and cold ones in the summer are beneficial to relieve severe pain of acute abscesses of external body parts (ibid., 8:35). Cataplasms are also therapeutic for severe intestinal colic (ibid., 9:91). For intestinal pain, the cataplasm should be made with millet (ibid., 9:92), as panicum milliaceum (see Ezekiel 4:9). A cataplasm prepared from wheat flour cooked in water and oil more rapidly extracts pus from an abscess than a cataplasm prepared with barley flour cooked in water in which hollyhock roots (radix altheae) have already been cooked (ibid., 21:95). [*See also* COMPRESSES]

———————

1. F. Rosner, *The Medical Aphorisms of Moses Maimonides* (Haifa: Maimonides Research Institute, 1989).

**CAUTERIZATION**—In his *Treatise on Poisons*,[1] Maimonides describes the value of cautery for snakebites when he states that cupping glasses with fire are more efficacious than those without fire. He also briefly discusses cautery in his *Treatise on Asthma*[2] and *Extracts from Galen*,[3] as well as his *Commentary on the Aphorisms of Hippocrates*,[4] in which he recommends cauterization for patients with pus between the chest wall and the lung (empyema?) (Chapter 6:27). Cautery is also used to treat cancer deep within the body (ibid., 6:38).

Further, cauterization is therapeutic to dry out viscous fluid in a dislocated, painful hip; otherwise, the patient becomes lame (ibid., 6:60). In his *Medical Aphorisms*,[5] Maimonides quotes Galen, who said that cauterization may be used as a last resort to eliminate certain illness-producing humors (Chapter 8:43). Cauterization with a red-hot iron or with corrosive medications should be employed at sites of virulent boils (ibid., 15:6), especially those in the chest (ibid., 15:7). Vitriol and arsenic are sharp medications that can be applied to malignant ulcers (ibid., 15:9). Cautery may also be used to stop bleeding from a wound (ibid., 15:39).

———————

1. F. Rosner, *Maimonides' Treatises on Poisons, Hemorrhoids and Cohabitation* (Haifa: Maimonides Research Institute, 1984), p. 40.
2. F. Rosner, *Moses Maimonides' Treatise on Asthma* (Haifa: Maimonides Research Institute, 1994), p. 114.
3. U.S. Barzel, *Maimonides' The Art of Cure. Extracts from Galen* (Haifa: Maimonides Research Institute, 1992), pp. 58 and 156.
4. F. Rosner, *Maimonides' Commentary on the Aphorisms of Hippocrates* (Haifa: Maimonides Research Institute, 1987).
5. F. Rosner, *The Medical Aphorisms of Moses Maimonides* (Haifa: Maimonides Research Institute, 1989).

**CESAREAN SECTION**—In his *Mishneh Torah*, Maimonides rules that if a woman dies in childbirth, it is permissible and perhaps mandatory to perform an immediate cesarean section, even on the Sabbath, in an attempt to save the baby (*Shabbat* 2:15). A child born by cesarean section is not considered a firstborn in relation to the laws of inheritance (*Nachalot* 2:11). If the child is a boy, he is exempt from redemption as a firstborn (*Bechorot* 11:16).

1. F. Rosner, *The Medical Aphorisms of Moses Maimonides* (Haifa: Maimonides Research Institute, 1989).

2. F. Rosner, *Moses Maimonides' Treatise on Asthma* (Haifa: Maimonides Research Institute, 1994).

3. F. Rosner, *Moses Maimonides' Three Treatises on Health* (Haifa: Maimonides Research Institute, 1990).

4. F. Rosner, "Milk and Cheese in Classic Jewish Sources," in *Medicine in the Bible and the Talmud*, augmented edition (Hoboken, NJ: Ktav and Yeshiva University Press, 1995), pp. 115–126.

**CHEESE**—In his *Medical Aphorisms*,[1] Maimonides quotes Galen, who said that the best type of fresh cheese is one made from milk whose fat has been removed (Chapter 20:45). Leaving churned milk in the sun sours and thickens it until it is what is known as white cheese (ibid., 23:107). Cheese sinks into the passages of the liver and obstructs them (ibid., 20:39), thereby harming patients with hydrops.

In his *Treatise on Asthma*,[2] Maimonides states that cheese is a fattening food and that salted cheese is detrimental to one's health. A similar statement about salted cheese is found in his *Mishneh Torah* (*Deot* 4:9). All types of cheese are said to be bad and thick; however, fresh, one-day-old white cheese without fat is good.[3] The Talmud also recommends one-day-old cheese (*Shabbat* 134a). Milk and cheese in classic Jewish sources is discussed elsewhere.[4]

**CHELMINSKY, ENRIQUE**—Chelminsky translated into Spanish Maimonides' *Treatise on Sexual Intercourse* (*Anales de Ars Medici*, Mexico, 5 (1961):240–248) as well as Maimonides' *Regimen of Health* (*Anales de Ars Medici*, Mexico, 5 (1961):303–344). The latter is titled *La Preservacion de la Juventud de Maimonides*, which coincides with H.L. Gordon's 1958 English version titled *The Preservation of Youth*, suggesting that Chelminsky translated Gordon's version into Spanish. The Spanish translation of Maimonides' *Treatise on Sexual Intercourse* was made from Gorlin's English version but his name was not mentioned.

**CHICKEN SOUP**—In the twentieth chapter of his *Medical Aphorisms*,[1] Maimonides states that boiled chicken soup neutralizes body constitution. Chicken soup is an excellent food, as well as a medication for the beginning of leprosy, and fattens the body substance of the emaciated and those convalescing from illness. Turtledoves increase memory, improve intellect, and sharpen the senses. The consumption of fowl, continues Maimonides, is beneficial for feebleness, hemiplegia, facial paresis, and the pain of edema. It also increases sexual potential. House pigeons that graze in the streets increase natural body heat. Soup made from the bird called *kanaber* loosens cramps of colic. Maimonides further states that chicken testicles provide excellent nourishment for a weakened or convalescent individual. Pigeon eggs are good aphrodisiacs, especially when cooked with onion or turnip. Finally, soup made from an old chicken is of benefit against chronic fevers that develop from white bile, and it also aids the cough that is called asthma.

In his *Treatise on Asthma*,[2] Maimonides advises the consumption of lean chicken meat for sufferers of asthma. Other small fowl, such as the turtledove, are also useful. The soup of chickens or fat hens is said to be an effective remedy for asthma. The method of preparation of the chicken soup and the ingredients are also described. An enema with sap of linseed, fenugreek, or both, with oil and chicken fat, with an admixture of beet juice, is strongly endorsed for the treatment of asthma.

In one of his treatises on health,[3] Maimonides recommends the meat of hens or roosters (or chickens or pullets) and their broth, because this type of fowl has the property of rectifying corrupted humors, especially the black humor (i.e., black bile, an excess of which was thought to cause melancholy), so much so that physicians mention that chicken broth is beneficial in leprosy. It thus seems evident that Maimonides, in the twelfth century, gave scientific respectability to what the proverbial Jewish mother has always known—that chicken soup can help cure a variety of ailments.[4]

1. F. Rosner, *The Medical Aphorisms of Moses Maimonides* (Haifa: Maimonides Research Institute, 1989), pp. 293–312.

2. F. Rosner, *Moses Maimonides' Treatise on Asthma* (Haifa: Maimonides Research Institute, 1994), p. 176.

3. J.O. Leibowitz and S. Marcus, *Moses Maimonides on the Causes of Symptoms* (Berkeley, CA: University of California Press, 1974), pp. 113–114.

4. F. Rosner, "Therapeutic Efficacy of Chicken Soup," *Chest*, 78 (1980): 672–674.

**CHILDBIRTH**—In his *Mishneh Torah*, Maimonides rules that a woman in labor is regarded as dangerously ill, and the Sabbath may be violated for her sake (*Shabbat* 2:11). A midwife or doctor may be summoned, and the umbilical cord may be cut and tied. If the mother asks for light or for a fire, one may provide it. Confinement and childbirth render a woman ritually unclean (*Issurei Biyah* 10:1).

In his *Medical Aphorisms,*[1] Maimonides quotes Galen, who says that the procreating and structure-forming forces dominate as long as the fetus is still in the uterus, while the nutritive and growth forces act as servants ministering to them. Following birth, the structure-forming force ceases to exist, and the growth force dominates until the end of adolescence (Chapter 1:73). If childbirth is difficult for a woman, complications such as abscess formation may occur (ibid., 16:33). After a woman gives birth and eliminates all the decayed blood that accumulated during the pregnancy, she should be fed nourishing foods such as barley gruel (ibid., 16:34). A birthstool is also described (ibid., 16:29), as are deformed newborns (ibid., 24:1). [*See also* CESAREAN SECTION]

1. F. Rosner, *The Medical Aphorisms of Moses Maimonides* (Haifa: Maimonides Research Institute, 1989).

**CHILLS**—In his *Medical Aphorisms,*[1] Maimonides quotes Galen, who said that repeated chill occurring during fever are grave prognostic signs because the body weakens through its perspiration and trembling (Chapter 6:64). Chills represent a sudden concentrated cold in the body owing to a cold humor (ibid., 7:43). Chills or shivering begin at the inception of tertian (ibid., 10:34) or quartan malarial fever (ibid., 7:45). Shivering patients may have great thirst (ibid., 7:46). Castoreum taken internally or applied externally both warms and dries, and is therefore therapeutic for shivering patients with chills (ibid., 7:40). Also therapeutic is diluted wine (ibid., 9:42). Two types of chills and their underlying causes are also described by Maimonides (ibid., 10:37). In his *Extracts from Galen,*[2] Maimonides writes that shivering and contraction of the skin may occur in a febrile patient with burning wastes in his body when he enters the bath or stands in the sun.

1. F. Rosner, *The Medical Aphorisms of Moses Maimonides* (Haifa: Maimonides Research Institute, 1989).

2. U.S. Barzel, *Maimonides' The Art of Cure. Extracts from Galen* (Haifa: Maimonides Research Institute, 1992), pp. 122–123.

**CHOKING**—A choking sensation during swallowing occurs in patients with synanche or angina tonsillaris. A variety of remedies for this condition, or for laryngitis or pharyngitis producing a choking sensation, are cited by Maimonides in his *Medical Aphorisms,*[1] based on the writings of Galen (Chapter 9:32–33). Narrowing of the passages of respiration with weakness of respiration may cause choking, which may be fatal (ibid., 7:47). Abscesses in the throat are of four varieties, three of which produce choking sensations (ibid., 23:77).

1. F. Rosner, *The Medical Aphorisms of Moses Maimonides* (Haifa: Maimonides Research Institute, 1989).

*CIRCUMCISION*—The laws and technical aspects of ritual circumcision are described by Maimonides in his *Mishneh Torah* (*Milah*). He describes the three major parts of the procedure: the incision of the prepuce, the tearing or cutting of the internal mucosa of the prepuce and its retraction over the glans, and the sucking of blood from the wound (*Milah* 2:2). He also describes the dressing to be applied and the care of the baby after the circumcision.

The reasons for ritual circumcision are explained by Maimonides in his *Guide for the Perplexed* (3:49), where he states that circumcision leads to physical, intellectual, and spiritual perfection and perpetuation of the belief in the unity of God.

Amazing is the recognition of the genetic transmission of hemophilia in the Talmud (*Yebamot* 64b) and subsequent rabbinic writings. The talmudic decree of Rabbi Judah that the sibling of two brothers who died of bleeding after circumcision may not be circumcised is codified by all rabbinic authorities of the last ten centuries. Modern rabbinic opinion extends this ruling to any child, even the firstborn, in whom a diagnosis of hemophilia can be established. Maimonides' discussion of the subject is as follows:

If a woman had her first son circumcised and he died as a result of the circumcision, which enfeebled his strength, and she similarly had her second son circumcised and he died as a result of the circumcision—whether the second child was from her first husband or from her second husband—the third son may not be circumcised at the proper time, on the eighth day of life. Rather, one postpones the operation until he grows up and his strength is established. One may circumcise only a child who is totally free of disease, because danger to life overrides every other consideration. It is possible to circumcise later than the proper time, but it is impossible to restore a single departed soul of Israel forever (*Milah* 1:18).

Maimonides may have been alluding to the mode of death when he stated "enfeebled his strength," that is, exsanguination. This conclusion may be unwarranted, however, as Maimonides may have lumped circumcision mortality from numerous causes, such as prematurity and anemia, with bleeding disorders. As a physician, his desire was to delay circumcision until health was established. Furthermore, whereas the Talmud does not state when circumcision can be performed in an afflicted child, Maimonides specifically sets a time limit—that is, circumcision may be performed at such time that the child is declared medically fit. Maimonides thus seems to feel that spontaneous remission or perhaps medical therapy can control, or even cure, hemophilia. Maimonides also recognized that a woman transmits the disease to all her male offspring, even if they were conceived by different fathers.

The conclusion to be drawn is that the sages of the Talmud in the second century and subsequent rabbinic authorities, including Maimonides, had a remarkable knowledge of the genetic transmission of a familial bleeding disorder, probably hemophilia. All recognized that females transmit the disease, but some thought that males can also do so. It is unclear, however, whether Maimonides and other rabbis were dealing only with hemophiliacs. Vitamin K deficiency—possibly determined by diet in certain families—or other bleeding disorders, such as congenital hypofibrinogenemia, may have been involved in some cases. Furthermore, the observations recorded in the Talmud by Maimonides and by other codifiers of Jewish law are incomplete. Although families with "loose blood"—that is, bleeding disorders—were recognized, the question of the circumcision of a child whose maternal uncles died of bleeding after circumcision is not considered. Such a woman, whose brothers bled to death after circumcision, might well be a carrier. Only the direct maternal transmission of the disease was recognized, whether demonstrated in siblings or in maternal cousins.

*CLIMATE*—In his *Treatise on Asthma*,[1] Maimonides writes that one can manage asthma properly only if one has a thorough knowledge of the patient's constitution and individual organs, the age and habits of the patient, the season, and the climate. The patient for whom this treatise was written asked whether a change in climate would be beneficial for his symptoms, which usually began with a common cold, especially in the rainy season, forcing him to gasp for air until phlegm was expelled. Maimonides explains the rules of diet and climate in general, and the rules specifically suited for asthmatics. He states that the dry Egyptian climate is efficacious for sufferers from this disease.

The last chapter of Maimonides' *Regimen of Health*[2] is devoted to his prescriptions relating to climate, domicile, occupation, bathing, sex, wine-drinking, diet, and respiratory infections. To cure depression, he advises elimination of all external irritants such as excessively warm climates or undesired company, and prescribes liquid refreshments such as oxymel, hydromel, and the famous "ox-tongue concoction." In the hot season, one should drink oxymel of roses or raisin oxymel upon awaking. In cool weather, one should engage in physical exercise and partake of foods that have a warming effect.

In his *Medical Aphorisms*,[3] Maimonides quotes Galen, who stated that the worst climate in any country is that which is closed to easterly winds and where raw and cold winds prevail. Galen also said that the climate is an uncontrollable external force that may contribute to loss of body weight and substance. Weather changes may lead to illness. Elsewhere,[4] Maimonides quotes Hippocrates, who said that if it is both hot and cold on the same day any time during the year, one should expect patients to develop diseases of autumn. He also said that the south wind induces dullness of hearing and dimness of vision, heaviness of the head, lethargy, and lassitude. He said further that autumn is a bad season for patients with consumption, which Maimonides explains is due to the cold and dry weather changes in that season. He also cites a long list of illnesses that are more common in the spring, the summer, and the rainy season, and offers explanations for them. Also described are the various winds and their characteristics: "Body secretions are less in the winter because the cold makes them rigid whereas in the summer they are plentiful because the heat dissolves them . . . semen and blood are of different constitutions in the summer and the winter. . . . The worst climate is . . . where raw and cold winds prevail." He thus repeatedly discusses seasonal and climatic influences on disease.

1. F. Rosner, *Moses Maimonides' Treatise on Asthma* (Haifa: Maimonides Research Institute, 1994).

2. F. Rosner, *Moses Maimonides' Three Treatises on Health* (Haifa: Maimonides Research Institute, 1990).

3. F. Rosner, *The Medical Aphorisms of Moses Maimonides* (Haifa: Maimonides Research Institute, 1989).

4. F. Rosner, *Maimonides' Commentary on the Aphorisms of Hippocrates* (Haifa: Maimonides Research Institute, 1987).

**COMA**—In his *Medical Aphorisms*,[1] Maimonides quotes Galen, who said that constipation can sometimes produce fever owing to thick humors that weaken the body, disturb mentation, and may even cause coma (literally, heavy sleep) (Chapter 8:27). If thick, cold, white phlegm increases in the brain, a headache develops from deep sleep without arousal, which is coma (ibid., 23:68). In his *Mishneh Torah*, Maimonides introduces the concept of a patient who appears dead but is in a deep stupor or coma. When one thinks that the soul of a person has departed, one should wait awhile and reexamine the patient, lest he is in a deep coma but still alive (*Avel* 4:5).

1. F. Rosner, *The Medical Aphorisms of Moses Maimonides* (Haifa: Maimonides Research Institute, 1989).

**COMMENTARY ON THE APHO-RISMS OF HIPPOCRATES**—Hippocrates was considered to be the father of medicine, and knowledge of the *Aphorisms of Hippocrates* was a requirement for physicians and medical students. Maimonides said that he saw greater value in these *Aphorisms* than in all the other books of Hippocrates, and therefore decided to write a commentary on them. He also said that some of the *Aphorisms of Hippocrates* are doubtful or require explanation; some are self-evident; some are repeated; some are not useful; and some are absolutely erroneous.[1]

Maimonides points out that Galen, who also wrote a commentary on the *Aphorisms of Hippocrates*, always attempted to justify the statements of Hippocrates even if they contradicted scientific fact. Whenever Maimonides feels that Galen's explanation of a Hippocratic aphorism is correct, he simply states, "This is clear." When he disagrees with Galen's explanation, Maimonides does not hesitate to indicate the inaccuracy and absurdity of Galen's pronouncement. Maimonides thus not only offers his own *Commentary on the Aphorisms of Hippocrates*, but critically analyzes and rebuts Galen's earlier commentary. For example, in the introduction to his *Commentary*, Maimonides says that "We find that Galen, in his commentaries on the writings of Hippocrates, explains certain statements in the opposite of their intended meanings in order to justify the correctness of the statement." In Section 2:36 of his *Commentary*, he states, ". . . this is the opinion of Galen. It is my opinion, however. . . ." He also criticizes Hippocrates where he believes it appropriate. Several times in his *Commentary*, Maimonides asserts that what Hippocrates states as a general rule is, in fact, the exception rather than the rule. Hippocrates saw one case of a certain disease and incorrectly generalized therefrom. Occasionally, Maimonides ridicules Hippocrates for making an absurd pronouncement, for example, "A male fetus matures better on the right side and a female fetus on the left side" (Section 5:48).

Maimonides was an original writer in medicine, as well as in philosophy, theology, mathematics, and rabbinics. He did not merely "copy" the medical writings of his predecessors, as some have accused. He did not hesitate to criticize even the fathers of medicine, Galen and Hippocrates. Such skepticism about the accuracy of their statements is also found in the last chapter of Maimonides' *Medical Aphorisms*,[2] which points out numerous inconsistencies and contradictions in Galen's writings.

---

1. F. Rosner, *Moses Maimonides' Commentary on the Aphorisms of Hippocrates* (Haifa: Maimonides Research Institute, 1987).

2. F. Rosner, *The Medical Aphorisms of Moses Maimonides* (Haifa: Maimonides Research Institute, 1989).

*COMPRESSES*—In his *Medical Aphorisms*,[1] Maimonides quotes Galen, who said that most hot compresses are useful when applied to abscesses arising from thin, watery blood. Irritating compresses (rubefacients) are helpful for dissolving thick viscous humors (Chapter 8:67). Cold compresses are applied to the head to treat nosebleeds (ibid., 9:5). Warm compresses applied to the teeth either inside or outside the mouth should be applied before meals on an empty stomach (ibid., 9:29). Warm compresses treat severe intestinal colic (ibid., 9:91). After incising a carbuncle, one applies a compress thereon made from watery barley flour (ibid., 15:51). Warming compresses made with millet are easy to make and are therapeutic (ibid., 21:94). In summary, compresses are of four types: moist, dry, irritating, and intermediate. Their preparation and uses are then described by Maimonides (ibid., 23:33). [ *See also* CATAPLASMS]

1. F. Rosner, *The Medical Aphorisms of Moses Maimonides* (Haifa: Maimonides Research Institute, 1989).

*CONSTIPATION*—Maimonides wrote a *Regimen of Health* for the Sultan al-Malik al-Afdal of Egypt, who suffered from constipation and melancholy. In the third chapter of this treatise,[1] Maimonides writes that the first principle of healthy living is to have soft stools. Constipation gives rise to "extremely bad gases which enter the heart and brain and corrupt the humors, disturb the vital pneumas, produce evil thoughts, confusion and melancholy, and prevent the expulsion of the superfluities of all the digestions. The best concoction for softening the stool is made of rhubarb with tamarind. An alternative remedy is lemon broth prepared with a fat chicken, saffron seeds, sugar, and beets. Meals should include vegetables spiced in sauce made from barley and good oil. After meals, one should suck on a quince, pear, apple, or pomegranate. All this is to prevent constipation.

If one suffers from constipation, the best remedy is cassia fistula prepared from ox tongue, licorice, maidenhair, barberry and althea seeds, fresh roses, and anethum. Other remedies for constipation are described in detail. In the ninth chapter of his *Treatise on Asthma*,[2] Maimonides also discusses constipation and again recommends regulation of one's bowels by the maintenance of a normal and regular diet. Enemas made with the sap of linseed, fenugreek, or both with oil, chicken fat, and beets are excellent preparations to evacuate wastes in constipated people without producing irritation or pain. For the elderly, one should add thereto a little honey or honeycake by mouth.

In his *Medical Aphorisms*,[3] Maimonides quotes Galen, who said that coldness of the outer organs leads to constipation (Chapter 7:64). Constipation may aggravate an illness (ibid., 8:27). Nausea is frequently associated with constipation (ibid., 9:47 and 55). Enemas for constipation are described (ibid., 13:40 and 13:43). Elderly people who suffer from constipation should be treated with certain plants together with barley gruel (ibid., 17:38). Other references to constipation, its causes, and its treatment are discussed by Maimonides in *Extracts from Galen*.[4]

---

1. F. Rosner, *Moses Maimonides' Three Treatises on Health* (Haifa: Maimonides Research Institute, 1990), pp. 53–72.

2. F. Rosner, *Moses Maimonides' Treatise on Asthma* (Haifa: Maimonides Research Institute, 1994), pp. 75–84.

3. F. Rosner, *The Medical Aphorisms of Moses Maimonides* (Haifa: Maimonides Research Institute, 1989).

4. U.S. Barzel, *Maimonides' The Art of Cure. Extracts from Galen* (Haifa: Maimonides Research Institute, 1992).

*CONTRACEPTION*—The Jewish attitude toward contraception by any method is a nonpermissive one if no medical or psychiatric threat to the mother or child exists. The duty of procreation—which is primarily a commandment on men—coupled with the wife's conjugal rights in Jewish law, militates against the use of the condom, coitus interruptus, or abstinence under any circumstances. Where pregnancy hazard exists, and where rabbinic sanction for the use of birth control is obtained, the most acceptable contraceptives are those that least interfere with the natural sex act and with the full mobility of the sperm and their natural course. "Oral contraception by pill enjoys preferred status as the least objectionable method of birth control."[1]

At least six methods of contraception are mentioned in the Bible and the Talmud.[2] The first one is coitus interruptus, which is unequivocally prohibited by Maimonides in *Mishneh Torah* (*Issurei Biyah* 21:18). The four contraceptive techniques discussed in the Talmud are the safe period (*Niddah* 31b); a twisting movement following cohabitation to expel the sperm (*Ketubot* 37a); an oral contraceptive potion (*Shabbat* 110a); and the use of an absorbent material during intercourse (*Yebamot* 12b).

Maimonides rules that it is forbidden to give a man an oral contraceptive, potion, or pill because he is commanded to propagate the race, whereas a woman is permitted to drink the potion in order not to conceive (*Issurei Biyah* 16:12). An ancient method of contraception is when a woman makes violent, twisting movements during or shortly after sexual intercourse in order to discharge the semen. This method, popular among harlots, was condemned by Rabbi Jose in the Talmud (*Ketubot* 37a). Maimonides codifies the talmudic rule (ibid., 72a) that if a man subjects his wife to a vow to make violent motions during intercourse to prevent conception, he must divorce her and pay her the *ketubah*, or marriage settlement (*Eeshut* 14:5).

1. D.M. Feldman, *Marital Relations, Birth Control and Abortion in Jewish Law* (New York: Schocken, 1974).

2. F. Rosner, *Modern Medicine and Jewish Ethics*, 2nd augmented ed. (Hoboken, NJ, and New York: Ktav and Yeshiva University Press, 1991), pp. 69–83.

*CORPSE*—In his *Mishneh Torah*, Maimonides rules that a human corpse conveys ritual uncleanness (*Tumat Met* 1:1), but only after the soul has departed. Maimonides provides considerable insight into Jewish practices with respect to the dead and their interment. In ancient and medieval times, in the absence of refrigeration, corpses were preserved by being placed on sand or salt until burial. It was believed that air entering the dead body through the nose, mouth, navel, rectum, or genitalia contributed to postmortem swelling and putrefaction of the body. Hence, rules Maimonides, when a person dies, one closes the eyes, binds the jaw, washes the body, stops up the organs of the lower body, rubs the body with various spices, cuts the hair, and dresses the body in simple shrouds sewn with white linen thread (*Avel* 4:1).

Facial features may change postmortem, making it difficult to identify a corpse. These changes may be delayed if the body is preserved in cold ocean water (*Gerushin* 13:21–22).

Self-mutilation in the form of tattooing, skin incisions, cutting the flesh as an expression of grief for the dead, or making a bald spot on the head are all prohibited as idolatrous practices (*Akum* 12:11–15). These practices are also forbidden in Judaism because of the prohibition against desecrating or mutilating a human body, whether alive or dead. Necrophilia, or having sexual intercourse with a corpse, as did Herod (*Baba Batra* 3b), is strictly forbidden. Cremation and embalming are strictly prohibited in Jewish law.[1] The obligation of burial is derived in the Talmud (*Sanhedrin* 46b) from a biblical verse (Deut. 21:23), and is so codified by Maimonides (*Sanhedrin* 15:8). Hence, the disposal of the body by cremation is contrary to Judaism. In fact, the Talmud (*Avodah Zarah* 1:3) considers the burning of a corpse to be an idolatrous practice. However, the burning of fragrant spices for deceased kings is specifically allowed by Maimonides (*Avel* 14:26) and others. [*See also* DEATH]

1. F. Rosner, "Embalming and Cremation," in *Modern Medicine and Jewish Ethics*, 2nd augmented ed. (Hoboken, NJ, and New York: Ktav and Yeshiva University Press, 1991), pp. 335–350.

**COUGH**—In his *Treatise on Asthma*, Maimonides recommends remedies to clear the lungs of moisture, ease respiration, and eliminate the cough of patients suffering from asthma.[1] Coughing, one of the classic symptoms of asthma, is necessary to expectorate phlegm. In his *Medical Aphorisms*,[2] Maimonides cites Galen, who describes cough with or without associated sputum production (Chapter 3:42). A malignant cough is one whose cause is either catarrh, which descends from the head, or a boil, ulcer, or inflammation in the organs of respiration. It is due to viscous sputum collected in the chest (ibid., 6:41). A benign cough is one secondary to bad lungs, or laryngitis or bronchitis. Such a cough may warm the sides of the chest and the lung and may increase fever and thirst (ibid.). The basic symptoms of pneumonia include fever; pleuritic chest pain; short, rapid breaths; serrated pulse; and cough associated mostly with sputum (ibid., 6:54). For severe cough, sedative and somniferant drugs are recommended (ibid., 18:38). Sometimes, musculoskeletal problems such as a bad constitution of the chest muscles can incite coughing (ibid., 9:36).

Maimonides also quotes Hippocrates, who said that a patient with fever and a dry cough is usually not thirsty, and that cold weather with snow and hail is harmful to the chest and may provoke coughing and bleeding from the lungs.[3] In his *Extracts from Galen*,[4] Maimonides again discusses blood expectorated from the lung during coughing. Treatment consists of bloodletting from the femoral vein to pull the blood away from the lungs, followed by medicines that "glue and close" with dilute vinegar or water in which quince or myrtle has been cooked. Other treatments for hemoptysis are also described. Wounds in the windpipe or in the lungs are best treated with milk, preferably sucked directly from a goat or mixed with honey before being imbibed. Although it is ordinarily prohibited to suck milk directly from an animal on the Sabbath, if one does so, he is exempt. But if he has a cough, he is permitted to suck because of his distress, even if there is no danger to his life (*Mishneh Torah, Shabbat* 21:14).

1. F. Rosner, *Moses Maimonides' Treatise on Asthma* (Haifa: Maimonides Research Institute, 1994).

2. F. Rosner, *The Medical Aphorisms of Moses Maimonides* (Haifa: Maimonides Research Institute, 1989).

3. F. Rosner, *Maimonides' Commentary on the Aphorisms of Hippocrates* (Haifa: Maimonides Research Institute, 1987), pp. 112 and 136.

4. U.S. Barzel, *Maimonides' The Art of Cure. Extracts from Galen* (Haifa: Maimonides Research Institute, 1992), pp. 63–70.

*CRUELTY TO ANIMALS*—Cruelty to animals is prohibited in Jewish law, a prohibition that the talmudic sages (*Baba Metzia* 31a) deduce from the Bible. Maimonides speaks of cruelty to animals in his *Mishneh Torah* when he asserts that whoever prevents an animal from eating by muzzling it while it is working is subject to punishment (*Sechirut* 13:2). Furthermore, if the animal is thirsty, he must water it (ibid., 13:3). However, if the thing at which the animal is working is bad for its stomach or injurious, or if the animal is sick and, if it eats of that thing, its stomach would become loose, it is permissible to prevent it from eating (ibid.).

Jewish law not only forbids cruelty to animals, but requires that we be kind to them, have compassion for them, and treat them humanely.[1] Thus, if one sees an animal collapsing under a heavy burden, one must unload it. In fact, one may not partake of any food until one has first fed one's animals. That animals may not work on the Sabbath is a rule enunciated in the Ten Commandments, indicating that care of and kindness to animals is of profound importance for our humanization.

These and other biblical and rabbinic moral and legal rules concerning the treatment of animals are based on the principle that animals are part of God's creation, for which humans bear responsibility. Maimonides offers an insight into these rules when he states that the prohibition of causing suffering to animals was set down with a view to perfecting humans so that we do not acquire moral habits of cruelty. Rather, we should not inflict pain gratuitously, but should be kind and merciful even with a chance or stray animal. The reason humans are forbidden to eat a limb cut from a living animal is that this act would make humans acquire the habit of cruelty. The same reason is given for the rule forbidding the slaughtering of an animal and its young on the same day and the commandment to release the mother bird before taking the young (*Guide for the Perplexed* 3:48). [*See also* ANIMAL EXPERIMENTATION]

1. F. Rosner, *Modern Medicine and Jewish Ethics*, 2nd ed. (Hoboken, NJ, and New York: Ktav and Yeshiva University Press, 1991), pp. 353–373.

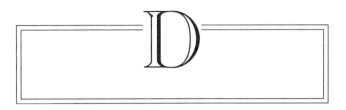

**DANGER TO LIFE**—In Judaism, life is of supreme value, and the preservation of life is a divine commandment. To save a human life, all biblical and rabbinic commandments except idolatry, murder, and forbidden sexual relations—such as incest—may be waived, if necessary. Thus, if physicians assert that a dangerously ill patient can be cured by the administration of a remedy that involves the violation of a biblical precept, it should be applied (Maimonides' *Mishneh Torah, Yesodei Hatorah* 5:6). To save a life, the Sabbath may be desecrated, nonkosher food may be consumed, and food may be eaten even on the Day of Atonement. The overriding consideration in suspending religious laws is the intrinsic value of human life, which transcends the moral worth of religious observance.

In Maimonides' *Mishneh Torah*, he deals with a variety of situations where Sabbath observance must be set aside in order to preserve and protect a human life (*Shabbat*, Chapter 2). The basis for this principle is the scriptural verse, "He shall live by them" (Leviticus 18:5), which teaches that Jews must live by the Torah, not die by it. If observance of one or more precepts would result in the loss of someone's life, that observance must be waived to preserve that life. This principle is applicable not only in cases of danger to life, but also in cases of potential or possible danger to life. A woman in confinement and shortly after delivery is considered to be in the category of someone dangerously ill, and all precepts are waived, if necessary, on her behalf (*Shabbat* 2:11). If a woman dies in labor, it is permissible and perhaps mandatory to perform an immediate cesarean section in an attempt to save the baby (ibid., 2:15). Even if the danger to life is not a physical illness but external danger, such as the case of a drowning victim or someone trapped in a burning house, one must do everything possible to rescue that person, including violating biblical or rabbinic laws. Dangerous or potentially dangerous mental or emotional illness is considered to be no different from physical illness, as shown by the case of the child accidentally locked in a room who might die of fright if not rescued (ibid., 2:17). A collyrium may be applied to an infected eye or a plaster to a wound on the Sabbath (ibid., 3:2). Because of possible danger to life, harmful reptiles such as snakes and scorpions may be captured on the Sabbath (ibid., 10:25). One may lance an abscess to drain the pus (ibid., 10:17). One may remove a dangerous obstacle in a public domain on the Sabbath to prevent it from injuring someone (ibid., 15:22).

Elsewhere in his *Mishneh Torah*, Maimonides rules that foods and beverages that were left uncovered overnight should not be consumed because a snake may have partaken of them and discharged poison into them (*Terumot* 12:13–14). Numerous talmudic and rabbinic references exist about the danger of drinking from uncovered water or wine.[1] Current scientific knowledge indicates that the danger of drinking from uncovered water or wine is extremely remote. Nevertheless, the point that Maimonides and others make is valid: One should avoid anything that is dangerous to one's life or injurious to one's health.

Since, in Judaism, life is of infinite value, and the preservation of life and health is a divine commandment, one must interrupt one's prayers if one is in mortal danger (*Tefillah* 6:9). Thus, if one sees deadly snakes and scorpions, one should first escape and then pray (ibid.). For the preservation of life, one may even eat forbidden food.

Thus, if a person is wandering in the wilderness and has nothing other than forbidden food to eat, it is permitted, because of the danger to life (*Maachalot Assurot* 14:13). If a pregnant woman develops an intense craving for forbidden food, such as swine's flesh, one may give her some of the gravy. If her craving is not thereby appeased, one may give her the meat until she is satisfied (ibid., 14:14). Similarly, if a sick patient develops a craving for a forbidden food, the same rule applies (ibid., 14:15). If a person is seized with an attack of morbid hunger (bulimia), he may be given forbidden things to eat at once, until his eyes brighten. One must not first search for permitted food, but should immediately give him whatever comes to hand because of the danger to his life (ibid., 14:16). Further discussion of this topic in Maimonides' *Mishneh Torah* can be found elsewhere.[2]

---

1. F. Rosner, *Medicine in the Bible and the Talmud*, 2nd ed. (Hoboken, NJ: Ktav and Yeshiva University Press, 1995), pp. 60–64.

2. F. Rosner, *Medicine in the Mishneh Torah of Maimonides* (New York: Ktav, 1984), pp. 109–122.

**DATES**—The date is one of the seven fruits with which the land of Israel is blessed, as described in the Torah (Deuteronomy 8:8). Nevertheless, in his *Mishneh Torah* (*Deot* 4:10), Maimonides advises against consuming dates to excess. In his *Treatise on Asthma*,[1] |Maimonides advises against the consumption of a variety of fruits and vegetables by asthmatic patients (Chapter 2:8). Among these are unripe dates because these are moist fruits, which are detrimental for asthmatics and may produce headaches (ibid., 2:9). Indian dates (tamarind), however, are a good ingredient in a beverage designed to maintain soft stools (ibid., 9:1). Dry dates effectively cool the stomach and strengthen it.[2] However, in his *Medical Aphorisms*,[3] Maimonides quotes Galen, who said that all kinds of date are difficult to digest and produce headache if one consumes a lot of them. They burn the mouth of the stomach and irritate it. Unripe dates fill the body with raw, unmetabolized liquids and produce shivering and horripilation (Chapter 20:54). Palm dates obstruct the liver because of an abundance of chymes. Fresh dates are even more detrimental, and may give rise to hemorrhoids (ibid., 20:75).

---

1. F. Rosner, *Moses Maimonides' Treatise on Asthma* (Haifa: Maimonides Research Institute, 1994).

2. U.S. Barzel, *Maimonides' The Art of Cure. Extracts from Galen* (Haifa: Maimonides Research Institute, 1992), p. 105.

3. F. Rosner, *The Medical Aphorisms of Moses Maimonides* (Haifa: Maimonides Research Institute, 1989).

**DEAF-MUTISM**—Often discussed together with the hermaphrodite and a person of indeterminate sex is the deaf-mute, whose legal status differs from theirs in some respects but resembles it in other respects. Wherever male or female deaf-mutes are mentioned, they signify persons who can neither hear nor speak. A person able to speak but not hear, or to hear but not speak, has the same status as any other person.

In his *Mishneh Torah*, Maimonides states that a deaf-mute priest (*kohen*) is disqualified from serving in the Temple (*Biyat Mikdash* 8:16). A deaf-mute is equated with the mentally deficient because he is not of sound mind and is not bound to observe the commandments (*Eydut* 9:11). The legal claims of a deaf-mute, a mentally incompetent person, and a minor are without legal effect (*Toan Venitan* 13:2). A guardian is appointed to handle their legal affairs (*Nachalot* 10:8). Among the ten classes of people ineligible to give testimony in court is a deaf-mute (*Eydut* 9:1). If a male deaf-mute marries a normal woman or if a female deaf-mute marries a normal man, their betrothal is completely valid—not according to the Torah, but according only to scribal law (*Eeshut* 4:9).

Maimonides also discusses deaf-mute marriages in his *Mishnah Commentary* (*Sanhedrin* 7:4). He also states that a deaf-mute is silent because of the deafness he developed in his mother's womb (*Terumot* 1:2). He also briefly mentions deafness in his *Medical Aphorisms*[1] and *Commentary on the Aphorisms of Hippocrates*.[2]

1. F. Rosner, *The Medical Aphorisms of Moses Maimonides* (Haifa: Maimonides Research Institute, 1989), p. 370.
2. F. Rosner, *Maimonides' Commentary on the Aphorisms of Hippocrates* (Haifa: Maimonides Research Institute, 1987), pp. 100 and 115.

**DEAFNESS**—In his *Medical Aphorisms*,[1] Maimonides quotes Galen, who said that deafness is when a person cannot hear a low voice at all and hears a loud noise with difficulty. The process progresses slowly over time until the patient becomes completely deaf (Chapter 23:73). In his *Commentary on the Aphorisms of Hippocrates*,[2] Maimonides cites Hippocrates, who said that if someone who is deaf develops diarrhea from an excess of red bile, the deafness ceases (Section 4:28). Later, he asserts that if a patient with acute fever develops deafness and blood flows from his nose, or if he develops diarrhea, the illness subsides (ibid., 4:60). Maimonides explains that Hippocrates' statements apply only to deafness that occurs suddenly, particularly if the time is near the acme of the illness. Maimonides implies that chronic deafness that is due to a malady of the ear is incurable, whereas acute deafness such as acute salpingitis of the Eustachian tube is reversible. [*See also* DEAF-MUTISM]

1. F. Rosner, *The Medical Aphorisms of Moses Maimonides* (Haifa: Maimonides Research Institute, 1989).
2. F. Rosner, *Maimonides' Commentary on the Aphorisms of Hippocrates* (Haifa: Maimonides Research Institute, 1987).

**DEATH, DEFINITION OF**—The definition of death as described in the Talmud (*Yoma* 85a) is codified by Maimonides in his *Mishneh Torah* as follows: "If, upon examination, no sign of breathing can be detected at the nose, the victim must be left where he is [until after the Sabbath] because he is already dead" (*Shabbat* 2:19). Maimonides does not seem to require examination of the heart, which is mentioned as a minority opinion in the Talmud. Cessation of respiration seems to be the determining physical sign for the ascertainment of death. At present, an intense debate exists among modern rabbinic authorities as to whether or not Jewish law recognizes total brain death with irreversible absence of spontaneous respiration. The affirmative view is described by Tendler and Rosner,[1] and the negative view is espoused by Bleich.[2]

1. F. Rosner, *Modern Medicine and Jewish Ethics*, 2nd ed. (Hoboken, NJ, and New York: Ktav and Yeshiva University Press, 1991), pp. 263–277.

2. J.D. Bleich, *Time of Death in Jewish Law* (New York: Berman, 1991).

### DEATH, LEGAL CONSEQUENCES OF

*DEATH, LEGAL CONSEQUENCES OF*—Maimonides provides considerable insight into Jewish practices with respect to the dead and their interment in his *Mishneh Torah* (*Shabbat* 26:20 and *Avel* 4:1ff). When a person dies, one closes the eyes, binds the jaw, washes the body, stops up the organs of the lower extremities, rubs the body with various spices, cuts the hair, and dresses the body in simple shrouds sewn with white linen thread.

A human corpse conveys ritual impurity (*Tumat Met* 1:1). Maimonides describes procedures for implementing the four methods of capital punishment (*Sanhedrin* 15:1–5) and the crimes for which each type of death is used (ibid., 15:10–13). He discusses the credibility of a woman's claim that her husband is dead (*Gerushin* 12:15), as well as the procedure to be followed if she claims that her husband died in war (ibid., 13:1–3) or in a mishap such as a collapsed building; was bitten by a snake or a scorpion (ibid., 13:4); died of hunger (ibid., 13:5); was slain by robbers (ibid., 13:6); or died by the plague (ibid., 13:7). If a man falls into the sea, he is not presumed to be dead unless part of his body, without which a person cannot survive, is recovered from the sea, because he may have emerged at another place (ibid., 13:16). Thus, his heirs do not yet inherit from him, nor can his wife remarry.

Metaphysical aspects of death are discussed by Maimonides in his *Guide for the Perplexed* (3:10) and his *Treatise on Resurrection*.[1]

---

1. F. Rosner, *Moses Maimonides' Treatise on Resurrection* (New York: Ktav, 1982).

### DEATH, MEDICAL CAUSES OF

*DEATH, MEDICAL CAUSES OF*—In medieval times, health was thought to require the proper mixture of the four body humors: white bile (phlegm), yellow bile, red bile (blood), and black bile (melancholy). An imbalance of these humors was thought to produce disease or even death. In his *Medical Aphorisms*, Maimonides quotes Galen, who said that "an extreme aggravation of the bad constitution of the heart" leads to death. A severe stroke, called apoplexy, produces death. Extreme weakness from lack of eating can cause a person's death. Sudden death and death by poisoning are also described.[1]

In his *Treatises on Health*, Maimonides describes remedies to save patients from death. Death can occur from excitement that is due to extreme joy or sadness. Death can also occur secondary to fear or because of a therapeutic error of the patient or physicians.[2]

1. F. Rosner, *The Medical Aphorisms of Moses Maimonides* (Haifa: Maimonides Research Institute, 1989).

2. F. Rosner, *Moses Maimonides' Three Treatises on Health* (Haifa: Maimonides Research Institute, 1990).

**DENTISTRY**—References to dentistry are found in Maimonides' medical and rabbinic writings.[1] He states that pain following a tooth extraction is due to the severance of the nerve that connects the tooth to the bone (i.e., jaw). Warm compresses should be applied. Various remedies are described, including sips of vinegar for a toothache, a suggestion already made in the Talmud (*Betzah* 18b and *Shabbat* 111a). Chewing mastic is said to remove mouth odors. Astringent medications harden and strengthen teeth. Maimonides discusses artificial teeth that replace missing ones, gold caps over teeth that have become discolored, and silver teeth.

1. F. Rosner, *The Medical Legacy of Moses Maimonides* (Hoboken, NJ: Ktav, 1998).

**DIABETES**—In his *Medical Aphorisms*,[1] Maimonides quotes Galen, who said that the illness diabetes (mellitus) occurs rarely and only exceptionally, and that he had seen only two such patients (Chapter 8:68). Maimonides responds as follows:

I, too, have not seen it in the West [Spain, where Maimonides was born, or Morocco, where he fled from the persecution of the Almochades] nor did any one of my teachers under whom I studied mention that they had seen it [diabetes]. However, here in Egypt, in the course of approximately ten years, I have seen more than twenty people who suffered from this illness. This brings one to the conclusion that this illness occurs mostly in warm countries. Perhaps the waters of the Nile, because of their suaveness, may play a role in this (ibid., 8:69).

Maimonides erroneously postulated the cause of diabetes to be the ingestion of the sweet waters of the River Nile. An apparent description of acidosis complicating diabetes seems to be the following: "Individuals in whom sweet white [humor] occurs are very somnolent [hyperglycemia]. Those who have an excess of sour white [humor] are hungry [hypoglycemia]. If an excess of salted white [humor] occurs, they become extremely thirsty [hypoglycemia]. When this white liquid is neutralized, the thirst disappears" (ibid., 6:9).

Diabetes insipidus, in which patients urinate a lot and have an intense thirst, is also accurately described. Such patients drink enormous quantities of fluid and rapidly void that which they drink (ibid., 23:94 and 24:39). Again Maimonides responds to Galen's statement about its rarity by asserting that he (Maimonides) saw no cases in Spain, but over a twenty-year period observed twenty-three such patients. He concludes that diabetes is rare in cold climates (i.e., Spain), but common in warm countries (i.e., Egypt), and is due to "the prevailing of heat which spreads over the kidneys" (ibid., 24:40).

---

1. F. Rosner, *The Medical Aphorisms of Moses Maimonides* (Haifa: Maimonides Research Institute, 1989).

*DIARRHEA*—In his *Treatise on Asthma*,[1] Maimonides states that overeating is one of the prime causes of many maladies, including diarrhea (Chapter 5:1). To stop diarrhea, one should not use strong medications, except upon the advice of a skilled physician (ibid., 9:5). In many cases, nature alone is sufficient to correct the diarrhea, and there is no need to resort to medicines (ibid., 12:5). In his *Regimen on Health*,[2] Maimonides describes astringent fruits such as quinces and pears as binding agents for patients with diarrhea (Chapter 1:13). Mild diarrhea is best left to nature to heal (ibid., 4:3). Strong purgatives can produce bloody diarrhea (ibid., 4:7).

In his *Extracts from Galen*,[3] Maimonides states that fever develops in many patients whose indigestion causes diarrhea and that gruel of parched barley with some vinegar should be given to the patient (pp. 104–105). The Talmud (*Shabbat* 156a) speaks of barley broth as a preventive against diarrhea. Numerous references to diarrhea are found in Maimonides' *Commentary on the Aphorisms of Hippocrates*.[4] For example, Maimonides states that children whose teeth begin to erupt may develop diarrhea because food is not properly digested (Section 3:25). Bloody diarrhea is said to be due to black bile (ibid., 4:24). Diarrhea that is due to tuberculous enteritis is evidence of the patient's extreme weakness and warns that death is near (ibid., 5:12). Stutterers are said to be prone to having loose stools or diarrhea (ibid., 6:32). Maimonides explains that a patient with diarrhea and an enlarged spleen filled with black bile benefits from expelling that thick humor (ibid., 6:43). Dropsy and diarrhea in a mad person remove the illness-producing material and may cure the patient (ibid., 7:5). Frothy diarrhea is due to a strong admixture therein of air (ibid., 7:30).

In his *Medical Aphorisms*,[5] Maimonides quotes Galen, who said that excessive, moist black humors can be eliminated from the body through diarrhea (Chapter 6:12) and thereby benefit the patient (ibid., 6:25). Bloody diarrhea may occur because of liver disease (ibid., 6:82). Severe diarrhea may lead to extreme weakness (ibid., 7:42) and should be treated with astringent foods such as quinces (ibid., 9:47). Diarrhea represents the rapid exit of unaltered food, whereas dysentery is the propulsion and immediate expulsion of the stools (ibid., 23:90).

---

1. F. Rosner, *Moses Maimonides' Treatise on Asthma* (Haifa: Maimonides Research Institute, 1994).

2. F. Rosner, *Moses Maimonides' Three Treatises on Health* (Haifa: Maimonides Research Institute, 1990).

3. U.S. Barzel, *Maimonides' The Art of Cure. Extracts from Galen* (Haifa: Maimonides Research Institute, 1992).

4. F. Rosner, *Maimonides' Commentary on the Aphorisms of Hippocrates* (Haifa: Maimonides Research Institute, 1987).

5. F. Rosner, *The Medical Aphorisms of Moses Maimonides* (Haifa: Maimonides Research Institute, 1989).

---

**DIENSTAG, JACOB ISRAEL**— Born in Austria in 1915, Dienstag is renowned as the world's leading Maimonidean bibliographer. From 1951 to 1970, he headed the Judaica library at New York's Yeshiva University, where he also served as professor of bibliography. Since 1974, he has been the editor of *Bibliotheca Maimonidica*. His numerous published bibliographies, as well as full-length books on Maimonides, include *Maimonides and the Kabbalists* (1956), *Maimonides' Book of Precepts* (1972), *Maimonides' Mishneh Torah* (1972), *Maimonides in Hasidic Literature* (1964), *Maimonides and the Tosafists* (1958), *Mai-*

*monides' Treatise on Resurrection* (1982), *Eschatology in Maimonidean Thought* (1983), *Christian Translators of Maimonides Mishneh Torah in Latin* (1974), *Maimonides' Shemonah Perakim* (1984), *Studies in Maimonides and Thomas Aquinas* (1974), *Bibliography of Maimonides' Guide for the Perplexed* (1986), *The Guide for the Perplexed in Poetry* (1986), and many more.

Specifically regarding Maimonides' medical writings, Dienstag has published a bio-bibliographical survey of translators and editors of Maimonides' medical works,[1] and bibliographies of Maimonides *Medical Aphorisms*,[2] Maimonides' *Three Treatises on Health*,[3] Maimonides' *The Art of Cure. Extracts from Galen*,[4] Maimonides' *Treatise on Asthma*,[5] Maimonides' *Glossary of Drug Names*,[6] and several medical works attributed to but not written by Maimonides, including the famous "Physician's Prayer."[7]

---

1. Dienstag J. I. in *Memorial Volume in Honor of Professor S. Muntner* (J.O. Leibowitz, edit.), Jerusalem, Israel Institute of the History of Medicine, 1983, pp. 95–135.

2. Dienstag J. I. in *The Medical Aphorisms of Moses Maimonides*. F. Rosner, edit. (Haifa: Maimonides Research Institute, 1989), pp. 455–471.

3. Dienstag J. I. in *Moses Maimonides' Three Treatises on Health*. F. Rosner, edit. (Haifa: Maimonides Research Institute, 1990), pp. 98–116, 163–174, and 222–245.

4. Dienstag J. I. in Maimonides' *The Art of Cure. Extracts from Galen.* U.S. Barzel, edit. (Haifa: Maimonides Research Institute, 1992), pp. 197–200.

5. Dienstag J. I. in *Moses Maimonides' Treatise on Asthma*. F. Rosner, edit. (Haifa: Maimonides Research Institute, 1994), pp. 161–170.

6. Dienstag, J. I. in *Moses Maimonides' Glossary of Drug Names*. F. Rosner, edit. (Haifa: Maimonides Research Institute, 1995), pp. 325–331.

7. Dienstag J. I. in *Six Treatises Attributed to Maimonides*. F. Rosner, edit. (Northvale, NJ: Jason Aronson, Inc. 1991), pp. 127–145.

*DIETARY LAWS*—Jewish dietary laws concern themselves with what animals, birds, and fish may be eaten; the way in which they must be prepared for consumption; and the fact that meat must not be cooked or consumed with any dairy product. Many attempts have been made throughout the centuries to explain the dietary laws from hygienic, sanitary, esthetic, folkloric, ethical, or psychological viewpoints. The Bible does not offer an explanation, but, in three separate passages (Exod. 22:30, Lev. 11:44–45, Deut. 14:21), the dietary laws are closely associated with the concept of holiness. The Talmud (*Yoma* 67b) states that dietary laws are divine statutes without explanation, and thus serve as aids to moral conduct.

In his *Guide for the Perplexed* (3:48), Maimonides gives hygienic and sanitary reasons for the dietary laws. He states that pork is more humid than is proper and contains much superfluous matter. It is prohibited because:

. . . it is very dirty and feeds on dirty things. . . . The law requires that one remove filth out of sight even in the field and in a military camp (Deut. 13:13–15), and all the more within cities. Now if swine were used for food, marketplaces and even houses would be dirtier than latrines . . . You know the dictum: The mouth of a swine is like walking excrement (*Berachot* 25a). . . .

As for the prohibition against eating meat boiled in milk, it is in my opinion not improbable that—in addition to this being undoubtedly very gross food and very filling—idolatry has something to do with it. Perhaps such food was eaten at one of the ceremonies of their cult or at one of their festivals.

These principles and commandments of Jewish dietary laws are codified by Maimonides in his *Mishneh Torah*, where he details the various dietary laws concerning milk, eggs, and cheese (*Maachalot Assurot* 3:1ff). One may not eat from an animal that died as a result of trauma or wounding or from illness (ibid., 4:1ff), nor may one consume a limb cut from a living animal (ibid., 5:1ff).

The consumption of blood is prohibited (ibid., 6:1). The salting of meat required by Jewish law (ibid., 6:10) is aimed at extracting the blood from the meat. Nevertheless, if one's teeth are bleeding, the blood may be swallowed without hesitation (ibid., 6:2). Various types of fat from animals are prohibited. These include the fat upon the entrails, upon the two kidneys; and upon the flanks (ibid., 7:5). Pericardiac fat is permissible (ibid., 7:9). There are two membranes on the kidneys, both of which are forbidden (ibid., 7:12). The sinew of the thigh vein must be removed before a ritually slaughtered animal may be eaten (ibid., 8:7). The prohibition of this sinew (ibid., 8:1) is based upon Genesis 32:33.

*DIGESTION*—In his *Medical Aphorisms*,[1] Maimonides subscribes to the three Galenical phases of digestion to explain the physiology of nutrition, and adds a fourth of his own. "The first stage is digestion in the stomach. . . . The second stage is the transition to the intestines where it adds to . . . the liver substance. The third stage . . . the metabolism that occurs in every one of the organs . . . there is an additional metabolic phase, a fourth, which is called assimilation" (Chapter 1:58). The quality, quantity, and frequency of stool excretion depends on the digestion of food in the stomach and intestines (ibid., 6:74). Foods that rapidly deteriorate or spoil interfere with normal digestion (ibid., 7:15) and may produce eructation (ibid., 7:52). If the stomach does not digest food properly, one should induce emesis prior to eating and drink sweet wine (ibid., 9:45). Soft food is most easily and rapidly digested (ibid., 20:6). Patients convalescing from illness should be fed frequent, small amounts of food (ibid., 20:8) so as not to overburden them (ibid., 20:9).

In his *Treatise on Asthma*,[2] Maimonides states that overeating interferes with digestion and gives rise to bad humors that cause acute illnesses (Chapter 5:3). Different foods have varying digestibility. A single food is best for digestion (ibid., 5:4). Resting after the meal helps digestion. Bad digestion may cause dyspepsia and a variety of other signs and symptoms (ibid., 5:6). A little wine helps digestion and has other beneficial effects (ibid., 6:1). To remain healthy, one must pay attention to normal digestion and proper elimination of wastes (ibid., 9:10). A variety of remedies are described to cleanse the stomach and improve digestion (ibid., 9:15).

Maimonides' *Regimen of Health*[3] was written for Sultan al-Malik al-Afdal, eldest son of Saladin the Great. The Sultan was a pleasure-seeking man subject to fits of melancholy or depression owing to his excess indulgences in feasting and sexual intercourse. He complained to Maimonides about constipation, indigestion, and dejection. In his four-chapter treatise, Maimonides criticizes people who overeat, underexercise, and drink lots of water after a big meal. Such behavior leads to serious indigestion that varies according to the different foods consumed and the constitution of the eater (Chapter 1:1). "When food is badly digested in the stomach, of necessity its second digestion in the liver is also bad. So, too, its third digestion in all the organs is also bad. This is mostly the cause of all types of illnesses" (ibid.). Numerous additional references to digestion are found in Maimonides' *Three Treatises on Health*[4] as well as in his *Extracts from Galen*.[5]

---

1. F. Rosner, *The Medical Aphorisms of Moses Maimonides* (Haifa: Maimonides Research Institute, 1989).

2. F. Rosner, *Moses Maimonides' Treatise on Asthma* (Haifa: Maimonides Research Institute, 1994).

3. F. Rosner, "The Regimen of Health," in *Moses Maimonides' Three Treatises on Health* (Haifa: Maimonides Research Institute, 1990).

4. F. Rosner, *Moses Maimonides' Three Treatises on Health* (Haifa: Maimonides Research Institute, 1990).

5. U.S. Barzel, *Maimonides' the Art of Cure. Extracts from Galen* (Haifa: Maimonides Research Institute, 1992).

**DIURETICS**—In his *Commentary on the Aphorisms of Hippocrates*,[1] Maimonides discusses the excretion of urine by medicinal means (Chapter 1:1). The emptying of "vessels," including the urinary bladder, can also occur spontaneously. In his *Medical Aphorisms*,[2] Maimonides quotes Galen, who said that diuretics should not be used if the patient is bleeding from the kidney, urinary bladder, or urethra (Chapter 3:105). The entire fifth chapter of this work is devoted to aphorisms pertaining to the examination of the urine. Diuretics are also described by Maimonides in his *Glossary of Drug Names*.[3] [*See also* UROLOGY] In his *Treatise on Asthma*,[4] he lists foods and spices that stimulate urination: lentils, borax, mint, anise, mastic, muscat, nuts, and nard.

---

1. F. Rosner, *Maimonides' Commentary on the Aphorisms of Hippocrates* (Haifa: Maimonides Research Institute, 1987).

2. F. Rosner, *The Medical Aphorisms of Moses Maimonides* (Haifa: Maimonides Research Institute, 1989).

3. F. Rosner, *Moses Maimonides' Glossary of Drug Names* (Haifa: Maimonides Research Institute, 1996).

4. F. Rosner, *Moses Maimonides' Treatise on Asthma* (Haifa: Maimonides Research Institute, 1994).

**DRUNKENNESS**—There are many references to drunkenness in the Bible and the Talmud,[1] some of which are codified by Maimonides and other rabbis. Drunkenness is said to bring poverty, woes, quarrels, wounds, strange visions, and much more (Prov. 20:1, 21:17, 23:19–21, 29:35, and 31:4–5), and causes kings to err in judgment (Prov. 31:4–5). Several narratives describe the disgrace—and sometimes death—of drunkards such as Noah

(Gen. 9:20–27), Lot (Gen. 19:31–38), Nabal (1 Sam. 25–36), Amnon (2 Sam. 13:28–29), Elah (1 Kings 16:9), Ben-Hadad (1 Kings 20:16), and Ahasuerus (Esther 1:10). The prophets frequently condemn drunkenness, particularly among the wealthy and the leaders (Isa. 28:1ff., 56:11–12), associating it with moral insensitivity (Isa. 5:11–12, 18) and forgetting God (Hos. 4:11–12). Drunkenness and gluttony are among the charges against the rebellious son (Deut. 21:20).

Excessive consumption of alcohol was also frowned upon in talmudic writings, and overindulgence was thought to be injurious to health, including its negative impact on the bones (*Niddah* 24b). Priests and judges, respectively, must refrain from alcohol before officiating or while hearing court cases or rendering decisions (*Erubin* 64a). The judges of the Sanhedrin had to abstain from wine during the entire hearing of a capital case (*Sanhedrin* 42a). A person should not pray in a state of drunkenness (*Berachot* 31b).

In his *Medical Aphorisms*,[2] Maimonides also states that habitual wine-drinking leads to confusion (Chapter 13:22) and that "it is not good for a person to drink more than a reasonable amount of wine because wine rapidly brings a person to anger, disgrace, and shame. Wine corrupts the thoughts of the psyche, and under-mines the sharpness and clarity of the intellect" (ibid., 17:26).

In his *Mishneh Torah*, Maimonides asserts that an inebriated person is still legally responsible for legal and business matters, unless he is drunk as Lot (Gen. 19:30ff), in which case he is exempt from responsibility and liability for punishment. Maimonides rules that an intoxicated priest (*kohen*) is unfit to minister in the Temple (*Biyat Mikdash* 1:1), whether he was drunk from wine or from any other intoxicating beverage (ibid., 1:2). An intoxicated person should not pray because he cannot concentrate (*Tefillah*, 4:17). An inebriated priest is not to pronounce the priestly benediction (ibid., 14:1).

The legal acts of a drunkard are valid unless he has reached the drunkenness of Lot, i.e., does not know what he is doing. Then his transactions are invalid and he has the status of an imbecile or of a minor less than six years of age (*Mechirah* 29:18). An intoxicated person who reaches the stage of Lot's drunkenness and declares himself to be a Nazirite is not obligated to observe Naziriteship because his words during such a state of drunkenness have no effect, and he is not responsible for his actions or for any transgression that he may commit (*Nezirut* 1:12).

Another example of a temporary mental disability during which a person is ineligible to act in legal matters is the condition known as *kordiakos*, which is probably an alcohol-induced confusion of the mind. Maimonides rules that a man seized by *kordiakos* cannot write a bill of divorce for his wife (*Gerushin* 2:14) until his mind is settled. The same is true of a drunkard whose intoxication reaches the degree of drunkenness of Lot (ibid.).

Maimonides further rules that if an intoxicated man betroths a woman, the betrothal is valid even if he is exceedingly drunk. If, however, he has reached the drunkenness of Lot (Gen. 19:31–38), his betrothal is invalid (*Eeshut* 4:18). The term *kordiakos*

appears several times in the Talmud (*Gittin* 67b), and its meaning has been the subject of recent controversy.[3]

1. F. Rosner (translator), *Julius Pruess' Biblical and Talmudic Medicine* (Northvale, NJ: Jason Aronson, 1993), pp. 570–572.

2. F. Rosner, *The Medical Aphorisms of Moses Maimonides* (Haifa: Maimonides Research Institute, 1989).

3. F. Rosner, "*Kordiakos* in the Talmud," in *Medicine in the Bible and the Talmud*, 2nd augmented ed. (Hoboken, NJ: Ktav and Yeshiva University Press, 1995), pp. 60–64.

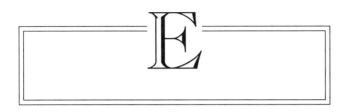

**EARS**—In his *Commentary on the Aphorisms of Hippocrates,*[1] Maimonides explains watery discharge from the ears to be due to superfluities of the brain that flow into the ears. In his *Medical Aphorisms,*[2] he quotes Galen, who also discusses discharges from the ears (Chapter 3:85–86), and recommends that those discharges that dissolve spontaneously should not be squeezed, nor should drawing salve be applied. However, if pus gathers, the abscess should be incised and drained (ibid., 4:86). Earache is treated by the instillation of warm drops into the ear (ibid., 9:27). In his *Extracts from Galen,*[3] Maimonides describes in detail the treatment of wounds of the ear and the need, at times, to prescribe analgesics for pain in the ear. Iron drops were cooked in vinegar and the viscous remedy applied to ear wounds.

In his *Mishneh Torah,* Maimonides describes various anatomical abnormalities of the ears such as nicks or slits (*Biyat Mikdash* 7:2–3), or extra-small or extra-large ears, pendulous ears, or unevenly-sized ears (ibid., 8:3). Anatomical defects of animal ears are also described (*Issurei Mizbeyach* 2:2). He also rules that a woman is permitted to go out into a public domain on the Sabbath with a plug of wool firmly stuffed in her ear (*Shabbat* 9:11). [*See also* HEARING]

---

1. F. Rosner, *Maimonides' Commentary on the Aphorisms of Hippocrates* (Haifa: Maimonides Research Institute, 1987).
2. F. Rosner, *The Medical Aphorisms of Moses Maimonides* (Haifa: Maimonides Research Institute, 1989).
3. U.S. Barzel, *Maimonides' The Art of Cure, Extracts from Galen* (Haifa: Maimonides Research Institute, 1992), pp. 65–66 and 140.

**EDEMA**—In his *Commentary on the Aphorisms of Hippocrates,*[1] Maimonides distinguishes between wet hydrops (edema) and dry hydrops (swelling that is due to air) (Section 4:9). He states that wounds do not heal well in edematous patients (ibid., 6:8). A patient with an enlarged spleen who has bloody diarrhea may develop dropsy (ascites) because of the weakened liver (ibid., 6:43). If a patient with dropsy develops a cough, it is a bad sign indicating watery humors in the bronchi (pulmonary edema?) (ibid., 6:35), and the patient may die (ibid., 7:47). Dropsy and diarrhea are ways in which the body rids itself of illness-producing material and humors (ibid., 7:5). Maimonides speaks of white humor as being the "dropsy of the flesh," i.e., anasarca, as opposed to ascites (ibid., 7:29).

In his *Medical Aphorisms,*[2] Maimonides quotes Galen, who said that a changing bad constitution may manifest itself as hydrops in the entire body or as local edema (Chapter 3:27). Hydrops of the flesh (anasarca?) is said to be caused by fluid accumulation within all solid body organs, which become soaked (ibid., 4:41). In all types of edema (e.g., ascites, anasarca, and the like), the liver is unable to transform liquids in the diet into blood because of a cold, bad mixture of humors that prevails over it (ibid., 9:65). Generalized edema is also called leukophlegmatia, and the white phlegm is also called hydrops (ibid., 23:50). Pitting and nonpitting edema are accurately portrayed (ibid., 23:52). Occasionally, a patient with hydrops is benefited by phlebotomy, but most are harmed by this procedure (ibid., 24:16).

1. F. Rosner, *Maimonides' Commentary on the Aphorisms of Hippocrates* (Haifa: Maimonides Research Institute, 1987).

2. F. Rosner, *The Medical Aphorisms of Moses Maimonides* (Haifa: Maimonides Research Institute, 1989).

**EGGPLANT**—Maimonides discusses numerous vegetables and their nutritional or medicinal value in many of his medical writings, as well as in his *Mishneh Torah* (*Deot* 4:9ff). In his *Regimen of Health,*[1] he enumerates eggplant as a bad nutrient for those who wish to preserve their health (Chapter 1:11). The reason is that eggplant heats the body and increases or aggravates bad digestion, hemorrhoids, headache, depression, and melancholy, all symptoms suffered by the Sultan for whom Maimonides wrote this work.

In his *Medical Aphorisms,*[2] Maimonides quotes Abu Merwan Ibn Zuhr, who said that eggplant (solanum melongena, or nigrum) strengthens the stomach and helps stimulate emesis, but is the worst of all foods since it gives rise to large quantities of black bile, which is the cause of melancholy (Chapter 20: 81). Apparently, a subcutaneous hematoma is being described when Maimonides states that if blood flows outside the blood vessels beneath the skin, that site resembles an eggplant (ibid., 24:13).

1. F. Rosner, Moses *Maimonides' Three Treatises on Health* (Haifa: Maimonides Research Institute, 1990).

2. F. Rosner, *The Medical Aphorisms of Moses Maimonides* (Haifa: Maimonides Research Institute, 1989).

**EGGS**—In both his *Medical Aphorisms*[1] and in his *Treatise on Cohabitation*,[2] Maimonides discusses the aphrodisiac properties of eggs, especially those from partridges, doves, pigeons, and other birds. All types of eggs help the libido, especially if they are cooked with onion or turnip. In his *Treatises on Health*, he states that chicken eggs, primarily their yolks, are wholesome, particularly if the eggs are soft-boiled.[3] He also confirms the asthmatic Sultan's habit of eating the yolks of five or six soft-boiled eggs together with a little cane sugar and salt.[4] In his *Extracts from Galen*,[5] Maimonides describes egg whites as one of many ingredients for a variety of medicaments. He also says that egg yolks are easier to digest than egg whites. Finally, in his *Mishneh Torah* (*Deot* 4:7), Maimonides asserts that if a person wishes to eat eggs and meat, he should eat the eggs first. [*See also* APHRODISIACS]

1. F. Rosner, *The Medical Aphorisms of Moses Maimonides* (Haifa: Maimonides Research Institute, 1989), p. 305.

2. F. Rosner, *Maimonides' Treatises on Poisons, Hemorrhoids and Cohabitation* (Haifa: Maimonides Research Institute, 1984), p. 167.

3. F. Rosner, *Moses Maimonides' Three Treatises on Health* (Haifa: Maimonides Research Institute, 1990), pp. 26 and 47.

4. F. Rosner, *Moses Maimonides' Treatise on Asthma* (Haifa: Maimonides Research Institute, 1994), p. 68.

5. U.S. Barzel, *Maimonides' The Art of Cure. Extracts from Galen* (Haifa: Maimonides Research Institute, 1992).

**EMACIATION**—In his *Medical Aphorisms*,[1] Maimonides quotes Galen, who said that emaciation may occur in seriously ill patients, particularly those with heart, liver, or stomach ailments (Chapter 9:60). A person whose body is emaciated is benefited by bathing after meals (ibid., 19:13). Some individuals are extremely emaciated, yet have much blood, and some fat people have little blood (ibid., 24:17). In his *Treatise on Asthma*,[2] Maimonides recommends that a healthy person should have a body midway between stoutness and leanness, but warns that it is not appropriate to be excessively thin. He agrees with Hippocrates that people who have become emaciated over a long period should be restored with food to normal corpulence slowly, whereas those who have become lean quickly should be rapidly restored.[3]

1. F. Rosner, *The Medical Aphorisms of Moses Maimonides* (Haifa: Maimonides Research Institute, 1989).

2. F. Rosner, *Moses Maimonides' Treatise on Asthma* (Haifa: Maimonides Research Institute, 1994), p. 51.

3. F. Rosner, *Maimonides' Commentary on the Aphorisms of Hippocrates* (Haifa: Maimonides Research Institute, 1987), p. 45.

**EMETICS**—The fourteenth chapter of Maimonides' *Medical Aphorisms* is devoted to emesis.[1] The onion of the narcissum (a member of the daffodil family) is characterized as a good emetic. Also useful for inducing vomiting is body movement that is compared to seasickness, where movement induces or contributes to emesis: "Body activity in the form of physical exercise after the imbibition of the emetic medication is helpful to the vomiting process because movement stimulates the liquids upwards as occurs to sea voyagers on ships in the ocean."

In his *Regimen of Health*, Maimonides says that regular vomiting twice monthly is good for remaining healthy, provided that the person does not have a weak chest, rapidly develop fullness of the head, or suffer from frequent headaches.[2] Vomiting also is not beneficial when it is very cold. In his *Treatise on Asthma*, Maimonides repeats the assertion that "vomiting is truly necessary for the preservation of health of all people." Its therapeutic application for asthma has also been verified.[3] He then describes various emetic concoctions such as those containing white radishes, dill, bees' honey, and vinegar. Numerous comments about emesis can also be found in his other medical writings.[4]

In his *Mishneh Torah* (*Shabbat* 21: 31), he rules that one may not induce vomiting on the Sabbath with emetic drugs, lest one be led to pound the ingredients. However, inserting one's finger into the mouth to cause vomiting is permitted.

---

1. F. Rosner, *The Medical Aphorisms of Moses Maimonides* (Haifa: Maimonides Research Institute, 1989), pp. 240–242.
2. F. Rosner, *Moses Maimonides' Three Treatises on Health* (Haifa: Maimonides Research Institute, 1990), p. 45.
3. F. Rosner, *Moses Maimonides' Treatise on Asthma* (Haifa: Maimonides Research Institute, 1994), pp. 80–82.
4. F. Rosner, *Maimonides' Commentary on the Aphorisms of Hippocrates* (Haifa: Maimonides Research Institute, 1987).

**EPILEPSY**—In his *Mishneh Torah*, Maimonides rules that an epileptic priest (*kohen*) is disqualified from serving in the Temple (*Biyat Mikdash* 8:16). During a fit, any epileptic— priest or not—is ineligible to serve as a witness, but during the interval between fits he is eligible, whether the paroxysms occur regularly or episodically without any regularity, provided that he is not mentally deranged all the time, for there are epileptics who are always confused in mind (*Edut* 9:9). Concerning epileptics and other people who are sane at times and insane at other times, the rule is that during the period of sanity, all their acts of sale and acquisition are valid (*Mechirah* 29:5). If a sold slave is found to be afflicted with epilepsy, the sale can be invalidated (ibid., 15:13).

In his *Medical Aphorisms*,[1] Maimonides quotes Galen, who states that epilepsy is due to thick, cold, viscous humors (Chapter 9:1) and that certain epileptics can be helped by physical exercise or a bland diet (ibid., 8:19). The immaturity of their nervous system predisposes children to convulsions (ibid., 3:10), but in them it is not dangerous. For childhood epilepsy, he recommends a liquid mixture of vinegar and honey after cleansing the body from its superfluities (ibid., 9:13). Muscle spasms and epilepsy are sometimes equated (ibid., 9:23). Epilepsy is also thought to result from a blow on the neck (ibid., 11:2) or a stomach ailment (ibid., 9:43). Maimonides criticizes Galen for contradictions in his writings about the onset of epileptic seizures (ibid., 25:45). Convulsions that are due to a brain abscess lead to a fatal outcome (ibid., 3:83). Tonic–clonic convulsive movements of grand mal epilepsy are described (ibid., 6:70). Venesection is said to be contraindicated in patients with convulsive disorders (ibid., 12:5), yet at times seems to be therapeutic (ibid., 12:22). This apparent contradiction is unexplained.

In his *Commentary on the Aphorisms of Hippocrates*,[2] Maimonides describes convulsive seizures in alcoholics (Section 5:5). Muscle spasms are sometimes reported as convulsions (ibid., 5:22), and may be induced by cold (ibid., 5:18 and 5:69). Convulsions represents an illness of black bile (ibid., 6:56) but may also occur because of a hemorrhage that weakens the brain (ibid., 7:9). Convulsions may also occur following ingestion of a poison (ibid., 5:1 and 7:25). Maimonides asserts that epilepsy and paralysis are both produced by cold, thick humors and are influenced by climatic and seasonal factors (ibid., 2:45). Thus, epilepsy occurs more in the spring (ibid., 3:20) and more in young people (ibid., 3:29). Finally, Maimonides explains that childhood epilepsy may improve as the patient gets older because the white, moist, cold humor causing the epilepsy improves in quality. Also of benefit are physical exercise, a drying diet, and appropriate medications (ibid., 5:7).

---

1. F. Rosner, *The Medical Aphorisms of Moses Maimonides* (Haifa: Maimonides Research Institute, 1989).
2. F. Rosner, *Maimonides' Commentary on the Aphorisms of Hippocrates* (Haifa: Maimonides Research Institute, 1987).

*EPISPASM*—Throughout history, periods of persecution against the Jews during which circumcision was forbidden, under penalty of death, were not uncommon. The first such prohibition was enacted under Antiochus Epiphanes (175–153 B.C.E.), son of Antiochus the Great (1 Macc. 1:48). Many mothers who had their sons circumcised suffered martyrdom (2 Macc. 6:10). Operations to reconstruct the prepuce surgically, either voluntarily or under coercion, were also performed. Maimonides mentions the case of a circumcised man whose prepuce had been drawn forward to cover up the corona (*mashuk*). Such a man must be recircumcised (*Terumot* 7:10).

During Hellenistic times, it is alleged that some Jews who wanted to participate nude in the Greek games in the gymnasia attempted to make their circumcision unrecognizable by methodically pulling the foreskin to the front. These epispastics (Greek, "to draw in"), according to Josephus (*Antiquities*, Book 12, Chap. 5:1), covered the circumcision of their penis so that even when they were naked, they could not be distinguished from the Greeks. Some authors believe that these Jews "underwent painful operations to obliterate the signs of circumcision (epispasm)."[1] In the course of the persecutions that preceded the Judean revolt led by Bar Koziba against Rome in 132 C.E., many Jews became epispastics by forcibly drawing their prepuces forward. After the liberation, many were recircumcised without any harm to their health or procreative ability, thus contradicting the assertion of R. Judah that to recircumcise an epispastic is dangerous (*Yebamot* 72a). Elsewhere

(*Sanhedrin* 44a), the Talmud states that Achan was an epispastic, based on the biblical passage in Joshua 7:11. The rabbinic exegetical work titled *Midrash Tanchuma*, in its commentary on the Book of Genesis, implies that Esau was also an epispastic. In his classic book on biblical and talmudic medicine,[2] Preuss cites several additional references to epispastics in ancient Hebrew writings. Maimonides rules that such epispastic priests may eat of heave-offerings (*Terumot* 7:10).

---

1. L.V. Snowman, "Circumcision," in *Encyclopedia Judaica*, Vol. 5 (Jerusalem: Keter), cols. 567–575.

2. F. Rosner (translator), *Julius Preuss' Biblical and Talmudic Medicine* (Northvale, NJ: Jason Aronson, 1993), pp. 240–248.

*EPISTAXIS*—In his *Medical Aphorisms*,[1] Maimonides quotes Galen, who says that epistaxis that occurs during apparent health is due to bad blood or an excess of blood. The treatment for epistaxis is to phlebotomize the antecubital vein of the forearm on the same side as the nasal bleeding. Then one should apply suction cups over the liver or spleen or below the loins on the contralateral side. If the epistaxis persists, one should apply a suction cup to the nape of the neck together with cold compresses to the head. An alternative way of treating epistaxis is to apply suction cups to both temples. If the nosebleeding does not stop, one should apply a suction cup to the occipital area of the skull. Epistaxis was thought to be the body's attempt to eliminate bad humors. Although bathing was said to be helpful in eliminating humors that poured into the stomach, bathing is bad for epistaxis in that it stimulates and irritates the bleeding nose.

Maimonides agrees with Hippocrates, who said that if epistaxis occurs as a mechanism to rid the body of that which should be excreted, then it is beneficial and easily tolerated.[2]

_____

1. F. Rosner, *The Medical Aphorisms of Moses Maimonides* (Haifa: Maimonides Research Institute, 1989).
2. F. Rosner, *Maimonides' Commentary on the Aphorisms of Hippocrates* (Haifa: Maimonides Research Institute, 1987).

**ERUCTATION**—In his *Commentary on the Aphorisms of Hippocrates,*[1] Maimonides states that acid eructations are evidence that food is remaining in the stomach sufficiently long to become partially changed (Section 6:1). Pleurisy was said to be rare in patients with acid eructations (ibid., 6:33), because pleurisy was thought to be caused by a thin humor and people with acid eructations have thick humors. In his *Treatise on Asthma,*[2] Maimonides relates that he observed gluttons who eructated and returned food to their mouths like ruminating animals (Chapter 5:3).

Overeating may lead to constant eructation. One should eat only when the stomach is empty, rather than consuming one meal after another. If one eructates and the taste of the previously eaten food is gone, one may eat again (ibid., 6:3).

In his *Medical Aphorisms,*[3] Maimonides quotes Galen, who said that constant eructation is a reflection of the power of the force that creates bad humors and various illnesses (Chapter 2:24). Eructation may cause acceleration of the pulse (ibid., 4:20). Digestion of food below the level of the stomach gives rise to eructation (ibid., 7:52). Eating foods that one is not accustomed to may produce distress that is relieved by eructation (ibid., 7:55). It is not clear whether the term "eructation" in Maimonides' writings refers to belching, heartburn, or pyrosis.

_____

1. F. Rosner, *Maimonides' Commentary on the Aphorisms of Hippocrates* (Haifa: Maimonides Research Institute, 1987).
2. F. Rosner, *Moses Maimonides' Treatise on Asthma* (Haifa: Maimonides Research Institute, 1994).
3. F. Rosner, *The Medical Aphorisms of Moses Maimonides* (Haifa: Maimonides Research Institute, 1989).

**ESOPHAGUS**—In his *Medical Aphorisms,*[1] Maimonides quotes Galen, who said that the esophagus is one of four organs that has two skins (Chapter 1:66). It stretches along the bones of the vertebral column and is painful when diseased (esophagitis?) (ibid., 6:56). A bad temperament in the esophagus may lead to powerful thirst (ibid., 7:57). Perhaps an early reference to tube-feeding in a comatose patient is the assertion that, for a person in stupor, liquid food is put into an instrument that is inserted in the mouth toward the base of the tongue so that the food pours into the esophagus (ibid., 9:11). Hemorrhage from the esophagus (from varices or from cancer?) is treated with viscous and astringent drugs (ibid., 9:37).

In his *Mishneh Torah*, Maimonides mentions a baby born with "an obstructed gullet" (*Issurei Biyah* 10:11), a clear reference to esophageal atresia.

***

1. F. Rosner, *The Medical Aphorisms of Moses Maimonides* (Haifa: Maimonides Research Institute, 1989).

**EXERCISE**—In his *Mishneh Torah* (*Deot* 4:2 and 15), Maimonides points out the importance of daily exercise and the dangers of leading a sedentary life. Although vigorous exercise on the Sabbath is prohibited (*Shabbat* 21:28), mild exertion such as walking is certainly permitted.

In his medical writings, Maimonides insists that general health measures for the preservation of health are superior to the powers of any medi-

cine. Among these measures is exercise, which he prescribes for both body and soul. He defines exercise as "strong or weak movement or a combination of both . . . as a result of which . . . the person begins to increase his breathing . . . extremely vigorous exercise is called exertion. Not everyone can tolerate exertion nor does he need it."[1] Daily walking or other physical exercise carried out within proper limits provides much strength and vitality. Maimonides repeatedly mentions the beneficial influence of physical exercise not only in his *Treatises on Health*, but also in his *Medical Aphorisms*,[2] and his *Treatise on Asthma*.[3]

***

1. F. Rosner, *Moses Maimonides' Three Treatises on Health* (Haifa: Maimonides Research Institute, 1990).

2. F. Rosner, *The Medical Aphorisms of Moses Maimonides* (Haifa: Maimonides Research Institute, 1989).

3. F. Rosner, *Moses Maimonides' Treatise on Asthma* (Haifa: Maimonides Research Institute, 1994).

**EXTRACTS FROM GALEN**—The *Extracts from Galen* is also known as the *Art of Cure* and the *Compendium of Galen*.[1] This Maimonidean book differs from the usual medieval presentation of medical subjects in an organ-oriented system, and deals with classifications of diseases, wounds, febrile disorders, and tumors. Galen's medical writings consist of over one hundred books. Maimonides therefore extracted what he considered to be Galen's most important pronouncements and compiled them in the *Extracts from Galen.*

Maimonides states that he was careful to prescribe only those treatment regimens and medications that he found by his own experience to be useful. The specific prescription for a treatment regimen for any condition took into account not only the nature of the illness, but also the constitution of the patient, his or her age and habits, geography, and climate—i.e., the town in which the patient lived, and the time of the year.

In contrast to some dated medical concepts, many principles enunciated by Maimonides in the treatment of injuries are still acceptable to surgeons today. For instance, he knew that a cut would heal if the parts were brought together by using one of several kinds of bandages. If the parts were separated by anything—be it air, pus, or bone—there would be no primary healing. Pus had to be dried with drying medication, and if a collection occurred, it had to be drained. If the edges of the wound appeared to become abnormal, they had to be excised to reach healthy tissues.

In all, the book enhances Maimonides' stature as a teacher of medicine. He was an observant and careful practitioner of medicine, well-versed in the art and science of medicine as it was understood in his day, and he used to advantage available resources for the care of his patients.

---

1. U.S. Barzel, *Maimonides' The Art of Cure. Extracts from Galen* (Haifa: Maimonides Research Institute, 1992).

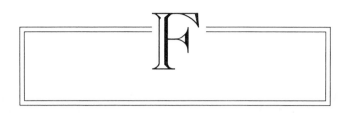

**FACIAL APPEARANCE**—In his *Medical Aphorisms*,[1] Maimonides asserts that if a patient's facial appearance closely resembles the normal, it is a favorable prognostic sign and signifies that nature is strong. If the facial appearance is far from normal, it is a sign of weakening of the overall reigning force in the body, and the patient's prognosis is poor (Chapter 6:94).

In his *Mishneh Torah*, Maimonides recognized that postmortem changes may distort the facial features of a person to make him nonrecognizable, and that these postmortem changes are delayed if the body is preserved in cold ocean water. These medical and pathological observations are described and codified by Maimonides as follows:

> If a slain man's facial features are sufficiently preserved to identify him as so-and-so, testimony may be given that he is dead (*Gerushin* 13:21).

---

1. F. Rosner, *The Medical Aphorisms of Moses Maimonides* (Haifa: Maimonides Research Institute, 1989).

**FASTING**—The subject of fasting on certain religious holidays such as Yom Kippur (the Day of Atonement) and Tisha B'Ab (the ninth day of the month of Ab) is discussed by Maimonides in his *Mishneh Torah* (*Shevisat Asor* and *Taanit*). In addition, the following are the afflictions for which a community should fast and sound an alarm: oppression of Israel by its enemies; war; pestilence; wild beasts; locusts; crickets; blasting of crops; mildew; collapse of buildings; epidemics; economic crises; and excess or deficiency of rain (*Taanit* 2:1). Maimonides then defines each of these.

If, after a second series of fast days, the community's prayers for rain or deliverance from other calamity are still unanswered, the court proclaims a sequence of seven fast days. On these seven fast days, even expectant and nursing mothers must fast; on other fast days, they need not do so (ibid., 3:5). However, when exempt from fasting, they should not pamper themselves with delicacies, but should eat and drink only that which is necessary to maintain the health of the child (ibid.).

The fast on the ninth day of Ab commemorates not only the destruction of both Temples, but several other related calamities (ibid., 5:3). Expectant and nursing mothers must fast all day on the ninth of Ab (ibid., 5:10). As on the Day of Atonement, it is forbidden to bathe in either warm or cold water, anoint oneself for pleasure, wear sandals, or have marital intercourse (ibid.).

Elsewhere in *Mishneh Torah* (*Deot* 3:1), Maimonides points out that people who constantly fast are not following a good path. Starvation may be associated with amenorrhea in young women (*Eeshut* 11:12). In fact, in his medical works, Maimonides warns against the danger of fasting, which "causes the development of fever."[1] Older people tolerate fasting better than young people.[2] Although fasting weakens body strength and diminishes it, fasting helps in the elimination of bad foods so that one does not become accustomed to them.[3]

---

1. U.S. Barzel, *Maimonides' The Art of Cure. Extracts from Galen* (Haifa: Maimonides Research Institute, 1992), p. 118.

2. F. Rosner, *Maimonides' Commentary on the Aphorisms of Hippocrates* (Haifa: Maimonides Research Institute, 1987), p. 30.

3. F. Rosner, *The Medical Aphorisms of Moses Maimonides* (Haifa: Maimonides Research Institute, 1989), pp. 103 and 293.

**FEVERS**—The tenth chapter of Maimonides' *Medical Aphorisms* is devoted entirely to fevers.[1] Maimonides recognizes that fever is only a symptom, not a disease, and that both symptom and underlying cause should be treated after careful search for the latter. "It is important to know the precise differentiation between the fever of a septic process and the cause for that septic process. It is important to know which remedy to use to treat a fever, which therapy to employ to treat a septic process and which medicine to use to treat the cause for the septic process. . . ." There is clear separation of fevers into tertian, quotidian, and quartan varieties, although the causes given for them are incorrect according to modern medical thought. Thus, Maimonides quotes Galen as follows: "Intermittent fevers which cease during specific intervals are of three types and these are: tertian fever, that which comes daily called permanent or quotidian, and quartan fever. Tertian fever occurs from red bile which putrefies. Quotidian fever is produced from biles which begin to decay and are of the white type. Quartan fever develops as a result of the deterioration of black bile." Various features of the three types of fever are then described. Much faith is placed in theriac as a therapeutic drink for quartan fevers preceded by the consumption of absinthium juice. Phlebotomy is recommended for chronic fevers.

Fever and its causes, types, and treatments are also discussed in considerable detail in Maimonides' other medical writings, including *Treatises on Health*[2] and *Asthma*,[3] *Extracts from Galen*,[4] and *Commentary on the Aphorisms of Hippocrates*.[5]

1. F. Rosner, *The Medical Aphorisms of Moses Maimonides* (Haifa: Maimonides Research Institute, 1989), pp. 184–203.
2. F. Rosner, *Moses Maimonides' Three Treatises on Health* (Haifa: Maimonides Research Institute, 1990).
3. F. Rosner, *Moses Maimonides' Treatise on Asthma* (Haifa: Maimonides Research Institute, 1994).
4. U.S. Barzel, *Maimonides' The Art of Cure. Extracts from Galen* (Haifa: Maimonides Research Institute, 1992).
5. F. Rosner, *Maimonides' Commentary on the Aphorisms of Hippocrates* (Haifa: Maimonides Research Institute, 1987).

*FIGS*—In his *Mishneh Torah* (*Deot* 4:11), Maimonides states that figs, grapes, and almonds are always good, whether fresh or dried, and that a person may eat therefrom as much as he requires. He asserts that fig cakes or dried figs spoil if put in brine (*Terumot* 11:3). Dried figs are used for their own sake, but also to flavor other food (*Tumat Ochlin* 1:8).

He quotes Galen, who said that figs and grapes are "like the princes of the other fruits,"[1] and that food for the elderly in the summer should include fresh figs, and in the winter dried figs.[2]

Dried figs dipped in grated and sifted anise aids the digestion, softens the stool, and alleviates bronchial inflammation in asthmatic patients.[3]

1. F. Rosner, *Moses Maimonides' Three Treatises on Health* (Haifa: Maimonides Research Institute, 1990), p. 29.
2. F. Rosner, *The Medical Aphorisms of Moses Maimonides* (Haifa: Maimonides Research Institute, 1989), p. 276.
3. F. Rosner, *Moses Maimonides' Treatise on Asthma* (Haifa: Maimonides Research Institute, 1994), p. 57.

*FISH*—In his *Medical Aphorisms*,[1] Maimonides recommends ocean fish that have a young body, little fat, and a pleasant taste, and white meat that can be separated to lessen its stickiness. These fish are helpful for asthmatics because they are easily digested and have little residue. River fish are not detrimental, provided that they come from a large river that has clean water. Also recommended for asthmatics are salt-water fish with scales, because of their tenderness and lightness. However, one should not consume a lot of these fish, so that they should not make the phlegm become sticky. Maimonides further recommends the consumption of fish known as *muglas* and also the salted, clefted, smooth fish that contain little salt, which are good if consumed once or twice a month.

In both *Regimen of Health*[2] and *Mishneh Torah* (*Deot* 4:10), Maimonides warns against excessive consumption of brine from small salted fish. In his *Medical Aphorisms*,[3] Maimonides quotes Galen, who said that *sela* fish is a good food to invigorate body strength and cleanse the respiratory passages of bad humors. Finally, in his *Extracts from Galen*,[4] Maimonides says that shallow-water fish are good, especially for patients with stomach disorders.

---

1. F. Rosner, *Moses Maimonides' Treatise on Asthma* (Haifa: Maimonides Research Institute, 1994), p. 54.
2. F. Rosner, *Moses Maimonides' Three Treatises on Health* (Haifa: Maimonides Research Institute, 1990), p. 85.
3. F. Rosner, *The Medical Aphorisms of Moses Maimonides* (Haifa: Maimonides Research Institute, 1989), p. 131.
4. U.S. Barzel, *Maimonides' Art of Cure. Extracts from Galen* (Haifa: Maimonides Research Institute, 1992), pp. 100 and 105.

**FOODS AND BEVERAGES**—The twentieth chapter of Maimonides' *Medical Aphorisms* deals with foods and beverages and their usages.[1] The second aphorism summarizes the importance of nutrition in both health and disease: "A knowledge of dietetics [literally, strengths of foods] is practically one of the most helpful things in the field of medicine because of the constant never-ending need for food during health as well as during illness." The remainder of the chapter elaborates at length on this prin-ciple. A few excerpts will suffice to impart the general flavor of the chapter: "Soft food is more easily and rapidly digested. . . . It is not proper for us to gorge ourselves full of food . . . the quantity consumed should not overburden [the patient]. Putrefied foods and beverages produce decay [i.e., toxins] similar to that produced by deadly poisons. Some foods soften the stool. . . . The most valuable and most appropriate bread for someone who does not perform any physical exercise or for the elderly is bread which has been well baked in the oven and which contains a large quantity of sourdough. Wine to which an equal quantity of water has been added warms the entire body and stimulates all limbs. . . . Drinking cold water before meals damages the food and the liver. Milk nourishes a defective body. . . . Cheese . . . harms patients with hydrops. Cow's milk is the thickest of all milks and the fattest of all."

A host of foods—including fruits, grains, meats, and others—their properties, and their characteristics are then enumerated. [*See also specific foods* (e.g., CHEESE, FIGS, HONEY) *and beverages* (e.g., MILK, WINE)]

---

1. F. Rosner, *The Medical Aphorisms of Moses Maimonides* (Haifa: Maimonides Research Institute, 1989), pp. 293–312.

**FORENSIC MEDICINE**—The Talmud describes a procedure for the application of seven substances on a garment to determine whether a red or brown stain is blood or colored dye (*Niddah* 63a). In his *Mishneh Torah*, Maimonides describes these substances (*Shabbat* 18:8) and supports the talmudic assertion about their efficacy in distinguishing a bloodstain from a dye (*Mishkav Umoshav* 4:13), perhaps the earliest reference to forensic pathology.

A bloodstain found on a woman's flesh or undergarment renders her ritually unclean (*Issurei Biyah* 9:6) unless it can be attributed to another cause, such as a wound or scratch (ibid., 9:19) or the handling of raw meat (ibid., 9:27). If doubt exists as to whether it is blood or red dye, the seven substances are to be applied in the prescribed sequence. If the stain disappears or grows faint, it is a bloodstain, and the woman is, therefore, unclean; if it remains as it was, it is a dye, and she is deemed clean (ibid., 9:37). Maimonides explains the source and preparation of the seven substances (ibid., 9:38). Regular soap washes out both blood and dye stains, and therefore would not resolve the question of ritual impurity.

Another item dealing with forensic medicine is a discussion by Maimonides[1] for estimating the amount of blood soaked into a garment (*Tumat Met* 4:13). A final item of interest to the forensic pathologist is a discussion dealing with the identification of a corpse and the postmortem changes that a body undergoes (*Gerushin* 13:21).

---

1. F. Rosner, "Forensic Medicine," in *Medicine in the Mishneh Torah of Maimonides* (New York: Ktav, 1984), pp. 287–290.

---

**FORGETFULNESS**—In his *Medical Aphorisms*,[1] Maimonides quotes Galen, who said that mental confusion and forgetfulness sometimes occur purely from senility or extreme weakness, and are due to cold humors or temperaments (Chapter 7:26). Amnesia for recent events is one of the signs of phrenesia (ibid., 6:37). Amnesia may also occur from a phlegmatic abscess in the membranes of the brain (meningitis?) (ibid., 23:60). Plucking of the hair with one's hand pulls the humors from the depths of the body to the surface, and may be beneficial to one who suffers from forgetfulness (ibid., 9:35).

---

1. F. Rosner, *The Medical Aphorisms of Moses Maimonides* (Haifa: Maimonides Research Institute, 1989).

---

**FREIMANN, ARON**—A bibliographer and historian, Freimann (1871–1948) served as editor of *Zeitschrift für Hebraeische Bibliographie.*[1] He also edited the facsimile reprint of Maimonides' *Regimen of Health* (c. 1480). Freimann's introduction to this work includes a bibliographical survey of the various editions and translations of this work. The facsimile was published in Heidelberg in 1931. Freimann also published a book of Maimonidean Responsa in 1934 (Jerusalem: Mekizei Nirdamim).

---

1. H. Oppenheimer and Aron Freimann. "Bibliographie (1893–1931)," in *Festschrift für Aron Freimann zum 60 Geburstage* (Berlin, 1935), 5–6.

*FRUITS*—Five species of fruit are mentioned in the Bible (grapes, pomegranates, figs, olives, and dates). In his *Mishneh Torah* (*Berachot* 8:1), Maimonides cites the blessing to be recited upon their consumption. Elsewhere in *Mishneh Torah* (*Deot* 4:11), Maimonides asserts that a person should abstain from fresh fruits of trees, and to consume them sparingly even when they are dried. Indeed, before fruits are completely ripe, they are like swords to the body. Carob pods (locust beans) are always injurious. All sour fruits are detrimental, and one should only eat a little of them, and only in the warm season and in warm climates. Figs, grapes, and almonds, however, are always good, whether fresh or dried. Maimonides repeats his warning against the consumption of fresh fruits in his *Treatises on Health*.[1] To stimulate the appetite and to soften the bowels, one may consume astringent fruits such as pears, quinces, and apples before meals. Maimonides cites Galen, who said that from the time he stopped eating fresh fruit he never again had any fever. One may consume dried fruits such as raisins, dried figs, and the kernels of pistachios or almonds, however. Fresh peaches and apricots should be avoided because they generate putrefied humors and fever. Similar statements about the harmful effects of most fresh fruits because they produce bad chymes or humors are found in Maimonides' *Medical Aphorisms*[2] where he also reiterates that figs, grapes, and almonds, especially dried ones, produce beneficial chymes. [*See also* specific fruits, *e.g.*, FIGS; *see also* NUTRITION and FOODS AND BEVERAGES]

---

1. F. Rosner, *Moses Maimonides' Three Treatises on Health* (Haifa: Maimonides Research Institute, 1990).
2. F. Rosner, *The Medical Aphorisms of Moses Maimonides* (Haifa: Maimonides Research Institute, 1989), p. 301.

*FUMIGATION*—In his *Treatise on Poisons*,[1] Maimonides states that fumigation with frankincense or other substances such as mustard, sulfur, nigella, or opium drives away poisonous animals, especially snakes. He therefore recommends that people take preventive measures and fumigate all places where poisonous animals may be found. In his *Treatise on Asthma*,[2] he states that the air in one's home should be kept dry at all times by sweet scents, fumigation, and drying agents. Inhaled fumigations to strengthen the brain and to dry humors in it and prevent their dripping may be beneficial to asthma sufferers. Such fumigations may also cleanse the lungs.

Elsewhere, Maimonides quotes Hippocrates, who said that fumigation with herbs promotes menstruation in women and may serve as a diagnostic test about a woman's fertility.[3] Maimonides adds that the fumigation should be performed with aromatic herbs such as galbanum, myrrh, and styrax. A similar statement is found in the Talmud (*Ketubot* 10b and *Yebamot* 60b, including the Rashi). He also says that fumigation is beneficial for warming cold places or for drying out humors, were it not for the fact that it fills the head.

An entire chapter in his *Treatise on Hemorrhoids*[4] is devoted to fumigations "beneficial in this illness." The following drugs used as fumigants, singly or compounded, are valuable for the flatulence that accompanies hemorrhoids: sandarac, leek seeds, snakeskin, colocynth, cottonseed, rue seeds, henbane seeds, herba sancta

seeds, long aristolochia, and roots of fenugreek. Maimonides describes the procedure for fumigation: Dig a hole in the ground and place a coal fire therein. Cover the hole with a large overturned earthen pot with a hole in its bottom (such a pot is described in *Kelim* 22:10 and in *Midrash, Deuteronomy Rabbah* 10:1). Cover the pot near the ground with a garment so that the vapors emerge only through the hole in the pot. Throw the fumigant medication on the fire through the opening in the pot. When the smoke rises, the patient should sit on the pot with his anus over the hole in the pot. When he feels that the smoke has finished, he should rise and add more drug to the fire, and again sit on the pot as he did before. This procedure should be done three times in one hour and repeated weekly.

---

1. F. Rosner, *Maimonides' Treatises on Poisons, Hemorrhoids and Cohabitation* (Haifa: Maimonides Research Institute, 1984), p. 76.

2. F. Rosner, *Moses Maimonides' Treatise on Asthma* (Haifa: Maimonides Research Institute, 1994).

3. F. Rosner, *Maimonides' Commentary on the Aphorisms of Hippocrates* (Haifa: Maimonides Research Institute, 1987), pp. 138 and 151.

4. F. Rosner, *Moses Maimonides' Treatises on Poisons, Hemorrhoids and Cohabitation*, pp. 148–149.

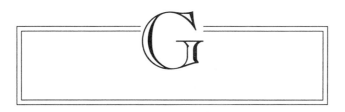

**GALEN, CRITICISM OF**—The twenty-fifth chapter of Maimonides' *Medical Aphorisms,* unlike the other chapters, does not deal with practical medicine, but contains a sharp attack on Galen, whose views were accepted as dogma throughout the Middle Ages. It demonstrates Maimonides' ability and courage as a profound critic, as well as his astounding knowledge of the spiritual world of the ancient Greeks. Aphorism 59 in this chapter is outstanding in this respect in that it presents Maimonides as a protagonist of the Aristotelian philosophy in its Arabic-Jewish garb conforming with the principles of Judaism. The peak of his greatness is revealed in aphorism 69, where he challenges conventional views in general, and exposes falsifications and errors of Galen, in particular. Maimonides demands research through experimentation and recognizes the influence of ecology on the human organism. He disputes Galen's views on life. He cannot comprehend how a man such as

Galen could pay attention only to "material" things to the exclusion of the spirit. Whereas to Galen knowledge without experience sufficed, to Maimonides, both are necessary to make a good physician. This final chapter of Maimonides' medical aphorisms is of such importance that the reader is referred to the full report[1] describing Maimonides' scholarly attack against dogmatic principles. An excerpt therefrom is as follows: ". . . if any man declares to you [that he has found] facts that he has observed and confirmed with his own experience, even if you consider this man to be most trustworthy and highly authoritative, be cautious in accepting what he says to you. If he attempts to persuade you to accept this opinion which is his viewpoint or any doctrine that he believes in, then you should think [critically] and understand [what he means] when he declares that he has observed it, and your thoughts should not become confused. . . . Rather, investigate and weigh this opinion or that hypothesis according to requirements of pure logic . . . [critically appraise] even a statement of the great sage Galen."

1. F. Rosner, *The Medical Aphorisms of Moses Maimonides* (Haifa: Maimonides Research Institute, 1989), pp. 401–454.

**GALLBLADDER**—In his *Medical Aphorisms*,[1] Maimonides quotes Galen, who describes the sphincter muscle, which controls the exit of bile from the gallbladder (Chapter 1:51), and the blood vessels that nourish it (ibid., 1:63). The spleen and the gallbladder are said to purify the blood (ibid., 2:9). The hepatic, cystic, and common bile ducts are described (ibid., 2:23). Red and black biles are attracted to the spleen and the gallbladder (ibid., 3:34). Extraction of a stone from the neck of the gallbladder is also mentioned (ibid., 24:54).

In his *Extracts from Galen*,[2] Maimonides asserts that the gallbladder lies on the spine posteriorly and that it may exude pus (empyema of the gallbladder?) (Chapter 13). Descriptions of the anatomy, the functions, and a variety of abnormalities of the gallbladder—including perforation, ectopic location, foreign objects, and wounds—are found in the Bible, the Talmud, and codes of Jewish law,[3] including Maimonides' *Mishneh Torah* (*Shechitah* 6:20), where he describes congenital absence or duplication of the gallbladder.

1. F. Rosner, *The Medical Aphorisms of Moses Maimonides* (Haifa: Maimonides Research Institute, 1989).

2. U.S. Barzel, *Maimonides' The Art of Cure. Extracts from Galen* (Haifa: Maimonides Research Institute, 1992).

3. F. Rosner, *Medicine in the Bible and the Talmud*, 2nd ed. (Hoboken, NJ: Ktav and Yeshiva University Press, 1995), pp. 107–112.

**GARLIC**—The Talmud (*Baba Kamma* 82a) asserts that garlic satiates, keeps the body warm, brightens the face, increases semen, and kills parasites in the bowels. Yet in *Mishneh Torah* (*Deot* 4:9) and *Treatises on Health*,[1] Maimonides says that garlic is detrimental to one's health. In his *Medical Aphorisms*,[2] he quotes Galen, who says that garlic may obstruct a cold body's openings. But if the body is warm, garlic helps to dissolve that which needs to be expelled. In an asthmatic patient, garlic may increase heat.[3] Garlic-containing compounded remedies applied to the site of a snake bite help to draw out the poison.[4] In his *Extracts from Galen*,[5] Maimonides states that garlic is one of the medicines that dissolves gases better than anything else and does not induce thirst. Garlic also reduces the swelling or pain caused by hard and viscous humor, and therefore is called the "theriac of the back." In his *Mishneh Torah* (*Tumat Ochlin* 14:3), he says that blocks of garlic were stored on the roof to preserve their freshness.

1. F. Rosner, *Moses Maimonides' Three Treatises on Health* (Haifa: Maimonides Research Institute, 1990), p. 28.
2. F. Rosner, *The Medical Aphorisms of Moses Maimonides* (Haifa: Maimonides Research Institute, 1989), pp. 320 and 330.
3. F. Rosner, *Moses Maimonides' Treatise on Asthma* (Haifa: Maimonides Research Institute, 1994), p. 53.
4. F. Rosner, *Maimonides' Treatises on Poisons, Hemorrhoids and Cohabitation* (Haifa: Maimonides Research Institute, 1984), p. 44.
5. U.S. Barzel, *Maimonides' The Art of Cure. Extracts from Galen* (Haifa: Maimonides Research Institute, 1992), p. 149.

*GLOSSARY OF DRUG NAMES*—
Maimonides' *Glossary of Drug Names* was discovered by Max Meyerhof, an Egyptian ophthalmologist, in the Aya Sofia library in Istanbul, Turkey, as Arabic manuscript 3711.[1] It is an alphabetical glossary of synonyms of medicinal drugs, as Maimonides explains in his brief introduction.[2] He defines his goal by declaring that he did not intend to describe simple remedies or to discuss their use, but to explain some—but not all—of their names, that is, to describe their synonyms. For this reason, he excluded from his list well-known drugs and, of course, those with only one name. As examples of these include camphor (*kāfūr*), ambergris (*'anbar*), musk (*misk*), violet (*banafsaǧ*), fig (*tīn*), and cantharides (*dararih*), which

are often described among the simple remedies in Maimonides' medical and theological works, but are omitted in his glossary of synonyms of drugs.

The book represents a type of work that was in vogue particularly in Maghrib, the west of the Musulman world. In fact, Maimonides mentions five extant works by Spanish authors that inspired him: four of the authors are Musulman, and one is Jewish. In general, Maimonides' work shows occidental inspiration. This is graphically illustrated in the concluding words of his introduction: "I have added thereto all that is reputed among the inhabitants of Maghrib. . . . I give preference to the interpretation which seems to me the one most accepted by us in Maghrib." This phrase "by us in Maghrib" is used repeatedly throughout the glossary. Maimonides frequently adds "the inhabitants of Egypt call it. . . ." It is, therefore, certain that he wrote this glossary in Egypt, where he wrote all his other medical writings.

By contrast, Maimonides' scientific thinking has its origin in the west, in Spain and in Morocco, where he spent his years of study. Maimonides is known for his philosophic, theologic, and other medical works. A book of medical lexicography such as the *Glossary of Drug Names* reveals a totally unknown or ignored aspect of the scientific activity and ability of Maimonides. Many works of this type appeared after Maimonides in both the eastern and western Musulman worlds. As in these other works of drug synonyms, the 405 articles of Maimonides' *Glossary of Drug Names* are of unequal length, sometimes comprising only a few words, other times occupying up to fifteen lines or nearly an entire manuscript page. Maimonides, in general, uses the best-known name of a drug as the title of an article and then follows it with synonyms in Arabic, ancient Greek, Syriac, Persian, Berber, and Spanish.

1. J. Meyerhoff, *Un Glossaire de Matière Médicale, Composé par Maïmonide (Sarh Asme al'Uqqar)* (Cairo: Memoires de l'Institut Egypte, 1940), vol. 41.
2. F. Rosner, *Moses Maimonides' Glossary of Drug Names* (Haifa: Maimonides Research Institute, 1996).

***GOLDSCHMIDT, ERNST DANIEL*** —A librarian and scholar of Jewish liturgy, Goldschmidt (1895–1972) edited an expanded transcript of Maimonides' *On the Causes of Symptoms* missing in the first edition of the Florence Latin incunable.[1] Goldschmidt's work was published in J.O. Leibowitz and S. Marcus, eds., *Moses Maimonides' On the Causes of Symptoms* (Berkeley: University of California Press, 1974), pp. 189–197. Goldschmidt also edited Maimonides' *Prayer Book* from an Ox-ford manuscript (*Seder Hatefilah shel Ha Rambam* (Jerusalem: Shocken, 5719), pp. 185–213).

1. E.E. Urbach and Daniel Goldschmidt, *Leo Baeck Institute Yearbook*, 19 (1974):175–180.

***GONORRHEA***—The term *zab* refers to a white seminal discharge from a man and is usually interpreted to refer to gonorrhea. In his *Mishneh Torah*, Maimonides refers to flux in a man as "semen that comes from the privy parts" (*Mechutrei Kaparah* 2:1). If a man suffers three consecutive emissions, he is called a man with flux, or *zab*. Continuous or intermittent dribbling is also discussed (ibid., 2:10). It seems likely that such genital discharge represents a venereal disease such as gonorrhea, in view of the rarity of spermatorrhea or benign urethral discharge. A *zab* was considered ritually impure for a variety of legal matters.

The difference between flux (gonorrhea) and sperm emission is that flux issues from a flabby penis, whereas sperm flows from an erect penis. Flux resembles the water of barley dough; it is pale or weak (ibid., 2:1) and resembles the white of incubated eggs. Sperm is bound and resembles the white of nonincubated eggs. Semen emission renders a man ritually unclean and conveys uncleanness by person and utensils by contact

(*Shar Avot Hatumah* 5:1). Red semen (hemorrhagic prostatitis, cystitis, or hematuria?) is deemed to be clean, until it grows white and is continuous (ibid., 5:3). A nocturnal emission is vividly described by Maimonides (ibid., 5:5). A healthy person shoots out his semen like an arrow (ibid., 5:7). Amazing is Maimonides' recognition that discharged sperm is viable for at least 36 hours (ibid., 5:12), and for much longer if it remains moist (ibid., 5:14). A similar assertion is found in the Talmud (*Shabbat* 86a and *Niddah* 7:1). In his *Mishnah Commentary* (*Zabim* 2:2), Maimonides states that flux in a man is an illness of the genitalia in which the retentive and digestive power has weakened, whereas the other powers of the body remain in their normal state. Then the sperm drips and issues forth "incompletely cooked," without pleasure and without erection; its appearance is a little reddish and it is thin in consistency. Often, dilute "uncooked" semen issues from the membrum after an issue of semen. People who indulge heavily in sexual intercourse suffer the most from this. They tell their physician that when they indulge excessively in sexual intercourse, their sperm issues from them extremely dilute in consistency and reddish in appearance, and they have pain (ibid., 2:3).

Certain causes of flux must be excluded before a man can be called a *zab*. For example, consuming certain foods and beverages, carrying heavy objects, jumping, and certain illnesses may lead to a genital discharge that does not render a man to be a *zab*. Sexually arousing thoughts and the observation of copulating animals may also induce semen emission that is not flux.[1,2]

1. F. Rosner, *Medicine in the Mishneh Torah of Maimonides* (New York: Ktav, 1984), pp. 134–143.
2. F. Rosner, "Medicine in Moses Maimonides' Commentary on the Mishnah," *Koroth* (Jerusalem), (1988):565–578.

***GORDON, HIRSCH L.***—A physician, orientalist, and writer, Gordon (1896–1969) contributed to various journals in seven languages.[1] His interest in Maimonidean medicine culminated in his translation into English of the sage's *Regimen of Health*. Gordon titled the volume *Moses ben Maimon. The Preservation of Youth* (New York: Philosophical Library, 1958).

1. J.I. Dienstag, "Contributions of Lithuanian Scholars to the Literature on the Mishneh Torah," *Abraham Colomb Jubilee Book* (Los Angeles, 1970), pp. 456–457 (Hebrew).

***GORLIN, MORRIS***—An American psychologist, Gorlin translated into English and published both authentic and spurious versions of Maimonides'

*Treatise on Sexual Intercourse* (Brooklyn, NY: Rambash Publishing Co., 1961). The translation, based mainly on Kroner's German version, is deficient in many respects, as Gorlin himself points out: "Some of the translations given have not been literal but paraphrased and excerpted . . . a considerable amount of errors have probably crept into this work. . . ." Gorlin's work, without mention of his name, was translated into Spanish by Enrique Chelminsky (Mexico: *Anales de Ars Medici*, 5 (1961), 5:240–248).

*GOUT*—In his *Medical Aphorisms*,[1] Maimonides quotes Galen, who said that the goal of therapy in gout (podagra) is to eliminate the damaging chymes (Chapter 9:121). Medications may not be able to eliminate the bad humors already in the painful joints, but may slow the accumulation there of more (ibid., 9:103). A cure for gout is the consumption of a decoctum of chickpeas with bee's honey for three successive days (ibid., 22:57).

In his *Commentary on the Aphorisms of Hippocrates*,[2] Maimonides writes that the alleviation of pain and subsidence of swelling of gouty joints by the pouring of cold water over them is due to the benumbing of one's sensation and the inhibition of pain-producing humor from going there. He quotes Hippocrates, who said that eunuchs do not develop gout, and that women do not develop gout unless their menses have stopped because women empty their gout-producing humors in the menstrual blood. Gout is also said to occur mostly in the spring and the autumn.

Gout in the Bible and the Talmud is discussed elsewhere.[3]

---

1. F. Rosner, *The Medical Aphorisms of Moses Maimonides* (Haifa: Maimonides Research Institute, 1989).

2. F. Rosner, *Maimonides' Commentary on the Aphorisms of Hippocrates* (Haifa: Maimonides Research Institute, 1987).

3. F. Rosner, "Gout," in *Medicine in the Bible and the Talmud*, augmented ed. (Hoboken, NJ: Ktav and Yeshiva University Press, 1955), pp. 58–59.

*GRAPES*—In his *Mishneh Torah* (*Deot* 4:11), Maimonides states that grapes, figs, and almonds are always good, whether fresh or dried, and that a person may eat therefrom as much as needed. Blessings to be recited before the consumption of fruits are discussed by Maimonides elsewhere in his *Code* (*Berachot* 8:1). In his *Treatise on Asthma*,[1] he recommends unripe grapes or dates as astringents for people with loose stools (Chapter 9:4). Grape juice is one of the ingredients of an opium potion that prevents catarrh, helps sleep, and assists in expectoration (ibid., 12:4). It is also beneficial when used as part of a concoction to cleanse the lungs, strengthen the brain, and stop catarrh (ibid., 12:5). In his *Regimen on Health*,[2] Maimonides quotes Galen, who said that figs and grapes are like the princes of fruits (Chapter 1:12), although no fruit is without some harm.

---

1. F. Rosner, *Moses Maimonides' Treatise on Asthma* (Haifa: Maimonides Research Institute, 1994).

2. F. Rosner, *Moses Maimonides' Three Treatises on Health* (Haifa: Maimonides Research Institute, 1990).

*GYNECOLOGY*—Chapter 16 of Maimonides' *Medical Aphorisms* is devoted to obstetrics and gynecology, or, in Maimonides' own term, "women."[1] Menstruation, pregnancy, amenorrhea, dysmenorrhea, anatomical features of the genitalia, and related subjects are discussed. The increased blood volume during pregnancy is recognized: "During pregnancy, the pulse is greater, the beat is stronger and also more rapid. However, other [body] functions remain in their condition." [*See also* ABORTION, BARRENNESS, CESAREAN SECTION, CHILDBIRTH, CONTRACEPTION, LACTATION, MENSTRUATION, PREGNANCY, PROCREATION, PUBERTY, VIRGINITY]

---

1. F. Rosner, *The Medical Aphorisms of Moses Maimonides* (Haifa: Maimonides Research Institute, 1989), pp. 262–270.

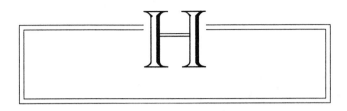

**HABITS**—In his *Mishneh Torah* (*Deot* 4:20), Maimonides codifies a regimen of health to which every person should become accustomed in order to remain healthy. In *Medical Aphorisms*,[1] he quotes Galen, who said that a person who rarely becomes ill should not change a single thing in his customary way of life, since such change of habits may produce illnesses (Chapter 3:73) and retard the period of convalescence and recovery (ibid., 8:23). Habit changes in regard to eating, drinking, and physical exercise may cause illness (ibid., 17:18), although a change in bad habits is sometimes beneficial (ibid., 17:37).

In his *Treatise on Asthma*,[2] Maimonides reiterates the harmful effects of bad habits in aggravating asthma and increasing the number of acute episodes (Chapter 1:1). Good eating habits are described (ibid., 6:1–3), as are those concerning sleep, bathing, massaging, and sexual intercourse (ibid., 10:1ff). In his *Regimen on Health*,[3] Maimonides again asserts that habit and regularity represent a fundamental principle for the maintenance of health and the cure of illnesses (Chapter 4:15). It is not proper for a person to change his healthy habits all at once, neither in eating or drinking, cohabitation, bathing, or exercise. Even if one's habits are unhealthy, one should change them gradually over a long period (ibid.). Similar statements are found in Maimonides' other medical writings. The talmudic sage Samuel also said that a change in one's habits leads to digestive disorders (*Ketubot* 110b).

1. F. Rosner, *Moses Maimonides' Treatise on Asthma* (Haifa: Maimonides Research Institute, 1994).

2. F. Rosner, *Moses Maimonides' Three Treatises on Health* (Haifa: Maimonides Research Institute, 1990).

3. F. Rosner, *The Medical Aphorisms of Moses Maimonides* (Haifa: Maimonides Research Institute, 1989).

**HAIR**—In his *Extracts from Galen*,[1] Maimonides states that alopecia and the falling out of hair are sicknesses that cause something natural to be lost. Nature books explain that hair grows because of a coarse vapory humor; loss or corruption of this humor causes loss of hair. The treatment is to cleanse the body of the bad humor. A variety of remedies for loss of eyelashes are described. In his *Medical Aphorisms,*[2] Maimonides quotes Galen, who said that the plucking of hair with one's hands pulls the humors from the depths of the body and benefits patients with forgetfulness or stupor, or those with joints afflicted by external influences (Chapter 9:35). Maimonides castigates Galen for suggesting that God commanded the hair of the eyebrow not to lengthen and that the hair complied (ibid., 25:61–65). In his *Mishneh Torah,* Maimonides vividly attributes baldness in man to a variety of causes:

> If all the hair of a man's head falls out because of sickness or because of a wound from which hair cannot grow again, or if he has eaten something that makes the hair fall out, or has smeared himself with something that makes the hair fall out—even though it may grow again afterward—since all the hair of his head is lost for the time, such a one is called "scalp bald" or "forehead bald." If his hair has fallen out from the crown downwards, sloping backward to the protruding bone in the neck, he is called "scalp bald"; and if it has fallen out from the crown downwards, sloping forward to the forehead, he is called "forehead bald"

(*Tumat Tzaraat* 5:8). Scalp baldness and forehead baldness attest uncleanness by two tokens—by quick flesh or by a spreading (ibid., 5:9).

Elsewhere in his *Mishneh Torah,* Maimonides speaks of depilatories. Although a Nazirite is forbidden to cut his hair, if he applies a depilatory to his head, causing the hair to fall out, he is not punished with flogging, although he made void a positive scriptural commandment (*Nezirut* 5:12).

Maimonides also rules that if one detaches hair from a human body on the Sabbath, he is liable for the prohibited work of shearing. Therefore, it is also forbidden to wash one's hands on the Sabbath with any substance that is certain to act as a depilatory, such as aloes and the like. It is, however, permissible to rub the hands with powdered frankincense, powdered peppers, powdered jasmine, and the like, and one need not be concerned that the powder might remove hair from the hands, because there is no intention that it should do so. If a sure depilatory is mixed with a nondepilatory, and the former constitutes the bulk of the mixture, it is forbidden to rub one's hand with it; otherwise it is permissible (*Shabbat* 22:13).

---

1. U.S. Barzel, *Maimonides' The Art of Cure. Extracts from Galen* (Haifa: Maimonides Research Institute, 1992), pp. 178–179.

2. F. Rosner, *The Medical Aphorisms of Moses Maimonides* (Haifa: Maimonides Research Institute, 1989).

**HA-MEATI, NATHAN**—Nathan Ha-Meati was a renowned thirteenth-century Italian translator of medical works from Arabic into Hebrew. His name Meati is probably derived from the Hebrew equivalent of cento (hundred), indicating that he was born in Cento in the Ferrara region. His most important Maimonidean translation is that of Maimonides' *Medical Aphorisms* (*Pirkei Moshe*), first published by Jides Rosnanes in Lemberg (Lvov) in 1804. In 1850, S. Zaks published the sections missing from the 1804 Lemberg edition. Ha-Meati's translation of Maimonides' *Medical Aphorisms* was again published in Vilna in 1888. The definitive critical edition is that of Suessman Muntner, published in 1959 by the Mossad Harav Kook in Jerusalem.

**HAND-WASHING**—In his *Mishneh Torah*, Maimonides devotes considerable discussion to Grace after Meals (*Berachot* 2:1ff). The five types of grain—wheat, barley, spelt, oats, and rye—are cited (ibid., 3:1), as are various foods prepared from them and the proper blessings to be recited by one who consumes them (ibid., 3:2ff). Washing one's hands is required before partaking of a meal (ibid., 6:2ff). The manner of hand-washing, the type of water and vessels to be used, and the drying of the hands are also described (ibid.). Various rules of etiquette and common sense at the dining table are also discussed. For example, the senior person washes his hands first (ibid., 7:1). One should avoid talking during the meal, lest one choke on the food (ibid., 7:6). Hand-washing is also required before one recites one's prayers (*Tefillah* 4:1ff).

**HASIDAH, MENACHEM ZEEV**—A scholar and editor of Hebrew manuscripts, M.Z. Hasidah (Botshan) (1888–1965) edited in Hebrew Maimonides' *Commentary on the Aphorisms of Hippocrates*. Hasidah printed this work in his mimeographed periodical *Ha Segulah* over a five-year period between 1934 and 1938.

**HEADACHE**—The most voluminous of Maimonides' medical treatises is the *Medical Aphorisms of Moses*, composed of fifteen hundred aphorisms based mainly on Greek medical writers such as Galen and Hippocrates.[1] Drawing heavily on the works of Galen, Maimonides speaks about the causes of headache as follows:

> Thick viscous humors cause headache. All thick black humors [i.e., black bile] cause headaches if they are retained in the passages of the

cavities of the brain [i.e., cerebral ventricular system]. If this [black humor] prevails and increases in the brain substance itself, black confusion [melancholy or manic depressive psychosis] ensues.

The reader is reminded of the medieval concept of the four body humors: white bile (phlegm), black bile (melancholy), red bile (blood), and yellow bile. Disease was thought to result from a disequilibrium of these humors, with one or more predominating over the others. Thus, an excess of black bile results in melancholy, and an excess of red bile in plethora. With this background, one can readily understand Maimonides' citations from Galen:

> If white, thick, cold phlegm which has not yet putrefied increases in the brain, a headache develops from deep sleep without arousal. . . . Severe headache occurs from heat or cold. On the other hand, headache produced by dryness is mild whereas moisture causes no [head] pain at all. However, if much moisture is present in the head, a heaviness is produced, not [true] pain, unless the illness called vertigo, otherwise known as scotodinia, ensues therefrom. Headache occurs proportional to the degree of obstruction. . . .

Maimonides seems to be describing the patient's inability to excrete "bad" humors or liquids thus resulting in headache. He also describes the location of headaches and discusses migraine headaches at length, includ-

ing a variety of remedies for them. He also recognized, as did the ancient Greek physicians, that headache may occur secondary to alcoholic intoxication.

Maimonides also suggests that people who suffer from headaches should refrain from physical exercise and other activities until the pain begins to diminish. For a mild headache, it is prudent not to take any medication, counsels Maimonides. Nature does well without help; a normal healthy conduct of life is quite sufficient. If one treats a mild headache, one's actions may be in error and aggravate the situation. Alternatively, medication may make nature lazy and become dependent on that medication.

Maimonides also speaks of headache in his legal code, where he rules that a man who has aches in his head is considered legally as in good health in regard to the validity of his buying, selling, and giving of gifts (*Mishneh Torah, Zechiyah Umatanah* 8:1).

Since most of Maimonides' pronouncements about headache in his *Medical Aphorisms* were derived from Greco-Roman medical writers such as Hippocrates and, especially, Galen, in regard to these statements Maimonides was merely a compiler, not an innovator. Some of his concepts about the causes of headaches being related to a disequilibrium of the body humors are clearly medieval in origin. Other statements demonstrate his concern with preventive medicine and the maintenance of a healthy regimen of daily living. Medications to treat illness should be used only if non-medicinal means such as diet and exercise are not effective.

More details about headache in the writings of Maimonides are found in a recent article.[2]

---

1. F. Rosner, *The Medical Aphorisms of Moses Maimonides* (Haifa: Maimonides Research Institute, 1989).

2. F. Rosner, "Headache in the Writings of Moses Maimonides and Other Hebrew Sages," *Headache*, 33 (1993): 315–319.

**HEARING**—In his *Medical Aphorisms*,[1] Maimonides states that the "best" and most beneficial of the senses is sight, followed by hearing (Chapter 6:94). The five senses, including hearing, distinguish humans and other living beings from plants (ibid., 7:73).

In his *Guide for the Perplexed*, Maimonides explains why hearing, sight, and smell are attributed to God, but not taste and touch (Part 1:47), and why the senses "are not always to be trusted" (Part 1:73) (e.g., we cannot hear at a distance). [*See also* EAR, TASTE, and SMELL]

---

1. F. Rosner, *The Medical Aphorisms of Moses Maimonides* (Haifa: Maimonides Research Institute, 1989).

**HEMORRHAGE**—In his *Commentary on the Aphorisms of Hippocrates*,[1] Maimonides asserts that fainting and even death may follow hemorrhage (Section 5:16). Hemorrhage may also interfere with brain function and produce confusion of the mind (ibid., 7:9). Cold water, snow, or ice should be applied near the site of hemorrhage (ibid., 5:23) as a hemostatic to stop the bleeding by causing vasoconstriction of the blood vessels. In his *Medical Aphorisms*,[2] Maimonides quotes Galen, who described hemorrhage that is due to amputation or incision of abscesses or gastrointestinal bleeding (hematemesis and melena) (Chapter 6:81). The treatment for massive epistaxis is elucidated (ibid., 15:46). The sealing-off of an artery to stop hemorrhage is suggested as a lifesaving measure (ibid., 15:46). Massive uterine bleeding is treated by applying suction cups next to the woman's breasts and on her knees and thighs (ibid., 16:11).

---

1. F. Rosner, *Maimonides' Commentary on the Aphorisms of Hippocrates* (Haifa: Maimonides Research Institute, 1987).

2. F. Rosner, *The Medical Aphorisms of Moses Maimonides* (Haifa: Maimonides Research Institute, 1989).

**HEMORRHOIDS**—In addition to his *Treatise on Hemorrhoids*, Maimonides discusses hemorrhoids in several of his other medical works. In *Treatise on the Causes of Symptoms*,[1] he suggests diet and local measures such as sitz baths, oils, and fumigation rather than surgical extirpation. Surgery was strongly advocated by Galen and Hippocrates, both of whom Maimonides quotes extensively. For example, in his *Medical Aphorisms*,[2] Maimonides cites Galen's assertion that black biles cause hemorrhoids (Chapter 2:25) and that they should be surgically excised (ibid., 15:21), although at times medications are preferable for treating hemorrhoids (ibid., 15:22). Eating fresh dates may also produce hemorrhoids (ibid., 20:79). A concoction of dried snakeroot, wheat flour, and sesame oil, kneaded, baked, and pulverized into a spiced honey drink, is said to obliterate hemorrhoids in three days (ibid., 22:62). Anal fistulas can be healed by suppositories made of olive and aloe resins kneaded in pear leaves' juice (ibid., 22:63).

In his *Commentary on the Aphorisms of Hippocrates*,[3] Maimonides states that black bile and, hence, hemorrhoids are more common in older people (Section 3:30). If the hemorrhoids bleed, they are attempting to excrete the black bile (ibid., 4:25). Hemorrhoids and asthma, the subjects of separate treatises by Maimonides, are not mentioned in *Extracts from Galen*.[4]

1. F. Rosner, *Moses Maimonides' Three Treatises on Health* (Haifa: Maimonides Research Institute, 1990).

2. F. Rosner, *The Medical Aphorisms of Moses Maimonides* (Haifa: Maimonides Research Institute, 1989).

3. F. Rosner, *Maimonides' Commentary on the Aphorisms of Hippocrates* (Haifa: Maimonides Research Institute, 1987).

4. U.S. Barzel, *Maimonides' The Art of Cure. Extracts from Galen* (Haifa: Maimonides Research Institute, 1992).

**HEPATITIS**—The clinical signs and symptoms of hepatitis are accurately described in Maimonides' *Medical Aphorisms*[1] as follows:

> The signs of liver inflammation include burning fever, thirst, complete anorexia, red tongue which turns black, biliary vomitus which turns dark green, pain on the right side which stretches up to the clavicle and down to the flanks (Chapter 6:55).

Venesection, or bloodletting, is recommended for the treatment of hepatitis (ibid., 12:22). In his *Commentary on the Aphorisms of Hippocrates*,[2] Maimonides explains in detail Galen's assertion that people with hepatitis have extremely hot skin (Section 4:48). Hiccough induced by hepatitis is a bad sign (ibid., 7:17). [*See also* HICCOUGH]

1. F. Rosner, *The Medical Aphorisms of Moses Maimonides* (Haifa: Maimonides Research Institute, 1989).

2. F. Rosner, *Maimonides' Commentary on the Aphorisms of Hippocrates* (Haifa: Maimonides Research Institute, 1987).

*HERMAPHRODITE*—The status of persons of indeterminate sex (*tumtums*) or with characteristics of both sexes (*androginos*, i.e., hermaphrodite) is discussed by Maimonides for the first time in relation to idolatry (*Mishneh Torah*, 12:4), although these types of persons are mentioned numerous times throughout the *Code*. Such persons are subject to the stringencies of both sexes and are bound to observe all obligations imposed on either sex. Maimonides defines hermaphrodites and individuals with indeterminate sex (*Eeshut* 2:24–25). Legally, the hermaphrodite is in an unfavorable position. He has all the obligations of a man, but not all his rights; he does not receive a portion of inheritance from his father, as do his brothers, nor is he supported from the inheritance, as are his sisters (*Nachalot* 5:1). Like women, he is unable to testify in court. If he is of priestly descent, he cannot partake of priestly gifts and allowances; he is also unfit to serve as a priest. He has all the religious (ceremonial) obligations of a man. He is subject to circumcision on the eighth day of life (*Milah* 1:7).

A person of doubtful sex and a hermaphrodite with flux are subject to both the stringencies affecting a man and the stringencies affecting a woman (*Mishkav Umoshav* 1:7). The law of the firstborn applies only to boys (*Bechorot* 1:1), but not to a hermaphrodite or one of indeterminate sex (ibid., 2:5). The inheritance of a child with indeterminate sex or a hermaphrodite is doubtful (*Nachalot* 5:1). A person of doubtful sex or a hermaphrodite is ineligible to sprinkle the water of purification on the red heifer (*Parah Adumah* 10:6).

If a person of indeterminate sex or a hermaphrodite betroths a woman or is betrothed by a man, the validity of the betrothal is in doubt, and the couple require a bill of divorce on account of this doubt (*Eeshut* 4:11). Congenital eunuchs and hermaphrodites are not subject to levirate marriage, or *chalitzah*, because they are unable to beget children (*Yibum Vechalitzah* 6:2). Other rules and regulations about hermaphrodites and *tumtums* are discussed in Maimonides' *Mishneh Torah*.[1]

-----

1. F. Rosner, *Medicine in the Mishneh Torah of Maimonides* (New York: Ktav, 1984), pp. 153–156.

*HERNIA*—In his *Medical Aphorisms*,[1] Maimonides quotes Galen, who said that a hernia in which the membrane covering the intestine, the stomach, and the momentum is caught is a serious illness, even though its size may not be large. A hernia that encloses water (hydrocele) is a mild illness, even if it becomes large. A hernia in which part of the intestines have descended (inguinal hernia?) also is not serious

(Chapter 9:102). The treatment for a hernia includes the application of plaster and a special diet of nourishing and pureed foods. Some patients also need bowel cleansing at the beginning of the therapy (ibid., 9:124). Later in this work, intestinal hernias, omental hernias, and varicoceles are again described (ibid., 23:57). Testicular hernias filled with water are also mentioned by Maimonides in his *Extracts from Galen.*[2]

---

1. F. Rosner, *The Medical Aphorisms of Moses Maimonides* (Haifa: Maimonides Research Institute, 1989).
2. U.S. Barzel, *Maimonides' The Art of Cure. Extracts from Galen* (Haifa: Maimonides Research Institute, 1992), p. 174.

**HICCOUGH**—In his *Commentary on the Aphorisms of Hippocrates,*[1] Maimonides states that hiccoughs are due to the overfilling of the body with humors and are cured by sneezing, since sneezing causes loss of fluids (Section 6:13). Redness of the eyes develops if hiccoughs do not cease after vomiting (ibid., 7:3). Hiccoughs occurring during intestinal colic (ibid., 7:10), from liver inflammation (ibid., 7:17), or following purgation (ibid., 7:41) are a bad prognostic sign. Hiccoughs may be cured by the drinking of diluted wine (ibid., 7:56). Hiccoughs that are due to liver inflammation or diaphragmatic disease was already recognized by the talmudic sages, who considered it a dangerous sign for which the Sabbath may be desecrated (*Abodah Zarah* 29a).

In his *Medical Aphorisms,*[2] Maimonides quotes Galen, who said that hiccoughs may produce a rapid and weak pulse (Chapter 4:20). Sneezing aborts hiccoughs (ibid., 6:48). Hiccoughs can also occur from coldness of the air (ibid., 9:40), from overeating, or from irritating humors (ibid., 9:52). Often, hiccoughs subside and disappear spontaneously (ibid., 24:19).

---

1. F. Rosner, *Maimonides' Commentary on the Aphorisms of Hippocrates* (Haifa: Maimonides Research Institute, 1987).
2. F. Rosner, *The Medical Aphorisms of Moses Maimonides* (Haifa: Maimonides Research Institute, 1989).

**HOARSENESS**—In his *Medical Aphorisms,*[1] Maimonides quotes Galen, who said that if the voice is weakened by catarrhs that descend from the head, hoarseness is produced (Chapter 3:66). Foreign substances, such as dust and smoke in the respiratory passages, may also cause hoarseness (ibid., 7:67). The remedy to relieve this hoarseness is to eat foods soaked and immersed in fat, soft, or viscous liquids (ibid.). Thus, dietary means, such as food cooked in butter, are prescribed.

1. F. Rosner, *The Medical Aphorisms of Moses Maimonides* (Haifa: Maimonides Research Institute, 1989).

(New York: Sepher Hermon, 1981), pp. 86–94.

*HOMOSEXUALITY*—In his *Mishneh Torah*, Maimonides clearly and emphatically prohibits homosexuality when he states:

> In the case of a man who lies with a man, or causes a man to have connection with him, once sexual contact has been initiated, the rule is as follows: If both are adults, they are punishable by stoning, as it is said, "Thou shalt not lie with a man" (Lev. 18:22), i.e., whether he is the active or the passive participant in the act. If he is a minor, aged nine years and one day, or older, the adult who has connection with him or causes him to have connection with him, is punishable by stoning, while the minor is exempt. It behooves the court, however, to have the adult flogged for disobedience, inasmuch as he has lain with a man, even though with one less than nine years of age (*Issurei Biyah* 1:14).

A similar discussion outlawing homosexuality is found in Maimonides' *Mishnah Commentary* (*Sanhedrin* 7:4). Although Maimonides unambiguously labels the practice of homosexuality as an abomination,[1] Judaism views the homosexual as mentally ill and deserving of medical and psychological assistance.

1. F. Rosner, *Maimonides' Commentary on the Mishnah, Tractate Sanhedrin*

*HONEY*—In his *Treatises on Health*,[1] Maimonides recommends adding honey to milk to make a nutritious beverage. Honey is an ingredient in a myrobalan electuary that improves digestion and strengthens the heart and stomach, as well as other organs. It is also an ingredient in the preparation of troches used to treat bad, hot temperaments. Bees' honey and fine white wine make the beverage known as hydromel. Honey and wine are said to be bad for children but salutary for the elderly, especially in the rainy season. In his *Treatise on Asthma*[2] and several other medical writings, Maimonides offers a honeyed drink (i.e., mead) seasoned with spices as a substitute for wine for Moslems to whom wine is forbidden. This honeyed beverage resembles wine in all its benefits except for the gladdening of the soul. Adding honey or cane sugar to fattening pastries is detrimental to the liver. Honey can also be used to prepare enema solutions for elderly people with constipation. Many other potions and concoctions containing honey for a variety of ailments are cited by Maimonides in this book, as well as in his *Extracts from Galen*[3] and *Medical Aphorisms*.[4] Quoting Galen, he asserts that honey-water is the best remedy for expectorating the thick humors of the body (*Aphorisms* 21:15). Milk mixed with honey is valuable for relieving pains in the chest and lung, but is harmful for the spleen and liver (ibid., 21:17). A mixture of butter and honey is exceptional in aiding expectoration from the lung in patients with pneumonia (ibid., 21:18).

In his *Mishneh Torah* (*Tumat Ochlin* 1:2), he rules that honey is one of the seven liquids that render foodstuffs such as bread, meat, grapes, olives, and the like susceptible to ritual uncleanness.

---

1. F. Rosner, *Moses Maimonides' Three Treatises on Health* (Haifa: Maimonides Research Institute, 1990).

2. F. Rosner, *Moses Maimonides' Treatise on Asthma* (Haifa: Maimonides Research Institute, 1994).

3. U.S. Barzel, *Maimonides' The Art of Cure. Extracts from Galen* (Haifa: Maimonides Research Institute, 1992).

4. F. Rosner, *The Medical Aphorisms of Moses Maimonides* (Haifa: Maimonides Research Institute, 1989).

## HUMAN EXPERIMENTATION

—Ten basic principles relate to the issue of human experimentation.[1] Human life is sacrosanct and of supreme and infinite worth (see Maimonides' *Mishneh Torah*, *Rotzeach* 2:6); any chance to save life must be pursued (*see* DANGER TO LIFE); the obligation to save a life devolves on anyone able to do so; every life is equally valuable, including that of a criminal and the handicapped; one must not sacrifice one life to save another; no one has the right to volunteer his life (see *Yesodei Ha Torah* 5:4); no one has the right to injure his own or anyone else's body, except for therapeutic purposes (see *Rotzeach* 1:4 and *Mamrim* 2:4); no one has the right to refuse necessary medical treatment; experimental treatment is permitted if standard therapy is not known or available; animal experiments are permissible for medical purposes (*see* ANIMAL EXPERIMENTATION). Other writings on human experimentation are available.[2,3] Based on classic Jewish sources, including Maimonides' legal code, the *Mishneh Torah*, human experimentation is permissible but not mandatory, and may be undertaken only if no standard treatments exist or are available.

---

1. I. Jakobovits, "Medical Experiments on Humans in Jewish Law," in *Jewish Bioethics* (F. Rosner and J.D. Bleich, eds.), (New York: Hebrew Publishing Co., 1979), pp. 377–386.

2. J.D. Bleich, "Experimentation on Human Subjects," ibid., pp. 384–386.

3. F. Rosner, "Modern Medicine, Religion and Law," *Human Experimentation: New York State Journal of Medicine*, 75 (1975):758–764.

## HUMORS

—Maimonides subscribed to the medieval concept of disease being caused by a disequilibrium in the quantity, quality, or mixture of the four body humors: white bile (phlegm), red bile (blood), black bile (melancholy), and yellow bile. An entire chapter in his *Medical Aphorisms* is devoted to body humors.[1] He quotes Galen, who said that all humors contain watery fluids that determine the thickness of the humors. Humors are also characterized as cold or warm and moist or dry. When food is digested in the liver, natural yellow bile is produced that is warm and dry. Black bile is cold and dry, and is considered the underlying cause of hemorrhoids in most instances.[2] Other illnesses that develop from black bile include cancer, lameness, psoriasis, quartan fever, confusion, and thickness of the spleen.

Humors are also discussed in detail in Maimonides' other medical writings. For example, in his *Treatise on Asthma*,[3] he again quotes Galen, who said that if bad humors are plentiful, many diseases result, some which can be prevented by regular exercise, proper diet, rest, attention to bowel function, and good moral virtues. Maimonides asserts that humors that move into abdominal locations produce pain in those organs. Elderly people are afflicted with illnesses because of cold humors.[4] His *Treatises on Health* are replete with references to the body humors, their abnormalities, and the illnesses they may cause.[5]

---

1. F. Rosner, *The Medical Aphorisms of Moses Maimonides* (Haifa: Maimonides Research Institute, 1989), pp. 26–34.

2. F. Rosner, *Maimonides' Treatises on Poisons, Hemorrhoids and Cohabitation* (Haifa: Maimonides Research Institute, 1984).

3. F. Rosner, *Moses Maimonides' Treatise on Asthma* (Haifa: Maimonides Research Institute, 1994).

4. F. Rosner, *Maimonides' Commentary on the Aphorisms of Hippocrates* (Haifa: Maimonides Research Institute, 1987).

5. F. Rosner, *Moses Maimonides' Three Treatises on Health* (Haifa: Maimonides Research Institute, 1990).

**HYGIENE**—In Maimonides' *Mishneh Torah*, the section titled *Deot* deals with human traits or temperaments and ethical tendencies. Particularly interesting is Chapter 4, which deals with a variety of hygienic and medical prescriptions for healthy living and for the prevention of illness. Among the many subjects discussed are normal bodily excretory functions; recommended times for eating; amounts and types of food to be consumed; beverage consumption; exercise; sleep habits; cathartics; climatic and weather effects on eating habits; detrimental and beneficial foods; fruits, meats, and vegetables; bathing; bloodletting; sexual intercourse; and domicile. The other chapters of this section are just as interesting, and deal with recommended moral traits and ethical standards of practice for which a person should strive.[1]

Elsewhere in his *Mishneh Torah*, Maimonides also discusses ethical conduct, personal hygiene and sanitation, and environmental health hazards. Good character and ethical conduct are essential features in a human being in his fulfillment of the divine precepts. Thus, a person should be scrupulous in his conduct, gentle in his conversation, and pleasant toward his fellow human beings; he should receive people in an affable and courteous manner, conduct his commercial affairs with integrity and honesty, and devote himself to the study of Torah (*Yesodei Hatorah* 5:11).

Eating should not be a purely biological function, as it is in animals. Rather, a person should eat in order to be able to study Torah and serve the Lord (*Talmud Torah* 3:6).

The treatise on "Forbidden Foods" in "The Book of Holiness" of Maimonides' *Mishneh Torah* concludes with a number of rules relating to personal hygiene and sanitation, as follows:

The sages have forbidden the consumption of food and drink of the kind that is revolting to most people, like food and drink contaminated with vomit, excrement, or putrid secretion, and their like. They have also forbidden eating and drinking out of filthy utensils that offend against one's natural fastidiousness, such as utensils used in the privy, the glass vessels used by barber–surgeons for bloodletting, and their like (*Maachalot Assurot* 17:29). Similarly, the sages forbade eating with grimy and dirty hands, or upon a soiled tablecloth, since all these things are included in the verse "You shall not make yourselves abominable" (Lev. 11:43). He who eats such revolting foods is liable to the flogging prescribed for disobedience (ibid., 17:30).

It is likewise forbidden to delay the normal evacuation of one's large or small orifices, and he who does so is counted among those who make themselves abominable, not to speak of the grave illnesses he may thereby bring upon himself, thus endangering his life. Man should, on the contrary, accustom himself to bowel movements at regular times, so that he would not make himself offensive in the presence of people nor render himself abominable (ibid., 17:31).

Indeed, he who is painstaking in these things gains exceeding sanctity and purity for his person, and purges his soul for the sake of the Holy One, blessed be He, as it is said, "You shall therefore sanctify yourselves and be holy, for I am holy" (Lev. 11:44) (ibid., 17:32).

Maimonides appears to be describing environmental hazards when he asserts that carcasses, graves, and tanneries must be kept fifty cubits from a town (*Shechenim* 10:3). A tannery may be set up only on the east side of the town, because the east wind is mild and reduces the unpleasantness of the odors produced by the tanning of the hides (ibid., 10:4). It is unclear whether the odor is harmful to health or simply a nuisance. Discomfort from smoke, the smell of a privy, dust, and the like, and shaking of the ground are grounds for the aggrieved party to sue his neighbor to compel him to move the damage-causing item to a proper distance (ibid., 11:4).

Maimonides also wrote two medical treatises on personal hygiene and health at the behest of the Egyptian Sultan al-Malik al-Afdal, eldest son of Saladin the Great.[2] These treatises are briefly described elsewhere in this encyclopedia. [*See also* TREATISES ON HEALTH and PREVENTIVE MEDICINE]

1. F. Rosner, *Medicine in the Mishneh Torah of Maimonides* (New York: Ktav, 1984), pp. 69–107.

2. F. Rosner, *Moses Maimonides' Three Treatises on Health* (Haifa: Maimonides Research Institute, 1990).

# I

IBN TIBBON, MOSES BEN
SAMUEL—A thirteenth-century
French rabbi, physician, astronomer,
mathematician, and translator from
Arabic into Hebrew, Ibn Tibbon was
a prolific author, but only his transla-
tions of Maimonides' medical works
are discussed here.[1] Ibn Tibbon's
Hebrew translation of Maimonides'
*Regimen of Health* was first published
by Bloch in *Kerem Chemed*, 3
(1838):31–39. It was then published
in 1883 by Pinchas Bleier, in 1885 by
Jacob Saphir, in 1886 by Jacob
Maharshak, and in 1957 by Suessman
Muntner (Jerusalem: Mossad Harav
Kook). Ibn Tibbon's Hebrew translation of Maimonides' *Treatise on
Poisons* was published by Suessman
Muntner in 1942 (Jerusalem: Reuben
Mass). Ibn Tibbon's Hebrew translation of Maimonides' *Commentary on
the Aphorisms of Hippocrates* was first
printed by Hasidah in mimeographed
form in the periodical *Ha Segullah*
(Jerusalem) over a five-year period
between 1934 and 1938. It was edited
and published by Suessman Muntner

twice, in 1943 (Jerusalem: Geniza)
and in 1961 (Jerusalem: Mossad
Harav Kook). Ibn Tibbon's father
Samuel translated Maimonides'
*Guide for the Perplexed* from Arabic
into Hebrew.

---

1. J.I. Dienstag, "Translators and
editors of Maimonides' Medical Works:
A Bio-bibliographical Survey," in *Memorial Volume in Honor of Prof. S. Muntner*,
J.O. Leibowitz, ed. (Jerusalem: Israel
Institute of the History of Medicine),
1983, pp. 95–135.

ILLNESS—In his *Mishneh Torah*,
Maimonides recommends the avoidance of illness by people's following
a healthy regimen of life, including exercise, diet, sleep, and moderate sex
(*Deot* 4:1ff) and conducting themselves according to ethical and moral
principles (*Deot* 1:1ff). In his *Treatise
on Asthma*,[1] he states that illnesses
which have exacerbations and remis-
sions such as gout, arthritis, kidney or
bladder stones, asthma, and migraine
cannot be cured but can be treated

(Chapter 1:1). If patients follow healthy regimens of life, the interval between attacks is prolonged and their severity is reduced; but if patients indiscriminately indulge their lusts, the attacks become more frequent and severe. Neurological diseases such as hemiplegia, facial paralysis, spasms, and tremors of the limbs are described in his *Regimen of Health*[2] (Chapter 4:16). The consumption of turtledoves heals illnesses of the nerves (ibid.).

In his *Medical Aphorisms*,[3] Maimonides quotes Galen, who said that the most important consideration in the causation of disease is the body constitution that becomes afflicted (Chapter 3:68). A change in the weather, overeating, excessive physical exercise, excessive bathing, and excessive sleep all can lead to illness in people with weak constitutions (ibid., 3:69). People with strong bodies remain healthy and free of disease for prolonged periods (ibid., 3:70). Bad humors may also cause illness (ibid., 3:74). Illnesses in children are more easily cured than those in adults (ibid., 3:76). An entire chapter in this book is devoted to aphorisms pertaining to the stages of illnesses and their crises. The four disease stages are onset, crescendo, acme, and decline (ibid., 11:1). The stages of various illnesses are then described, as are the signs to recognize the transition from one stage to another. Acute illnesses are said to run a rapid course and may

be life-threatening (ibid., 11:24). The duration of the stages of different illnesses depends on the nature of the illness, the patient's constitution, the season of the year, and the excrements from the body such as urine, stool, sweat, and sputum (ibid., 11:25). For example, white-bile-induced arthritis has a long onset, and much time elapses until the acme of the disease is reached (ibid.). Another long chapter in Maimonides' *Medical Aphorisms* is devoted to specific disease entities such as epilepsy (ibid., 9:1); epistaxis (ibid., 9:2); migraine (ibid., 9:4); upper respiratory infections (ibid., 9:7); headaches (ibid., 9:9); insomnia (ibid., 9:10); melancholy (ibid., 9:16), brain abscess (ibid., 9:17); laryngitis (ibid., 9:33); hemoptysis (ibid., 9:42); bulimia (ibid., 9:53); jaundice (ibid., 9:60); liver abscess (ibid., 9:62); cirrhosis (ibid., 9:72); pneumonia (ibid., 9:83); intestinal parasites (ibid., 9:93); kidney abscess (ibid., 9:95); emaciation and wasting (ibid., 9:100); obesity (ibid., 9:101); gout (ibid., 9:103); leprosy (ibid., 9:107); and many more. Remedies for many of these illnesses are also discussed. In the last chapter, Maimonides describes diseases of the mind or soul and the interrelationship between physical illness and mental illness (ibid., 25:59). This early description of psychosomatic medicine is also found in the third chapter of his *Regimen of Health.*

In his *Commentary on the Aphorisms of Hippocrates*,[4] Maimonides points out that, for chronic illnesses, an adequate and appropriate diet is essential (Section 1:4). However, for patients with extremely acute illnesses, the diet should be restricted, depending on the severity of illness, so as not to burden nature with food digestion at a time when it is attempting to rid the body of the humors that produced the illness (ibid., 1:8). Pneumonia and head abscess (brain abscess or meningitis?) are characterized as extremely acute illnesses, whereas hydrops and phthisis (tuberculosis?) are said to be chronic illnesses (ibid., 1:12).

Legal aspects of illness and the waiving of biblical and rabbinic laws to treat life-threatening illnesses are discussed by Maimonides in his *Mishneh Torah* (*Shabbat* 2:1ff and 21:14ff). A discussion of illnesses in animals in Maimonides' writings is found in the section VETERINARY MEDICINE. Human illnesses described by Maimonides in *Mishneh Torah* are summarized elsewhere.[5]

---

1. F. Rosner, *Moses Maimonides' Treatise on Asthma* (Haifa: Maimonides Research Institute, 1994).

2. F. Rosner, *Moses Maimonides' Three Treatises on Health* (Haifa: Maimonides Research Institute, 1990).

3. F. Rosner, *The Medical Aphorisms of Moses Maimonides* (Haifa: Maimonides Research Institute, 1989).

4. F. Rosner, *Maimonides' Commentary on the Aphorisms of Hippocrates* (Haifa: Maimonides Research Institute, 1987).

5. F. Rosner, *Medicine in the Mishneh Torah of Maimonides* (New York: Ktav, 1984), pp. 156–159.

*IMMUNIZATION*—Immunization against disease is strongly suggested by the following citation from Galen in Maimonides' *Medical Aphorisms*: "Someone who is about to undertake a long journey should drink an amount of theriac [almost pulverized in diluted wine] equal to a large bean in six ounces of warm water prior to eating, in order to immunize against [literally, repulse or expel] the damage of [toxic] waters [that he might drink on the road]." Furthermore: "A knowledgeable physician once related to me that once a devastating pestilence occurred . . . and he recommended to people to take this theriac because no medicine was effective against the aforementioned illness. . . . He who drank it [prophylactically] prior to the onset of the illness was saved from developing it. This is not surprising because this medication is an antidote against all [types of] poison."[1] Theriacs were antidotes to poisons in ancient and medieval times as described by Maimonides in his *Treatise on Poisons*.[2] In the belief that repetitious consumption of small doses of a specific theriac conferred immunity against a specific poison, various complex theriacs were developed in the hope of their providing lasting immunity against human or animal poisoning. The most famous of these were the Theriac of Mithridates (King of Pontus from 120 to 63 B.C.E.) and the Electuary of Theodoretus (c. 110 C.E.), both containing numerous ingredients. They are cited frequently by Maimonides.[3]

1. F. Rosner, *The Medical Aphorisms of Moses Maimonides* (Haifa: Maimonides Research Institute, 1989), pp. 321–322.

2. F. Rosner, *Maimonides' Treatises on Poisons, Hemorrhoids and Cohabitation* (Haifa: Maimonides Research Institute, 1984), pp. 1–115.

3. F. Rosner, *Moses Maimonides' Three Treatises on Health* (Haifa: Maimonides Research Institute, 1990), p. 45.

INFLAMMATION—In his *Medical Aphorisms*,[1] Maimonides quotes Galen, who said that bladder inflammations make the pulse hard (Chapter 1:65). Skin inflammation that expands to become an abscess may exude pus (ibid., 3:48). The inflammation called *chumra* probably refers to erysipelas (ibid., 3:110). An inflammation below the diaphragm may represent a subphrenic abscess (ibid., 6:53). Inflammation and abscess formation owing to a carbuncle that arises at a site that appears as though branded with fire may lead to fever and great danger (ibid., 15:2).

In his *Commentary on the Aphorisms of Hippocrates*,[2] Maimonides discusses inflammation in the rectum or uterus, which may produce urinary

symptoms such as strangury (Section 5:58). If inflammation ascends to the brain, madness ensues (ibid., 5:65). The inflammation called *chumra* (erysipelas?) is again mentioned (ibid., 6:25 and 7:20). Inflammation of nerves may cause hiccoughs (ibid., 7:3). Chronic abdominal pain may be due to stomach inflammation (gastritis or peptic ulcer?) (ibid., 7:22). Inflammations of organs and nerves secondary to trauma and the remedies for them are discussed by Maimonides in *Extracts from Galen*[3] (Chapter 6). Broken bones should be doubly bandaged to try to prevent inflammation at the site (ibid.). Warm compresses are helpful at sites of inflammation and abscess formation (ibid.).

1. F. Rosner, *The Medical Aphorisms of Moses Maimonides* (Haifa: Maimonides Research Institute, 1989).

2. F. Rosner, *Maimonides' Commentary on the Aphorisms of Hippocrates* (Haifa: Maimonides Research Institute, 1987).

3. U.S. Barzel, *Maimonides' The Art of Cure. Extracts from Galen* (Haifa: Maimonides Research Institute, 1992).

INSOMNIA—In his *Medical Aphorisms*,[1] Maimonides quotes Galen, who said that insomnia, or lack of sleep, is of two types. One is that which follows any occurrence that disturbs sleep and leaves no permanent difficulty. The other type occurs without any external cause and is due to waning of strength, loss of appetite, and weakness of digestion and other natural functions. One of the symptoms of phrenesia is insomnia. Insomnia weakens body strength. Maimonides says that pain and insomnia may lead to dissolution of life spirits. This theme is repeated several times in his *Medical Aphorisms.* Insomnia may also occur because of cold or hot brain abscesses. Insomnia also develops if red bile prevails in the head. Severe insomnia is a contraindication to bloodletting.

In his *Treatise on Asthma,*[2] Maimonides asserts that insomnia is one of a multitude of symptoms that may develop as a result of bad digestion. Elsewhere,[3] he says that insomnia and other symptoms of illness are usually milder at the beginning of the illness and then become more severe until the climax of the illness, when all symptoms begin to abate. Additional references to sleeplessness are found in his *Extracts from Galen.*[4]

1. F. Rosner, *The Medical Aphorisms of Moses Maimonides* (Haifa: Maimonides Research Institute, 1989).

2. F. Rosner, *Moses Maimonides' Treatise on Asthma* (Haifa: Maimonides Research Institute, 1994), p. 65.

3. F. Rosner, *Maimonides' Commentary on the Aphorisms of Hippocrates* (Haifa: Maimonides Research Institute, 1987).

4. U.S. Barzel, *Maimonides' The Art of Cure. Extracts from Galen* (Haifa: Maimonides Research Institute, 1992).

**INTESTINES**—In his *Medical Aphorisms,*[1] Maimonides quotes Galen, who describes the various phases of digestion and food assimilation in the stomach and intestines (Chapter 1:58). He also depicts the muscles (ibid., 1:74 and 7:65) and the blood vessels (ibid., 3:36) of the intestines. Diseases of the intestines are usually not life-threatening (ibid., 3:89). Colitis and duodenal ulcer are described (ibid., 3:93 and 7:53). Suction cups are recommended to draw out pus from intestinal abscesses (ibid., 3:105–106). If the intestines become afflicted with black bile (cancer?), there is no cure (ibid., 6:72). Laxatives should not be given to patients with intestinal ulcerations (ibid., 8:50). Colitis can be treated with therapeutic enemas (ibid., 13:34 and 36). The symptoms of colitis include tenesmus, increased peristalsis, and slimy stools (ibid., 23:91).

In his *Treatise on Asthma,*[2] Maimonides lists the symptoms resulting from bad digestion. They include epigastric and intestinal pain, anorexia, and stool abnormalities (Chapter 5:6). He recommends periodic emptying of the intestines by enemas for the preservation of health (ibid., 9:6). He states that Divine Providence provided yellow bile to cleanse the intestines (ibid., 9:10), a rare reference to God by Maimonides in his medical writings.

In his *Regimen on Health,*[3] Maimonides suggests that various remedies, including barberry seeds, strengthen the intestines (Chapter 3:4 and 3:8). Catarrhs that descend into the intestines may produce irritation (enterocolitis?), which is difficult to cure (ibid., 4:12). In his *Mishneh Torah*, Maimonides rules that one should not drink much water during meals, but should wait until the food begins to be digested in the intestines (*Deot* 4:2). He then describes a variety of fruits that purge the intestines and others that bind the intestines (*Deot* 4:6). Numerous additional references to the treatment of intestinal disorders are found in his *Extracts from Galen*,[4]

and his *Commentary on the Aphorisms of Hippocrates.*[5]

1. F. Rosner, *The Medical Aphorisms of Moses Maimonides* (Haifa: Maimonides Research Institute, 1989).

2. F. Rosner, *Moses Maimonides' Treatise on Asthma* (Haifa: Maimonides Research Institute, 1992).

3. F. Rosner, *Moses Maimonides' Three Treatises on Health* (Haifa: Maimonides Research Institute, 1990).

4. U.S. Barzel, *Maimonides' The Art of Cure. Extracts from Galen* (Haifa: Maimonides Research Institute, 1992).

5. F. Rosner, *Maimonides' Commentary on the Aphorisms of Hippocrates* (Haifa: Maimonides Research Institute, 1987).

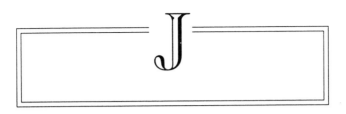

**JOHN OF CAPUA**—A thirteenth-century Italian translator from Hebrew into Latin, John of Capua (1262–1278) was an apostate from Judaism whose original name is unknown. A Latin translation of Maimonides' *Regimen of Health* made at the request of the papal physician, William Corvi, is attributed to John of Capua. Of interest is his apologetic introduction freely translated by Bar Sela et al.[1] It is not clear whether this translation is identical to the seven Latin editions of this work printed between 1477 and 1535. According to Bar Sela et al., Maimonides' *Treatise on Poisons* was also translated by John of Capua, not by Armengaud Blasius, as was claimed by Muntner. It was never printed, but is extant in several manuscripts. Bar Sela et al. also claim, without citing proof, that the Latin translation of Maimonides' *Medical Aphorisms* titled *Aphorismi Secundum Doctrinam Galeni* is also by John of Capua.

---

1. A. Bar Sela, H.E. Hoff, and E. Faris, "Introduction to *Maimonides' Two Treatises on the Regimen of Health*," *Transactions of the American Philosophical Society*, new series, 54:4 (July 1964), pp. 7–12.

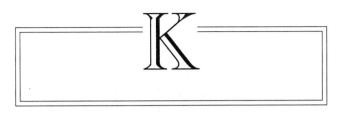

**KAHLE, PAUL ERNST**—An Orientalist, Masoretic scholar, and German minister, Paul E. Kahle (1875–1964) translated into German Maimonides' introduction to his *Medical Aphorisms*. It was published in Kahle's *Opera Minora* (Leiden: E.J. Brill, 1956), pp. 157–166.

**KLEIN-FRANKE, FELIX**—A Latinist and Arabic scholar, Felix Klein-Franke has been Professor at the Hebrew University in Jerusalem since 1976. He prepared a critical edition of the Latin manuscripts of Maimonides' *Causes of Symptoms*, which are lacking in the incunable and sixteenth-century printed Latin versions.[1] He thus edited the heretofore unpublished part of the Latin text of this work. He also pointed out that in recommending wine to the Sultan, Maimonides was safeguarding the free choice of the patient and respecting his conscience.[2]

---

1. F. Klein-Franke, in *Moses Maimonides on the Causes of Symptoms*, J.O.

Leibowitz and S. Marcus, eds. (Berkeley: University of California Press, 1974), pp. 198–212.

2. F. Klein-Franke, "Der hippokratische und der maimonidische Arzt," *Freiburger Zeitschrift für Philosophie und Theologie*, 17 (1970):442–449.

**KORDIAKOS**—The term *kordiakos* appears several times in the Talmud, and its meaning is the subject of considerable controversy.[1] The Talmud states that *kordiakos* means being overcome by new wine from the vat and that the demon that causes the dizziness is called *kordiakos* (*Gittin* 67b). Most of the Commentaries on the Talmud state that *kordiakos* is an alcohol-induced confusion of the mind. In his *Mishnah Commentary* (*Gittin* 7:1), Maimonides interprets the term *kordiakos* to refer to "an illness that occurs as a result of filling of the chambers of the brain, and the mind become confused therefrom; it is one of the varieties of falling sickness [i.e., epilepsy]." Elsewhere in the Talmud (*Gittin* 70b), a man with *kordiakos* is compared to one who is asleep or to a madman.

In two separate discussions ( *Gittin* 7:1; *Terumot* 1:1 ), the Jerusalem Talmud clearly distinguishes an idiot or fool from someone afflicted with *kordiakos.* An idiot or fool is a person suffering from temporary and reversible insanity or madness caused by imbibing fresh wine from a vat (i.e., undiluted). The syndrome is characterized by confusion, dizziness, and mental incompetence, and is treated with red meat and dilute wine. Whether one identifies *kordiakos* as chronic alcoholism, delirium tremens, or a form of epilepsy—as does Maimonides—is not of great consequence, since all three can be reconciled as a single entity. That is, following indulgence in alcoholic beverages, a chronic alcoholic may develop epileptic seizures in the course of delirium tremens. Convulsions from alcoholic excess (i.e., withdrawal seizures) are also described by Maimonides in his *Commentary on the Aphorisms of Hippocrates,*[2] where he explains them as follows: Convulsions when a drunken person suddenly loses his speech is because of the overfilling of the nerves from the wine or alcohol (Section 5:5).

---

1. F. Rosner, *Medicine in the Bible and the Talmud,* 2nd ed. (Hoboken, NJ: Ktav and Yeshiva University Press, 1995), pp. 60–64.

2. F. Rosner, *Maimonides' Commentary on the Aphorisms of Hippocrates*

(Haifa: Maimonides Research Institute, 1987).

**KRONER, HERMANN**—Hermann Kroner (1870–1930) was Rabbi in Oberdorf-Bopfingen, a small town in South Germany, from 1900 until his death. He devoted much of his life to collecting Arabic and Hebrew manuscripts of Maimonides' medical works. He edited, translated, and wrote commentaries on Maimonides' treatises on sexual intercourse and hemorrhoids, *Regimen of Health,* and *Causes of Symptoms.* He is considered one of the great Maimonidean scholars of the twentieth century, laying the foundation for the important subsequent contributions to Maimonidean scholarship of Leibowitz, Muntner, and Rosner.

Kroner's critical edition of both authentic and spurious versions of Maimonides' *Treatise on Sexual Intercourse* was first published in 1906 in Hebrew and German.[1] Ten years later, he published the true short version from the original Arabic manuscript in Granada.[2] In 1911, Kroner published a critical edition of Maimonides' *Treatise on Hemorrhoids* in Arabic, Hebrew, and German.[3] Between 1923 and 1925, his critical edition of Maimonides' *Regimen of Health* in Arabic text with Hebrew and German translations appeared in a Dutch medical journal.[4] In 1914, Kroner had already published the all-important third chapter of Maimonides' *Regimen of Health*, which dealt with psychosomatic medicine, under the title "Hygiene of the Soul."[5] In 1928, he published Arabic, Hebrew, and German versions of Maimonides' *Causes of Symptoms*. Kroner titled it "Maimonides' Swan Song,"[6] as it was thought to be the last of his medical works, having been written in the year 1200, four years before his death.

---

1. H. Kroner, *Ein Betrag zur Geschichte der medizin des XII Jahrhunderts an der Hand Zweier Medizinischer Abhandlungen des Maimonides auf Grund von 6 unedierten Handschriften* (Oberdorf-Bopfingen: Itzowski, 1906), 116 pp. (Ger.), 28 pp. (Heb.).

2. H. Kroner, "Eine Medizinische Maimonides Handschrift aus Granada. Ein Beitrag zur Stilistik des Maimonides und Charakteristik der Hebraischen Ueberzetzungsliteratur," *Janus* 21 (1916):203–247.

3. H. Kroner, "Die Haemorrhoiden in der Medizin des XII und XIII Jahrhunderts," *Janus* 16 (1911):441–456 and 644–718.

4. H. Kroner, "*Fi tadbir as sihhat.* Gesundheitsanleitung des Maimonides fur den Sultan al-Malik al-Afdhal," *Janus* 27 (1923):101–116, 286–330; 28 (1924): 61–74, 143–152, 199–217, 408–419, 455–472; 29 (1925):235–238.

5. H. Kroner, *Die Seelenhygiene des Maimonides. Auszug aus dem 3. Kapital des diatetischen Sendschreibens des Maimonides an den Sultan al Malik Alafdahl (ca. 1198)* (Frankfurt A.M.: J. Kauffmann, 1914), 18 pp. (Ger.), 8 pp. (Heb. and Arab.).

6. H. Kroner, "Der Medizinische Schwanengesang des Maimonides," *Janus* 32 (1928):12–116.

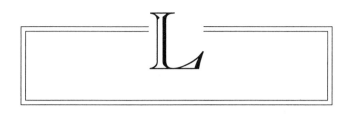

**LACTATION**—In his *Mishneh Torah*, Maimonides states that the usual lactation period is twenty-four months.[1] A wife who is nursing her child should work less than usual and consume more than usual of foods and beverages that are beneficial for lactation. If she gives birth to twins, she may not be compelled to nurse both of them; rather, she should nurse one of them, and the husband should hire a wet-nurse for the other. The nursing of a child by a divorcee is also discussed.

In his *Medical Aphorisms*, Maimonides asserts: "Milk of the mother is the proper nutrition for the newborn infant, because its composition is the same as the blood from which he was created. If the milk ceases, then one should choose [another] suitable milk for him."[2]

The Talmud (*Shabbat* 53b) also discusses lactation in a man (galactorrhea), which is a rare medical disorder. The case concerned a man whose wife died and left a child to be suckled. He could not afford to pay a wet nurse, whereupon a miracle occurred: His breasts opened like the two breasts of a woman, and he suckled his infant himself. This man certainly had galactorrhea, albeit by divine intervention.

---

1. F. Rosner, *Medicine in the Mishneh Torah of Maimonides* (New York: Ktav, 1984), pp. 279–280.
2. F. Rosner, *The Medical Aphorisms of Moses Maimonides* (Haifa: Maimonides Research Institute, 1989), p. 268.

**LAXATIVES**—An entire chapter in Maimonides' *Medical Aphorisms* is devoted to "emptying the body by means of laxative medications and enemas."[1] Galen is quoted as saying that all laxative medications are harmful to the stomach, and that aromatic drugs to neutralize this effect without altering the laxative action should be added. Maimonides says that various kinds of spurge and scammony plants purge as soon as they are absorbed, whereas laxative resins such as opop-

*133*

anax, galbanum, and wild sagapenum purge only after a long time period. He also recommends chicken soup after the laxative action has been successful to rinse any residual laxative medication out of the stomach prior to the person's ingestion of food. He criticizes Galen and Hippocrates for advising the regular use of barley gruel and barley soup immediately after purgation because they produce nausea. He therefore suggests warm julep or warm water in which roots or seeds of marshmallow plants were boiled together with fresh fennel wine, anise, cinnamon, or the like to combine viscosity with fluidity, nutritiousness, and a pleasant taste.

Many more aphorisms dealing with purgation by means of cathartics, emetics, or enemas are cited by Maimonides from Greek (Galen) and Persian or Arabic (Ibn Zuhr, Abu Merwan, Al Tamimi) writers. For example, purgation should be used only for patients who need emptying urgently. Thick humors should first be diluted and dissolved, and then expelled. Various laxative medications and concoctions and their indications and contraindications are described. High fever is a contraindication to the use of cathartic drugs. In that case, emptying by bloodletting is preferred. Icterus, psoriasis, chronic pain, and other ailments can be successfully treated with purgation. Colitis is best treated with clysters or salt-water enemas containing astringent medica-

tions. For weak patients, suppositories or troches are preferable. Milk clysters are used to treat women with boils or sores on their wombs. Maimonides even describes antidotes for overzealous purgation with toxic medications such as colocynth meat, or turpethum.

Purgation with laxatives or enemas is also discussed in several other medical works of Maimonides.[2,3,4]

---

1. F. Rosner, *The Medical Aphorisms of Moses Maimonides* (Haifa: Maimonides Research Institute, 1989), pp. 226–239.
2. F. Rosner, *Moses Maimonides' Treatise on Asthma* (Haifa: Maimonides Research Institute, 1994).
3. U.S. Barzel, *Maimonides' The Art of Cure. Extracts from Galen* (Haifa: Maimonides Research Institute, 1992).
4. F. Rosner, *Moses Maimonides' Three Treatises on Health* (Haifa: Maimonides Research Institute, 1990).

---

*LEIBOWITZ, JOSHUA O.*—A native of Vilna, Poland, and educated in Germany (M.D., University of Heidelberg), Joshua Leibowitz (1895–1993) was Professor of the History of Medicine at Hebrew University in Jerusalem from 1959 till his death, and also visiting medical historian and lecturer at Yale and Johns Hopkins medical schools in the United States and the Wellcome Institute in England. His classic book is *The History of Coronary Heart Disease* (London: Wellcome Institute, 1970).

Leibowitz also contributed various studies and reviews on Maimonides and Maimonidean scholarship, including a new Hebrew translation of the Physician's Prayer attributed to Maimonides, which Leibowitz proves was actually written by Marcus Herz in 1783.[1] Together with Shlomo Marcus, Leibowitz published a critical edition of Maimonides' *Causes of Symptoms* in which the text is presented in four languages (Arabic, Hebrew, Latin, and English) and is accompanied by a running commentary, explanatory essays, and a comprehensive catalogue of drugs.[2] He also wrote articles about Maimonides' medical writings,[3,4] discussed the Latin translations of Maimonides' *Aphorisms*,[5] and commented on Maimonides' responsum on longevity.[6]

---

1. J.O. Leibowitz, "Hateffillah Hameyucheset Le Rambam," *Dapim Refuim*, 13 (1954):77–81.

2. J.O. Leibowitz and S. Marcus, *Moses Maimonides on the Causes of Symptoms* (Berkeley: University of California Press, 1974).

3. J.O. Leibowitz, "Rabbenu Moshe ben Maimon: Chiburov Birefuah," *Encyclopedia Ha Ivrit*, vol. 24, 1972 (5732): 563–564.

4. J.O. Leibowitz, "Maimonides in the History of Medicine," *Ariel*, 41 (1976):37–52.

5. J.O. Leibowitz, "The Latin Translations of Maimonides' Aphorisms," *Koroth*, 6 (1973):273–281 (Heb.) and XCIII–XCIX (Eng.).

6. J.O. Leibowitz, "A Responsum of Maimonides Concerning the Termi-

nation of Life," *Koroth* 1969; 5:I–VI. [*See also Kiryat Sefer* 29 (1953): 67–68].

**LEPROSY**—The Hebrew biblical term *tzaraat* probably is not limited to true leprosy, but is a collective or generic name, embracing many different skin diseases including leprosy. A detailed discussion of *tzaraat* and its medical and other interpretations is found in Preuss's classic book *Biblical and Talmudic Medicine*.[1]

In his *Mishneh Torah* (*Tumat Tzaraat* 1:1ff), Maimonides analyzes the details prescribed in Scripture (Leviticus, Chapters 13 and 14) for the detection of leprosy in men, garments, and houses; the procedures to be followed when these are certified unclean; and the ceremonies of purification required after they are pronounced clean. Maimonides concludes his legal treatise on leprosy with an overall clarification of this "medical" illness as being divine punishment for speaking slander, as befell Miriam (Numbers 12:10), who spoke against her brother Moses. Maimonides explains the matter as follows:

> Now this change in garments and in houses which Scripture includes under the general term "leprosy" was no normal happening, but was a portent and a wonder among the Israelites to warn them against slanderous speaking. For if a man repented, the house would again become clean. But if he continued

in his wickedness until the house was torn down, leather objects in his house on which he sat or lay would suffer a change. If he repented they would again become clean. But if he continued in his wickedness until they were burnt, his skin would suffer a change and he would become leprous and be set apart and exposed all alone until he should no more engage in the conversation of the wicked, which is raillery and slander (*Tumat Tzaraat* 16:10).

In commenting on the curious character of this so-called leprosy and its effects on humans, garments, and houses, Maimonides does not attempt to rationalize the biblical descriptions or to suggest that they need not all be taken literally. However, leprosy is thus thought to result from slanderous talk and grossness of spirit.

In his treatise *The Medical Aphorisms of Moses Maimonides*, Maimonides speaks of amputating leprosy and maiming leprosy, in which limbs fall off. A good diet and nutrition with barley gruel and milk soup; vegetables such as marshmallow, African rue, pigweed, and gourds; and fish or fowl meat are recommended for those who suffer from maiming leprosy.[2] Greater details about Maimonides' pronouncements concerning leprosy are found elsewhere.[3]

2. F. Rosner, *The Medical Aphorisms of Moses Maimonides* (Haifa: Maimonides Research Institute, 1989), pp. 53, 167, 169, and 350.

3. F. Rosner, *Medicine in the Mishneh Torah of Maimonides* (New York: Ktav, 1984), pp. 273–280.

*LESBIANISM*—Lesbianism is prohibited by Maimonides in his *Mishneh Torah* when he states that women are forbidden to engage in lesbian practices with one another, these being "the doings of the land of Egypt" (Lev. 18:3), against which we have been warned: "What did they do? A man would marry a man, or a woman a woman, or a woman would marry two men . . . such an act is forbidden" (*Issurei Biyah* 21:8).

In his *Mishnah Commentary* (*Sanhedrin* 7:4), he states that the abominable practice of lesbianism between women who lie one with the other is a disgraceful practice. However, there is no punishment therefor, either biblical or rabbinic. Neither of such women is called a prostitute, and neither is prohibited to her husband. Nor is such a woman forbidden to marry a priest. These are women that the sages have called *mesolelot* (lesbians), from the word *maslol* (Isaiah 35:8), which is the manner of practicing lewdness one with the other.[1]

1. F. Rosner (translator), *Julius Preuss' Biblical and Talmudic Medicine* (Northvale, NJ: Jason Aronson, 1993), pp. 323–374.

1. F. Rosner, *Maimonides' Commentary on the Mishnah, Tractate Sanhedrin* (New York: Sepher Hermon, 1981), pp. 86–94.

*LETHARGY*—In his *Medical Aphorisms*,[1] Maimonides quotes Galen, who said that weakness may be prolonged during convalescence from illness, particularly if intercurrent complications damage body strength (Chapter 8:40–41). A cold brain abscess known as lethargos is associated with lethargy and requires aggressive intervention including phlebotomy and the application of oil-of-roses-and-vinegar compresses to the head to remove the damaging humors (ibid., 9:17 and 23:68). Weakness may be caused by a faulty body constitution of humors (ibid., 23:13). Weak bodies cannot digest large amounts of food, even if it is healthy food. Therefore, feed a patient according to his strength and choose the food according to the constitution of the body (ibid., 20:12). Lethargic slumber or lethargy in which the patient falls into profound sleepiness is discussed by Maimonides in his *Extracts from Galen*.[2] It is caused by a bad humor and is treated by inhalation of the fumes of thyme or mint cooked in vinegar in order to dissolve the coarse humor in the brain.

---

1. F. Rosner, *The Medical Aphorisms of Moses Maimonides* (Haifa: Maimonides Research Institute, 1989).

2. U.S. Barzel, *Maimonides' The Art of Cure. Extracts from Galen* (Haifa: Maimonides Research Institute, 1992), pp. 161–162.

*LIEBER, ELINOR*—Physician and Hebrew medical historian at Oxford University, Elinor Lieber has published several articles on Maimonides including "Maimonides, Philosopher as Physician" [*Bulletin of the History of Medicine* 53 (1979):268–265] and "The Medical Works of Maimonides: a Reappraisal" (in *Moses Maimonides, Physician, Scientist and Philosopher*, ed., F. Rosner and S.S. Kottek, Northvale, NJ: Jason Aronson, Inc. (1993), pp. 13–24).

*LIVER*—Quoting Galen in his *Medical Aphorisms*,[1] Maimonides states that blood is formed in the liver (Chapter 2:1). The liver is nourished by thick red blood (ibid., 3:35) and is innervated by small nerves (ibid., 3:62). He describes abscesses in the liver (ibid., 3:82 and 92) and therapy for them (ibid., 9:62 and 73). Other ailments and illnesses of the liver are also discussed (ibid., 5:11 and 23:88). Perhaps most interesting is his accurate description of hepatitis: "The signs of liver inflammation are eight in number as follows: high fever, thirst, complete anorexia, a tongue which is initially red and then turns black, biliary vomitus . . . pain on the right side which ascends to the clavicle . . . a mild cough and a sensation of heaviness. . . ."

In his *Treatises on Health*,[2] Maimonides again quotes Galen, who said that "the health of our liver is our life." Vinegar-containing medications irritate the liver and weaken it. Adding raisins neutralizes this harmful effect. Maimonides describes an exudate in the liver (hepatitis?). He criticizes the suggestion of placing sandalwood on the liver, and recommends measures to regulate the temperament of the liver so that good blood is produced.

In his *Treatise on Asthma*,[3] he reiterates the damaging effect of vinegar on the liver and the beneficial effect of raisins, again discusses inflammation of the liver, recommends chicory for both cold and warm livers, and warns against excessive bloodletting because it may lead to severe weakness of the liver. Many more references to the liver are found in his other medical works.[4,5] In his *Mishneh Torah* (*Shechitah* 8:12), Maimonides recognizes that total absence of the liver in an animal is incompatible with life and that, if only a small portion of the liver remains, an animal can live normally.

1. F. Rosner, *The Medical Aphorisms of Moses Maimonides* (Haifa: Maimonides Research Institute, 1989).

2. F. Rosner, *Moses Maimonides' Three Treatises on Health* (Haifa: Maimonides Research Institute, 1990).

3. F. Rosner, *Moses Maimonides' Treatise on Asthma* (Haifa: Maimonides Research Institute, 1994).

4. U.S. Barzel, *Maimonides' The Art of Cure. Extracts from Galen* (Haifa: Maimonides Research Institute, 1992).

5. F. Rosner, *Maimonides' Commentary on the Aphorisms of Hippocrates* (Haifa: Maimonides Research Institute, 1987).

**LONGEVITY**—A responsum of Maimonides dealing with the duration of life is not included in most Maimonidean Responsa collections. This responsum on longevity was edited and published in Arabic and German in 1953 by Gotthold Weil.[1] It was also translated into English[2] and French.[3] The basic question to which Maimonides addresses himself is whether or not a person's life span is predetermined. He cites evidence from both medical and Jewish religious sources in giving a negative answer to this question. Medical proof that human life span is not predetermined is discussed in relation to the medieval concept of the disruption of the normal equilibrium between the four body humors: blood (red bile), phlegm (white bile), choler (yellow bile), and melancholy (black bile). Maimonides states that causes detrimental to innate body heat can be external and produce deterioration of the organs of warmth, or that these bad influences can cause qualitative or quantitative deterioration of the warmth itself. Each of these three possibilities is exemplified separately. Maimonides concludes from all the physiologic information that "if a person is careful concerning these causes [or premature accidental death or those causes leading to disequilibrium of innate body heat] that we have presented . . . the person will more readily attain his natural life's end."

Classic biblical and rabbinic writings are then presented by Maimonides to support his contention that life span is not predetermined, or that, if it is, it can be altered. Several commandments affecting human life are cited (Numbers 35:11–12; Deuteronomy 19:5–6, 20:7, and 22:8) that prove that the termination of life is not fixed, and that precautionary measures can pre-vent premature death. Other scriptural verses and religious writings that support this thesis are also discussed. [*See also* GERIATRICS]

1. G. Weil, *Maimonides. Uber die Lebensdauer* (Basel: S. Karger, 1953), pp. 1–59.

2. F. Rosner, "Moses Maimonides' Responsum on the Duration of Life," *Geriatrics,* 23 (1968):170–178.

3. F. Rosner, "Responsum sur la Longévité de Moise Maïmonide (1135–1204)," *Revue d'Histoire de la Médécine Hebraïque,* 27 (1974):71–78.

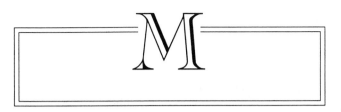

**MARCUS, SHLOMO**—A retired librarian and a medical and scientific historian, Shlomo Marcus was affiliated with the Hebrew University Library and Hadassah Medical School in Jerusalem, and specialized in the study of Hebrew medical manuscripts. Marcus and Joshua Leibowitz published *Moses Maimonides on the Causes of Symptoms* (Berkeley: University of California Press, 1974), in which Marcus supplied corrections and annotations to the Hebrew text and a catalogue of the materia medica in that treatise (pp. 213–248). He also published an article on Maimonides' attitude toward music (*Koroth* 5 (1972):819–822).

**MARTINI, UMBERTO DE**—Umberto de Martini issued an Italian translation of the two *Treatises on Sexual Intercourse* originally published by Kroner in 1906, one of which (the longer one) is wrongly attributed to Maimonides. De Martini's work, titled *Segreto dei Segreti*, was published in 1960 by the Institute of the History of Medicine of the University of Rome.

**MASSAGE**—In his *Treatise on Asthma*,[1] Maimonides recommends seven hygienic principles: clean air, correct eating and drinking, regulating one's emotions, exercise and rest, sleep and wakefulness, excretion or retention of wastes, and bathing and massaging. Chapter 10 deals with the effects of sleeping, waking, bathing, massage, and coitus on asthma. Massaging the body upon awakening in the morning and before going to bed at night is highly recommended. Several types of massage are described, as are certain forms of exercise for the young and for the elderly.

In his *Medical Aphorisms*,[2] Maimonides quotes Galen who said that palpation and light massage of the abdomen can help diagnose the cause of abdominal spasm (Chapter 6:66). Moderate massaging, as a general therapeutic measure for a variety of illnesses (ibid., 8:2 and 8:21), is most helpful if applied during periods of quiescence of illness (ibid., 8:60). Massaging with oil is beneficial after bathing (ibid., 19:33). Massage is also recommended to help bring on sleep, although too much sleep is also not good.[3] In his *Mishneh Torah*, Maimonides rules that the abdomen may be anointed and massaged on the Sabbath, provided that both actions are performed simultaneously, so as to constitute a departure from the normal weekday procedure (*Shabbat* 21:28).

---

1. F. Rosner, *Moses Maimonides' Treatise on Asthma* (Haifa: Maimonides Research Institute, 1994).
2. F. Rosner, *The Medical Aphorisms of Moses Maimonides* (Haifa: Maimonides Research Institute, 1989).
3. U.S. Barzel, *Maimonides' The Art of Cure. Extracts from Galen* (Haifa: Maimonides Research Institute, 1992).

*MASTURBATION*—Masturbation is prohibited by Jewish law. Maimonides enunciates this rule using very expressive language in his *Mishneh Torah*.

> It is forbidden to expend semen to no purpose. Consequently, a man should not thresh within and ejaculate without [i.e., coitus interruptus] . . . as for masturbators, not only do they commit a strictly forbidden act, but they also expose themselves to a ban. It is to them that Scripture refers in saying,

"Your hands are full of blood" (Isa. 1:15), and a masturbator's act is regarded as equivalent to killing a human being (*Issurei Biyah* 21:18).

Similarly, a man should not bring about an erection deliberately or by unchaste thoughts (ibid., 21:19), by gazing at animals when they are mating (ibid., 21:20) or by gazing at women "while they are bending over their washing" (ibid., 21:22).

Further condemnation of the practice of masturbation is discussed by Maimonides in his *Mishnah Commentary* (*Sanhedrin* 7:4), where he asserts that the sages strongly warned against licentious thoughts and things that provoke them. They spoke at length that a man should fear and be afraid of intentionally producing an erection and of emitting semen for naught (*Niddah* 13a–b), and they explained that all such acts are prohibited; however, they did not impose flogging as a penalty for any of them.[1]

---

1. F. Rosner, *Maimonides' Commentary on the Mishnah, Tractate Sanhedrin* (New York: Sepher Hermon, k1981), pp. 86–94.

*MEAT*—In his *Mishneh Torah*, Maimonides rules (based on *Chullin* 84a) that a person should not eat meat regularly, save when he desires it, as it is written: "because thy soul desireth to eat flesh" (Deuteronomy 12:20). A healthy person should do so once weekly. However, if he is rich enough to eat meat every day, he may do so (*Deot* 5:10). If a person wishes to eat fowl meat and cattle meat together, he should first consume the poultry meat, because it is lighter (*Deot* 4:7). In his *Regimen on Health*,[1] Maimonides states that the best meats are those of a kid, a one-year-old lamb, chicken, and pheasant (Chapter 1:6). These are preferable to cattle or sheep meat (ibid., 1:7). The best sorts of game meat are gazelle and rabbit (ibid., 4:17). In his *Causes of Symptoms*, Maimonides advises against venison or salted meat for a patient suffering from dejection and melancholy. He also recommends that one always try to eat the meat of chickens or pullets and to drink its broth because this type of fowl improves harmful humors. Advice concerning the preparation of meat is also provided.

In his *Treatise on Asthma*,[2] Maimonides warns against the consumption of fattening meat, such as that from cattle, goats, and grown sheep, because it is difficult to digest and thick humors are produced that may obstruct body vessels or passages (Chapter 3:3). He again recommends fowl, except water fowl such as geese and duck (ibid., 3:4). Cattle meat, if consumed, should be lean (ibid., 3:6). Gazelle, deer, and rabbit are highly recommended (ibid., 3:7). In his *Medical Aphorisms*,[3] Maimonides quotes Galen, who said that elderly people with weak bodies should eat only cooked meat, whereas young people and those with strong bodies may also eat fried or roasted meat (Chapter 17:34). Fowl is easily digested (ibid., 20:20); roasted meat strengthens the body more than cooked meat; boiled meat strengthens more than any other cooked dish (ibid., 20:21). Maimonides also quotes Abu Merwan Ibn Zuhr, who said that chicken soup equilibrates body constitution and is an excellent food (ibid., 20:68). Turtle doves increase memory, improve intellect and sharpen the senses (ibid.). The consumption of fowl is beneficial for a variety of illnesses, and it increases sexual potential (ibid., 20:69). Kid meat is considered to be exceptionally good, more so than the meat of any other animal (ibid., 20:70). The meat of young deer increases the appetite, strengthens those who are weak, and heals one who has fainted from excessive purgation (ibid.).

1. F. Rosner, *Moses Maimonides' Three Treatises on Health* (Haifa: Maimonides Research Institute, 1990).

2. F. Rosner, *Moses Maimonides' Treatise on Asthma* (Haifa: Maimonides Research Institute, 1994).

3. F. Rosner, *The Medical Aphorisms of Moses Maimonides* (Haifa: Maimonides Research Institute, 1989).

**MEDICAL APHORISMS**—The *Medical Aphorisms of Moses Mai-*

*monides* is the most voluminous of his ten authentic medical treatises. The book is composed of fifteen hundred aphorisms based mainly on Greek and Arabic medical writers. There are twenty-five chapters, each dealing with a different area of medicine, including anatomy; physiology; pathology; symptomatology; diagnosis and etiology of diseases; therapeutics; fevers; bloodletting; laxatives; emetics; surgery; gynecology; hygiene; exercise; bathing; diet; drugs; and medical curiosities.[1] At the end of each aphorism, Maimonides cites his source. He did not do this in his earlier theological and philosophical writings, an omission for which he was severely criticized both during his lifetime and for many years thereafter. Most aphorisms are annotated and commented upon by Maimonides, and a significant number are original with him. Maimonides' own statements always begin with "Moses says."

The *Aphorisms of Moses* was originally written in Arabic, as were all of Maimonides' medical works. The reason for writing the aphorisms, the format used, the source material available at the time, and a general outline of the contents of the book are given by Maimonides in his foreword to the book. The book is a rich collection of medical rules and regulations in which Maimonides displays an exemplary knowledge and erudition of contemporary and less recent medical litera-

ture. What others could not express in lengthy treatises, he clarifies in concise and lucid phrases. With the systematic exactitude and meticulous methodology characteristic of all his writings—medical and otherwise—Maimonides attempts to eradicate preformed opinions and dictated dogmas in medicine from the minds of students and physicians alike. He encourages them to experiment and observe for themselves, and to develop an attitude of keen criticism and skepticism toward accepted traditions and teachings, even if these originate from as renowned a medical scholar or authority as Galen. Maimonides takes issue with many of Galen's views in the important twenty-fifth treatise of this book. The book is based almost entirely on rational medicine, independent observation, and the scientific method. Rule-of-thumb, guesswork, and superstition have no place in this work or in Maimonides' thinking, although an occasional "specific therapy" he advocates has no rational basis.

Chapter 2 is devoted to the ancient concept of physiology, dealing with the four humors: blood, white bile (phlegm), red bile (blood), yellow bile, and black (melancholy) bile. The sites of production of these various substances are described and their various characteristics are outlined. Red bile is considered the best, and black bile the worst. Disease consists of derangements in the normal qualities, quantities, or interrelationships of the body humors. Maimonides, quoting Galen, states: "The illnesses which occur as a result of black bile are: cancer, elephant skin, psoriasis, quartan fever, confusion [depression], and thickness of the spleen."

The last chapter does not deal with practical medicine, but contains a sharp attack on Galen, whose views were accepted as dogma throughout the Middle Ages. It shows Maimonides' ability and courage as a profound critic and demonstrates his astounding knowledge of the spiritual world of the ancient Greeks. Aphorism 59 in this chapter is outstanding in that it presents Maimonides as a protagonist of the Aristotelian philosophy in its Arabic-Jewish garb conforming with the principles of Judaism. The peak of his greatness is revealed in aphorism 69, where he challenges conventional views, in general, and exposes falsifications and errors of Galen, in particular. Maimonides demands research through experimentation and recognizes the influence of ecology on the human organism. He disputes Galen's views on life. He cannot comprehend how a man such as Galen could pay attention to "material" things to the exclusion of the spirit. Whereas to Galen knowledge without experience sufficed, to Maimonides, both are necessary to make a good physician.

1. F. Rosner, *The Medical Aphorisms of Moses Maimonides* (Haifa: Maimonides Research Institute, 1989).

**MEDICAL CURIOSITIES**—Chapter 24 of Maimonides' *Medical Aphorisms* comprises aphorisms on medical curiosities, strange occurrences, and unusual and rare happenings.[1] One example is the statement that, following a complete solar eclipse in Sicily, women gave birth to bicephalic monsters. Another is the remarkable description of teratomas: "Inflammations that are called 'tumors' are found to be of varying types when cut open. Sometimes, objects resembling mud, urine, feces, honey, excrement, stone, teeth, and flesh are found therein. Sometimes one even finds living creatures therein that arise from putrefaction." The last sentence seems to indicate the belief in spontaneous generation, an accepted fact in the Middle Ages, which Spallanzani disproved in the eighteenth century [*see* SPONTANEOUS GENERATION].

Maimonides also cites the eggplant (Solanum melongena, or *bading'an* in Arabic) from one of Galen's works, but which Galen had not yet known. Maimonides adds that this word crept into the book of Galen only as a conjecture on the part of the translator or copyist who thought that a black and reddish fruit could be nothing but eggplant. Many interesting customs and qualities of various peoples

*145*

are described in this chapter, where we hear of Greeks, Romans, Scythians, Germans (Slavs), and Berbers. We also hear of diseases in Rome, Athens, Ethiopia, Alexandria (Egypt), and Maimonides' Spanish homeland when he states: "In our land. . . ." Famous physicians encountered in this chapter include Galen, Hunain Ibn Yitzchak, Ali Ibn Rodhwan, Hippocrates, Batrik, Aristedes of Mysia, and Plato.

---

1. F. Rosner, *The Medical Aphorisms of Moses Maimonides* (Haifa: Maimonides Research Institute, 1989), pp. 383–400.

**MEDICAL INSTRUMENTS**—In his *Mishneh Torah*, Maimonides describes various instruments used by physicians and allied health personnel.[1] These include a barber's nail used for bloodletting (*Kelim* 10:3), physicians' tongs (ibid., 11:12), a scalpel (ibid., 11:17), a knife (ibid., 11:8), scissors (ibid., 11:9), a needle to remove splinters (ibid., 8:4), a hide that a physician lays on his knees when pricking ulcers (ibid., 24:1), a midwife's labor stool (ibid., 25:2), and a cripple's stump or artificial limb (ibid., 25:19). He also speaks about circumcision instruments, including flints and glass, but rules that a knife is preferred (*Milah* 2:1). All these instruments and implements are susceptible to ritual uncleanness as utensils.

In his *Medical Aphorisms*, Maimonides discusses splints for the stabilization of bone fractures.[2] Cutting with a knife at the site of a snakebite is recommended in his *Treatise on Poisons*.[3] A scalpel is cited in the *Regimen of Health*,[4] and ligatures and bandages are mentioned in the *Extracts from Galen*.[5]

In his *Mishnah Commentary*,[6] Maimonides speaks of a physician's drill used by surgeons to incise swollen wounds, i.e., abscesses (*Oholot* 2:3); a box in which physicians store their medications (*Eduyot* 3:9); a large ladle used by physicians to remove solid and liquid medicines from jars (*Kelim* 17:12); a basket or box used by physicians to store their bandages (ibid., 12:3), the cover of which was used to prepare the bandages; and a bloodletter's lancet (ibid., 12:4).

---

1. F. Rosner, *Medicine in the Mishneh Torah of Maimonides* (New York: Ktav, 1984), p. 66.
2. F. Rosner, *The Medical Aphorisms of Moses Maimonides* (Haifa: Maimonides Research Institute, 1989), pp. 256–257.
3. F. Rosner, *Maimonides' Treatises on Poisons, Hemorrhoids and Cohabitation* (Haifa: Maimonides Research Institute, 1984), p. 39.
4. F. Rosner, *Moses Maimonides' Three Treatises on Health* (Haifa: Maimonides Research Institute, 1990), p. 80.
5. U.S. Barzel, *Maimonides' The Art of Cure. Extracts from Galen* (Haifa: Maimonides Research Institute, 1992), pp. 26–27.

6. F. Rosner, "Medicine in Moses Maimonides' Commentary on the Mishnah," *Koroth* (Jerusalem), 9 (1988): 565–578.

*MEDICAL WRITINGS*—Maimonides wrote ten medical treatises and books.[1] All were originally written in Arabic. Several were composed at the behest of members of the royal family of Saladin the Great, ruler of Egypt at the time of the Crusades. All ten of these works are described individually in this encyclopedia. They are the *Extracts from Galen*, the *Commentary on the Aphorisms of Hippocrates*, the *Medical Aphorisms of Moses (Maimonides)*, the *Treatise on Asthma*, the *Treatise on Poisons and Their Antidotes*, the *Treatise on Sexual Intercourse*, the *Regimen of Health*, the *Causes of Symptoms*, the *Treatise on Hemorrhoids*, and the *Glossary of Drug Names*. Several other medical works, including the *Book of Remedies* and the famous *Physician's Prayer* are attributed to Maimonides, but are spurious and were not written by him.[2]

Maimonides' medical writings are varied, comprising extracts from Greek medicine, a series of monographs on health in general and several diseases in particular, and a more recently discovered pharmacopoeia demonstrating Maimonides' extensive knowledge of Arabic medical literature and his familiarity with several languages. Some people believe that Maimonides' medical writings are not as original as his theological and philosophical writings; however, his medical works demonstrate the same lucidity, conciseness, and formidable powers of systemization and organization so characteristic of all his writings. The *Book on Poisons*, the *Regimen of Health*, and the *Medical Aphorisms of Maimonides* became classics in their fields in medieval times. Bibliographies of Maimonides the physician and his medical writings are available for the interested reader.[3]

1. F. Rosner and S.S. Kottek, *Moses Maimonides: Physician, Scientist, and Philosopher* (Northvale, NJ: Jason Aronson, 1993), pp. 3–12.
2. F. Rosner, *Six Treatises Attributed to Maimonides* (Northvale, NJ: Jason Aronson, 1991).
3. F. Rosner, "Maimonides the Physician. A Bibliography," *Bulletin of the History of Medicine*, 43 (1969): 221–235; ibid., *Clio Medica*, 15 (1980): 75–79.

*MEDICATIONS*—Chapter 21 of Maimonides' *Medical Aphorisms* is devoted entirely to medications.[1] It is a veritable pharmacopoeia of materia medica. Several hundred drugs, simple and compounded, are described. The value of alcohol in the form of wine as a diuretic and a soporific is mentioned at the outset. Milk mixed with honey is said to be "valuable against pains in the chest and lung. However, it is . . . harmful . . . for the spleen and liver." The benefits and contraindications of oxymel (a mixture of honey and vinegar) are outlined. Astringents such as extracts of blackberry bushes or wine bushes are recommended for stomach ailments. Regarding exogenous poisons and endogenous toxins, Maimonides states: "Milk, garlic, boiled [distilled] wine, vinegar, and salt are of value against [animal] poisons or against substances that develop [in the body] that are similar to poisons." Caper is reported to be an appetite stimulant and a purgative. The actions and indications for a variety of medications such as saffron, Ceylon cinnamon, spikenard, andropogon, aromatic calamus, spicknel, aloe, wormwood, bdellium, and many others are stated.

Next follows a classification and categorization of drugs according to various parameters. Sweetness, saltiness, bitterness, and sharpness are indicators of different drug effects. The properties of drugs that are astringent, sour, sharp, bitter, tasteless, sweet, or oily are described. The remainder of this chapter enumerates hundreds of drugs that fit into these various categories. This list is by no means exhaustive, as Maimonides himself states: "I, therefore, [only] intend to describe the properties of drugs that are universally commonly used, whose names

are well known and which are employed internally." A sample excerpt from one of these aphorisms describing one group of medicaments states: "Cooling drugs that moisten to the first degree are ten [in number]. These are pears, spinach, violets, chicory, lotus, fenugreek, wormwood, marigold, mallow, and liquiricia." This lengthy chapter supplements and complements Maimonides' *Glossary of Drug Names*, a work devoted entirely to the description of 405 drugs, herbs, and medicaments and their various therapeutic indications and uses.[2] Additional discussions of many drugs and medications for a variety of ailments are found in his other medical works, especially his *Treatises on Health*.[3]

---

1. F. Rosner, *The Medical Aphorisms of Moses Maimonides* (Haifa: Maimonides Research Institute, 1989), pp. 313–341.

2. F. Rosner, *Moses Maimonides' Glossary of Drug Names* (Haifa: Maimonides Research Institute, 1996).

3. F. Rosner, *Moses Maimonides' Three Treatises on Health* (Haifa: Maimonides Research Institute, 1990).

*MELANCHOLY*—Maimonides' *Regimen on Health*[1] was written for a member of the royal family in Egypt, a young Sultan subject to fits of melancholy or depression owing to his excessive indulgences in wine and women and to his warlike adventures against his own relatives in the Crusades. He complained to his physician of constipation, dejection, bad thoughts, and indigestion. Maimonides' prescription is for public and private hygiene for the preservation of the health of the body and the soul. This book shows Maimonides not only as a scholar and physician, but also as a healer of the mind. He clearly asserts that physical and mental well-being are interdependent, one of the earliest descriptions of psychosomatic medicine.

In his *Commentary on the Aphorisms of Hippocrates*,[2] Maimonides points out that melancholy is caused by black bile, as opposed to epilepsy, which is caused by white bile (Section 3:20). He explains melancholy to represent confusion of the mind (ibid., 6:11). Fright and despondency without any apparent reason is also a type of melancholy (ibid., 6:23). In his *Medical Aphorisms*,[3] Maimonides quotes Galen, who said that delirium or confusion of the mind may be caused by pain in the temporal muscles (Chapter 3:77). Melancholic confusion is also called phrenesia (ibid., 6:11) or black confusion (ibid., 9:16). Such patients have real or imaginary fears (ibid., 6:15) or restlessness and anxiety (ibid., 6:52). Mental confusion and forgetfulness can also occur from senility, and even from red bile (ibid., 7:26). The treatment for melancholy is venesection (ibid., 12:22).

1. F. Rosner, *Moses Maimonides' Three Treatises on Health* (Haifa: Maimonides Research Institute, 1990).

2. F. Rosner, *Maimonides' Commentary on the Aphorisms of Hippocrates* (Haifa: Maimonides Research Institute, 1987).

3. F. Rosner, *The Medical Aphorisms of Moses Maimonides* (Haifa: Maimonides Research Institute, 1989).

**MELONS**—In his *Treatise on Asthma*,[1] Maimonides considers pomegranate (Punica granatum) juice beneficial for the chest (Chapter 3:9). Pomegranates are also astringent and therefore useful for patients with loose stools (ibid., 9:4). Melons in season also help a person in whom vomiting must be induced (ibid., 9:13). A pomegranate electuary is also described that is "among the healing medications" (ibid., 13:46). In his *Treatise on Poisons*,[2] Maimonides recommends, for bee or wasp stings, the drinking of a pomegranate beverage in cold water. In his *Regimen on Health*,[3] he discusses the yellow melon (Cucumis melo), which is extensively consumed by all people and "cools the body, stimulates urine flow, and cleanses the blood vessels" (Chapter 1:11). He recommends "a pomegranate with its seeds" after one finishes the meal (ibid., 3:2). A barley distillate made with pomegranate seeds may be imbibed after a bath (ibid., 4:11). The astringent property of pomegranates is also reiterated (ibid., 4:14).

In his *Treatise on the Causes of Symptoms*, Maimonides advises the consumption of apples and quinces and the sucking of pomegranate seeds after the meal for all people, for the maintenance of good health in general (Section 9). He warns, however, against the consumption of a variety of fresh fruits, including melons, as foods since they are rapidly transformed into harmful humors (ibid., 11). In his *Mishneh Torah*, he allows the ingestion of melons before the meal if a laxative is needed, or the ingestion of pomegranates after the meal if a constipating agent is needed (*Deot* 4:6). In either case, "One should not eat excessively thereof." Stems and rind of watermelon are said to have no food value (*Terumot* 11:10). Melons are usually cut into sections before being served (*Bikkurim* 6:6).

In his *Medical Aphorisms*,[4] Maimonides quotes Abu Merwan Ibn Zuhr, who said that a sweet pomegranate has a wonderful quality when eaten with bread because it prevents illness in the stomach (Chapter 20:76). Numerous additional references to pomegranates are found in Maimonides' *Extracts from Galen*.[5]

In his *Glossary of Drug Names*,[6] Maimonides describes the wild pomegranate tree that has no fruits (drug no. 243). He also discusses melons and watermelons (drug no. 54), as well as pumpkins (drug no. 332).

1. F. Rosner, *Moses Maimonides' Treatise on Asthma* (Haifa: Maimonides Research Institute, 1994).

2. F. Rosner, *Maimonides' Treatises on Poisons, Hemorrhoids and Cohabitation* (Haifa: Maimonides Research Institute, 1987), p. 64.

3. F. Rosner, *Moses Maimonides' Three Treatises on Health* (Haifa: Maimonides Research Institute, 1990).

4. F. Rosner, *The Medical Aphorisms of Moses Maimonides* (Haifa: Maimonides Research Institute, 1989).

5. U.S. Barzel, *Maimonides' The Art of Cure. Extracts from Galen* (Haifa: Maimonides Research Institute, 1992).

6. F. Rosner, *Moses Maimonides' Glossary of Drug Names* (Haifa: Maimonides Research Institute, 1995).

**MENSTRUATION**—The physiology of menstruation and its effects on the health of a woman are described in some detail by Maimonides in Chapter 16 of his *Medical Aphorisms*, which was devoted entirely to gynecology.[1] He discusses amenorrhea and drugs that increase menstrual flow. He portrays the results of hypermenorrhea. Menstruation and menstrual blood are also discussed in his other medical writings.

In his *Mishneh Torah*, Maimonides recognized that vaginal bleeding can occur following trauma, such as jumping; or from sexual excitation, such as if a woman sees animals copulating (*Issurei Biyah* 5:1). Only blood derived from the uterus renders a woman ritually unclean (ibid., 5:2); vaginal blood from a local sore does not (ibid., 5:5). Hematuria and melena do not render a woman ritually unclean (ibid., 5:17); neither does virginal blood (ibid., 5:18). To help decide on the origin of blood, Maimonides provides a detailed and vivid anatomical description of the female genitalia (ibid., 5:13).

Maimonides then describes the various shades and hues of blood. Five varieties of woman's blood render her ritually unclean: red; black; the shade of bright crocus; the shade of water mixed with earth, and the shade of wine diluted with water (ibid., 5:7). Each of these is defined quite precisely (ibid., 5:8ff). A white or green fluid issuing from the womb does not render a woman ritually unclean (ibid., 5:6). Whether or not Maimonides is referring to a venereal or other infectious endometritis is unclear. Clear, however, is the assertion that the blood of a menstruant, the blood of a woman with flux, the blood of labor, the blood of a woman in childbirth, and postpartum blood are all the same species of blood and emanate from the uterus (ibid., 6:1). Blood of labor is defined as that which commences to flow before parturition, when the pregnant woman begins to experience distress and is seized with birth pangs (ibid., 7:1). Regular and irregular menses are mentioned (ibid., 8:1). Symptoms at or just prior to the onset of menstruation may include sneezing, yawning, pain in the pit of the stomach and in the lower part of the abdomen, hair upon the woman's flesh standing up, or her flesh becoming heated (ibid., 8:2).

Menstrual blood, the blood of parturition, and other types of blood are also discussed in Maimonides' *Mishnah Commentary* (*Eduyot* 5:4 and *Niddah* 2:5). Seven substances applied to a garment can determine whether a stain is blood or dye (*Niddah* 9:6–7). The laws of ritual impurity related to a woman's menses and intermenstrual spotting or bleeding are discussed in detail in *Mishneh Torah*.[2]

---

1. F. Rosner, *The Medical Aphorisms of Moses Maimonides* (Haifa: Maimonides Research Institute, 1989), pp. 262–270.

2. F. Rosner, *Medicine in the Mishneh Torah of Maimonides* (New York: Ktav, 1984), pp. 134–143.

**MEYERHOF, MAX**—An ophthalmologist, medical historian, and German native, Max Meyerhof (1874–1945) spent most of his life in Cairo, where he headed the Khedivial Ophthalmic Clinic. He was a prolific writer with a bibliography of over three hundred books, monographs, papers, and treatises on ophthalmology and medical history.[1] In 1937, he co-authored in Arabic and English part of the last chapter of Maimonides' *Medical Aphorisms*,[2] in which Maimonides criticizes Galen. In another article three years later, Meyerhof again discussed this Maimonidean criticism of

Galen.[3] Meyerhof's major Maimonidean work is his critical edition in Arabic and French translation with extensive commentaries, bibliographies, and indices of Maimonides' *Glossary of Drug Names*.[4] This was a previously unknown work of Maimonides that Meyerhof discovered in the Aya Sofia library in Istanbul, Turkey, as Arabic manuscript 3711. In connection with the preparation of Maimonides' *Glossary*, Meyerhof published several studies (see *Bulletin de L'Institut d'Egypte*, 17 (1935):223–235 and *Mélanges Maspero*, 3 (1935–40):1–7). He also wrote an article on "The Medical Work of Maimonides" in Salo Baron's *Essays on Maimonides* (New York: Columbia University Press, 1941), pp. 265–299.

1. J.I. Dienstag, "Translators and Editors of Maimonides' Medical Works: A Bio-bibliographical survey," in J.O. Leibowitz, ed., *Memorial Volume in Honor of Prof. S. Muntner* (Jerusalem: Israel Institute of the History of Medicine, 1983), pp. 95–135.

2. J. Schacht and M. Meyerhof, "Maimonides Against Galen on Philosophy and Cosmogeny," *Bulletin of the Faculty of Arts of the University of Egypt* 5(Part 1) (1937):53–88.

3. M. Meyerhof, "Maimonides Criticizes Galen," *Medical Leaves* 3 (1940):141–146.

4. M. Meyerhof, "*Sarh Asma Al-Uqqar* (L'Explication des Noms de Droges)," *Un Glossaire de Matière Médicale, Composé par Maïmonide*, Cairo: Mémoires Présentés à l'Institut d'Egypte, 41 (1940).

**MIGRAINE**—In his *Treatise on Asthma*,[1] Maimonides gives general advice concerning illnesses that are characterized by acute attacks such as arthritis, migraine, asthma, and kidney stones. He characterizes migraine as an "illness affecting half the head" (Chapter 1:1). In his *Medical Aphorisms*,[2] he quotes Galen, who said that some people with unilateral headaches called migraine feel the pain outside the membranes of the brain, whereas others feel it into the depths of the brain. In either event, the pain extends only to the linea mediana, which separates the two halves of the head (Chapter 6:35). Migraine is caused either by biliary humors or by an excess of humors whose vapors ascend to the brain (ibid.). Some, but not all, patients with migraine derive benefit from bloodletting from the pulsating arteries behind the ears (ibid., 15:14). In the final chapter of his *Medical Aphorisms*, Maimonides criticizes Galen for making contradictory statements about the causes and consequences of migraine headaches (ibid., 25:52).

1. F. Rosner, *Moses Maimonides' Treatise on Asthma* (Haifa: Maimonides Research Institute, 1994).

2. F. Rosner, *The Medical Aphorisms of Moses Maimonides* (Haifa: Maimonides Research Institute, 1989).

**MILK**—In his *Mishneh Torah*, Maimonides uses the word "milk" over one hundred times, mostly in codifying various biblical and talmudic assertions about milk.[1] In his treatise on poisons,[2] Maimonides recommends that a person who ingested poison should be made to vomit and then consume milk because it neutralizes the effect of the poison. In his *Medical Aphorisms*,[3] he quotes Galen, who states that a mother's milk is the proper nutrition for a newborn infant because its composition is the same as the blood from which the infant was created (Chapter 16:37). He further writes that:

Milk nourishes a malnourished body and revives it and destroys the badness of the detrimental humors by weakening them and softening the stool . . . milk is more nourishing than wheat . . . milk is the best of all chymes. The liquid watery portion in camel's and donkey's milk prevails, the cheesy part dominates in sheep's milk, and the buttery part in cow's milk. The milk which is most beneficial is that obtained from a healthy and well nourished animal. If one drinks it immediately after milking, it is proper to add honey and some salt thereto to counteract its becoming cheese. . . . Cow's milk is the thickest and fattest of all milks. Camel's milk is the most watery of all milks and the least fat of all. After camel's milk is horse mare's milk, and after that is donkey's milk. Goat's milk is intermediate between thick and thin and sheep's milk is thicker than the latter. All milks are good and suitable for [illnesses in] the

chest or lung but are not appropriate for a head[ache] even if it is very severe (ibid., 16:39ff).

Numerous other references to milk are found in Maimonides' *Medical Aphorisms*, as well as in his other medical books, especially the *Treatises on Health*[4] and *Extracts from Galen*.[5]

---

1. F. Rosner, "Milk and Cheese in Classic Jewish Sources," in *Medicine in the Bible and the Talmud*, augmented ed. (Hoboken, NJ: Ktav and Yeshiva University Press, 1995), pp. 115–126.

2. F. Rosner, *Maimonides' Treatises on Poisons, Hemorrhoids and Cohabitation* (Haifa: Maimonides Research Institute, 1984).

3. F. Rosner, *The Medical Aphorisms of Moses Maimonides* (Haifa: Maimonides Research Institute, 1989), pp. 26–34.

4. F. Rosner, *Moses Maimonides' Three Treatises on Health* (Haifa: Maimonides Research Institute, 1990).

5. U.S. Barzel, *Maimonides' The Art of Cure. Extracts from Galen* (Haifa: Maimonides Research Institute, 1992).

**MUNTNER, SUESSMAN**—A physician, humanitarian, and medical historian, Suessman Muntner (1897–1973), born in Poland and educated in Berlin, dedicated himself to editing, publishing, and disseminating the medical writings of Moses Maimonides. He lived and practiced medicine in Jerusalem for most of his life, and it is there that most of his works were published. Muntner's indefatigable zeal in making all the unpublished Hebrew translations of Maimonides' medical works available was awesome, and has become legendary. It was also Muntner's aspiration and scholarly obsession to see that these works were translated into as many western languages as possible.[1] For a decade, he collaborated with Fred Rosner of New York in the English translations of Maimonides' medical works.[2] He published German translations of Maimonides' *Regimen of Health* and *Causes of Symptoms*,[3] and translated but never published several other Maimonidean works into German, including his *Medical Aphorisms* and his *Commentary on the Aphorisms of Hippocrates.* He also collaborated with Isidor Simon of Paris in a French translation of Maimonides' *Treatise on Asthma.*[4]

Muntner was a gifted translator and editor. He translated Musaeus's *Hero and Leander* from the original Greek into Hebrew hexameters. He also translated into Hebrew verses the writings of German classical writings such as Goethe and Schiller. He compiled an 80,000-word Hebrew medical lexicon, which he unfortunately never published. He edited the medical works of Asaph[5] and Donnolo,[6] Jewish physicians from the sixth and tenth centuries, respectively. In addition to his more than twenty books, several hundred articles by Muntner appeared in Hebrew, German, French, English, and Spanish medical and scientific periodi-

cals. He was thus a multilingual prolific writer. He wrote about seventy sections for the *Encyclopedia Judaica.* Together with Joshua O. Leibowitz and David Margalith, Muntner cofounded and edited, until his death, the Israeli medical historical journal *Koroth.*

Muntner's lasting legacy, however, is the series of Hebrew edited and published medical works of Maimonides, based on numerous medieval Arabic and Hebrew manuscripts. Muntner's works include Maimonides' *Treatise on Asthma* (Jerusalem: Reuben Mass, 1940; 2nd ed., Jerusalem Genizah, 1963; reprinted by Mossad Harav Kook, 1965); *Treatise on Poisons* (Jerusalem: Rubin Mass, 1942); *Commentary on the Aphorisms of Hippocrates* (Jerusalem: Genizah, 1943; reprinted by Mossad Harav Kook, 1961); *Regimen of Health* (Jerusalem: Mossad Harav Kook, 1957); *Medical Aphorisms* (Jerusalem: Mossad Harav Kook, 1959); *Treatise on Hemorrhoids* and *Treatise on Sexual Intercourse* (Jerusalem: Mossad Harav Kook, 1965); and *Glossary of Drug Names* (Jerusalem: Mossad Harav Kook, 1969).

Muntner, who was probably the twentieth century's greatest authority on the medical writings of Maimonides, received numerous honors for his contributions to Maimonidean scholarship and Jewish medical history. A memorial volume in his memory was published ten years after his death.[7]

1. J.I. Dienstag, "Translators and Editors of Maimonides' Medical Works: A Bio-bibliographical Survey, in J.O. Leibowitz, ed., *Memorial Volume in Honor of Prof. S. Muntner* (Jerusalem: Israel Institute of the History of Medicine, 1983).

2. F. Rosner, "Suessman A. Muntner, M.D. 1897–1973," *New York State Journal of Medicine*, 78 (1978):119–121.

3. S. Muntner, *Maimonides' Regimen Sanitatis oder Diaetetik fur die Seele und den Korper mit anhang der Medizinischen Responsen und Ethik des Maimonides* (Basel: S. Karger, 1966).

4. S. Muntner, I. Simon, "Le Traité de l'Asthme de Maïmonide (1135–1204)," *Revue d'Histoire de la Médecine Hebraïque*, 16 (1963):171–186; 17 (1963):5–13; 18 (1964):83–97, 127–139, 187–196; 18 (1965):5–15.

5. S. Muntner. *Introduction to the Book of Asaph the Physician*. Jerusalem, Geniza, 1957 (Hebrew).

6. S. Muntner. *Rabbi Shabtai Donnolo*, Jerusalem, Mossad Harav Kook, 1949 (Hebrew).

7. J.O. Leibowitz (Edit.). *Memorial Volume in Honor of Prof. S. Muntner*, Jerusalem, Israel Institute of the History of Medicine, 1983.

**MUSCLES**—In his *Medical Aphorisms*,[1] Maimonides quotes Galen, who said that every muscle has a sensory and motor nerve originating from the brain and spinal cord (Chapter 1:1). The diaphragm is innervated by the phrenic nerve (ibid., 1:2). Muscle is said to be a structure for mobility only, not an organ for sensation (ibid., 1:13). Muscles contract and stretch (ibid., 1:24). During sleep, the muscles are idle and inactive (ibid., 1:27), except for the chest muscles, which continue unimpeded (ibid., 1:32). The muscles of the arms, urinary bladder, and diaphragm are all round and are under voluntary control (ibid., 1:28). Stretching of the diaphragm facilitates the inhalation of air (ibid., 1:29). Synergistic movements occur in hand, feet, and head movements, which involve many muscles contracting and relaxing (ibid., 1:70–71). If skin overlying a muscle loses its sensation, the movement of that muscle is not abolished, because the skin and the muscles have separate nerves (ibid., 3:54). Pain or an affliction of both temporal muscles may lead to convulsions, fever, stupor, and delirium owing to their proximity to the origin of nerves (ibid., 3:77). Muscle fibrillation originates from air vapors pouring into the heart (ibid. 7:38). Cramps are due to stretching and contraction of muscles where the nerves insert (ibid., 7:39). Yawning is produced by feebleness of the muscles that move the jaw (ibid., 9:42).

In his *Extracts from Galen*,[2] Maimonides asserts that cutting a muscle spoils its movements and makes it idle. Muscle injuries require bandaging or sewing together (Chapter 4). The treatment of a swelling caused by a strike or a blow that affects a muscle is achieved with a medicine that ripens, dissolves, and constipates (Chapter 14).

---

1. F. Rosner, *The Medical Aphorisms of Moses Maimonides* (Haifa: Maimonides Research Institute, 1989).
2. U.S. Barzel, *Maimonides' The Art of Cure. Extracts from Galen* (Haifa: Maimonides Research Institute, 1992).

*MUSIC THERAPY*—Music therapy is defined as the planned and controlled use of music to achieve therapeutic aims, and differs from music used in recreation and entertainment. In one of his medical treatises addressed to the Sultan al-Malik al-Afdal, Maimonides recommends sleep induced by slowly fading music, since that "endows the soul with a good nature, greatly widens it and thereby improves its direction over the body."[1] In his psychological and ethical treatise *The Eight Chapters* (*Shemonah Perakim*), Maimonides asserts that one who suffers from melancholy may rid himself of it by listening to singing and all kinds of instrumental music, by strolling through beautiful gardens, and by other things that enliven the mind and dissipate gloomy moods. The purpose of all this is to restore the body to health so that the real object of obtaining wisdom—acquiring knowledge of God—can be striven for.

In his *Treatise on Eternal Bliss* (*Pirkei Ha-hatzlachah*), Maimonides reiterates this theme when he states that the perfect soul is helped by listening to beautiful music and musical instruments, and then becomes like a bride with her accompanying musical instruments. In his *Guide for the Perplexed* (3:46), Maimonides suggests a reason for the musical accompaniment to some of the sacrificial offerings in the Temple when he asserts that music is most agreeable to the psychic faculty, the source of which is in the brain. Also in his *Guide* (3:45), he states that pleasantness of sound is a precondition for its effect on the soul.

Singing by the Levites in the Temple was an essential part of the offering of certain sacrifices, accompanied by the playing of musical instruments. In his *Mishneh Torah* (*Kelei Hamikdash* 3:3–6), Maimonides describes the Levites and their ministering, chanting, and playing of musical instruments including lyres, flutes, harps, trumpets, and cymbals. He also describes the chambers where the Levites kept their musical instruments (*Bet Ha-bechirah* 6:6–8), as well as the officers in the Temple appointed over the singers and over the instruments (ibid., 7:1). Finally, he provides a vivid portrayal of the rejoicing in the Temple during the Festival of Tabernacles, when fifes sounded and harps, lyres, and cymbals were played (*Lulav* 8:12–15), accompanied by singing, foot-stomping, hand-clapping, leaping, and dancing. This rejoicing was a supreme act of divine worship in accordance with Leviticus 23:40.

Maimonides discusses the prohibition against secular music now in effect, which was primarily imposed to limit joy since the destruction of the Temple and also to prevent frivolity and lewdness. He also wrote a lengthy responsum on music[2] in which he permits music therapy for medical therapeutic purposes and religious music for religious services, but prohibits music if used solely for secular purposes such as recreation and entertainment.

In summary, Maimonides prohibits listening to vocal and instrumental music as a sign of mourning following the destruction of the Temple, and because secular music leads to inappropriate gaiety, frivolity, and debauchery. Exceptions to this ban on music include festive occasions of a religious nature, such as weddings or the celebration of the Festival of Tabernacles. Another exception is the singing of praises and hymns to God, since the goals of such singing are to approach the Creator and to strive for moral perfection to know God.

On the other hand, Maimonides prescribes music therapy for the preservation of body health and for the cure of psychiatric illness such as melancholy. He recognizes the relationship of the soma to the psyche, and asserts that mental and physical health are dependent upon each other. Both are necessary to obtain wisdom and to strive for the acquisition of the knowledge of God. If music therapy is needed to achieve that goal, Maimonides permits it. He thus foresaw the modern medical demonstration that music therapy is useful for the treatment, rehabilitation, education, or training of people suffering from physical, mental, or emotional disorders.

---

1. F. Rosner, *Moses Maimonides' Three Treatises on Health* (Haifa: Maimonides Research Institute, 1990), pp. 117–174.

2. F. Rosner, "Moses Maimonides on Music Therapy and His Responsum on Music," *Journal of Jewish Music and Liturgy* XVI (1993–1994):1–16.

**MUSTARD**—In his *Mishneh Torah*, Maimonides considers mustard to be a detrimental food that should be consumed only in small amounts during the winter season (*Deot* 4:9). Yet, in his *Medical Aphorisms*,[1] he quotes Galen, who listed mustard among the humor-thinning vegetables (20:49). In his *Regimen on Health*,[2] hedge-mustard seeds are among many ingredients in a famous myrobalan electuary known as the Great Itrifal (Chapter 3:10–11). In his *Treatise on Asthma*,[3] Maimonides explains in detail the preparation of mustard into which bread may be dipped as a popular food in Spain (Chapter 4:6).

In his *Glossary of Drug Names*,[4] Maimonides describes the seed of black mustard (drug no. 400), which is used in medicine as a rubefacient and an irritant, and in cooking as a condiment. Wild mustard (drug no. 218) is said to be a type of culinary mustard. Another mustard's seed (drug no. 322) was extracted by means of vinegar and used medicinally as a rubefacient, irritant, and stimulant.

1. F. Rosner, *The Medical Aphorisms of Moses Maimonides* (Haifa: Maimonides Research Institute, 1989).

2. F. Rosner, *Moses Maimonides' Three Treatises on Health* (Haifa: Maimonides Research Institute, 1990).

3. F. Rosner, *Moses Maimonides' Treatise on Asthma* (Haifa: Maimonides Research Institute, 1994).

4. F. Rosner, *Moses Maimonides' Glossary of Drug Names* (Haifa: Maimonides Research Institute, 1995).

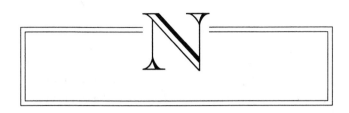

NATURE—Maimonides interprets "And the tables were the work of God" (Exod. 32:16) to mean that they were the product of nature, not art (*Guide for the Perplexed* 1:66) because all natural things are the work of the Lord, as in Psalms 107:24 and 104:16 and 24. In drawing a parallel between the universe and man, Maimonides writes that:

> In man there is a certain force which unites the members of the body, controls them, and gives to each of them what it requires for the conservation of its condition, and for the repulsion of injury—the physicians distinctly call it the leading force in the body of the living being; sometimes they call it "nature." The Universe likewise possesses a force which unites the several parts with each other, protects the species from destruction, maintains the individuals of each species as long as possible, and endows some individual beings with permanent existence. Whether this force operates through the medium of the sphere or otherwise remains an open question (*Guide* 1:72).

Maimonides quotes Aristotle, who says that none of the products of nature are due to chance (ibid., 2:20). In his introductory remarks to his exposition of the reasons for all the divine commandments (ibid., 3:34), Maimonides states that the Torah is a divine institution. Just as, in nature, the various forces produce benefits that are general but in some solitary cases may cause injury, so, too, the Torah is founded on that which is the rule, not the exception. It ignores the injury that may be caused to a single individual through a certain divine precept. There are people who are not perfected by the Torah, just as there are people who do not receive from nature all that they require.

NAUSEA—In his *Causes of Symptoms*,[1] Maimonides states that coriander consumed by itself after meals causes nausea and "destruction" of the food. If combined with other food, coriander apparently does no harm. In his *Medical Aphorisms*,[2]

Maimonides quotes Galen, who said that certain stomach ailments are associated with nausea (Chapter 2:21) and a rapid pulse (ibid., 4:20). A liver abscess may produce marked nausea (ibid., 6:57). To avoid nausea in both stomach and liver ailments, one should eat moderate-size portions so as not to overburden the stomach (ibid., 9:41). Marked nausea may also precede epileptic convulsions (ibid., 9:43). Other patients with nausea have illnesses of the spleen in which rust-colored humors pour from the spleen into the stomach (ibid., 9:44). Nausea associated with severe diarrhea should be treated with a diet containing astringent foods (ibid., 9:47). Nausea also develops in association with constipation. In that case, the patient should consume vegetables scented with oil and myrrh followed by pears, asparagus, or pomegranates (ibid., 9:55). [*See also* EMETICS]

1. F. Rosner, *Moses Maimonides' Three Treatises on Health* (Haifa: Maimonides Research Institute, 1990).

2. F. Rosner, *The Medical Aphorisms of Moses Maimonides* (Haifa: Maimonides Research Institute, 1989).

**NOSE**—In *Medical Aphorisms,*[1] Maimonides quotes Galen, who said that the nostrils represent the first organ for respiration (Chapter 3:22a). Nasal polyps are considered a chronic illness (ibid., 3:76) and sometimes require surgical excision (ibid., 15:23). Nasal polyps are also referred to as hemorrhoids of the nose (ibid., 23:74). If the nasal bone is broken, it should be bandaged, and it heals and unites in ten days (ibid., 15:62). A mucous discharge from the nose should be treated with inhalation medications (ibid., 9:6). Catarrh of the nose (coryza) is also discussed by Maimonides in *Regimen on Health,*[2] where he warns people to be careful about such nasal catarrhs (Chapter 4:12–13).

In *Mishneh Torah*, Maimonides enumerates several physical blemishes of the nose that render priests unfit to serve in the Temple, such as a pierced, slit, or nicked nose (*Biyat Mikdash* 7:6). Other such blemishes include a flat nose (see Leviticus 21:18), a nose protruding upward, a nose tip turned downward, a nose bent sideways, or an excessively small or large nose (*Biyat Mikdash* 8:7). Certain nasal blemishes also render animals unfit to be offered in the Temple (*Issurei Mizbe'ach* 2:2).

Nosebleeding is discussed in the section EPISTAXIS. [*See also* SNEEZING]

1. F. Rosner, *The Medical Aphorisms of Moses Maimonides* (Haifa: Maimonides Research Institute, 1989).

2. F. Rosner, *Moses Maimonides' Three Treatises on Health* (Haifa: Maimonides Research Institute, 1990).

*NUTRITION*—In his *Medical Aphorisms*, Maimonides, citing Galen, devotes an entire chapter to foods and beverages and their usages.[1] He begins by summarizing the importance of nutrition in both health and disease, and then elaborates on the efficacy of certain foods. He continues with descriptions of the properties and characteristics of many foods, such as fruits, grains, meats, and others. Then follows a lengthy quotation on dietetics from Abu Marwan Ibn Zuhr, one of Maimonides' teachers, in which the therapeutic efficacy of chicken, chicken soup, and other fowl is described.[2] Maimonides states that chicken soup neutralizes body constitution. Chicken soup is not only an excellent food, but also a medication for the beginning of leprosy, and it fattens the body substance of the emaciated and those convalescing from illness. Turtledoves increase memory, improve the intellect, and sharpen the senses.

In his *Treatise on Poisons*,[3] Maimonides recommends soups made from bread, oil, and butter for someone who has swallowed poison. The victim should also eat figs, nuts, pistachios, hazelnuts, garlic, onions, and rice. He also prescribes a dietary regimen for someone bitten by a snake or a rabid dog. Nutritional advice and dietary guidelines are found throughout Maimonides' medical treatises, especially *Treatises on Health*.[4]

In his legal code, the *Mishneh Torah*, he says that fig cakes or dried figs spoil if put in brine (*Terumot* 11:3). Boiling wine reduces it (ibid., 11:4). Soaking onions in vinegar spoils the vinegar (ibid.). Stems of figs and watermelon rinds have no food value (ibid., 11:10). Fenugreek and bitter vetch are unfit for human consumption (ibid., 12:7). The various fruits and vegetables that require tithing are enumerated by Maimonides (*Maaser* 2:5). First fruits must be brought to the Temple (*Bikkurim* 2:1). If one is seriously ill, another person may bring them to Jerusalem (ibid., 4:8).

Any foodstuff that is set apart as human food, such as bread, meat, grapes, olives, and the like, is susceptible to uncleanness (*Tumat Ochlin* 1:1) if it is first rendered moist by one of the following seven liquids: water, dew, oil, wine, milk, blood, or honey (ibid. 1:2). Flavors and spices, such as costus, amomum, crowfoot, asafetida, black pepper, and lozenges of safflower, do not contract uncleanness because they are not foodstuffs, but merely add flavor to food (ibid., 1:6). Dill is eaten for its own sake, but is also used to flavor other foods (ibid., 1:7); the same applies to dates or dried figs (ibid., 1:8). Many other foods and flavorings are cited by Maimonides, including mustard, lupines, olives, and other pickled foodstuffs (ibid., 1:15–16).

Finally, in his *Mishnah Commentary*,[5] Maimonides states that vegetables such as cabbage and beets may be eaten cooked or raw (*Berachot* 6:1). People drink brine to counteract the constipating effect of certain foods and fruits (ibid., 6:7). Meat cooked with turnips, but not other vegetables, imparts its taste to the turnips (*Chullin* 7:4), but nerves cooked with meat do not give any taste to the meat (ibid., 7:5).

Maimonides asserts that Jews eat garlic on Fridays because it is an aphrodisiac (*Nedarim* 3:8, 4:8, and 8:6). Fish, milk products, and spiced eggs were withheld from the High Priest on the eve of the Day of Atonement because these foods increase semen production and may stimulate an erection. Maimonides also speaks of oats, eggs, cucumbers, and other cooked dishes that have nutritional value (*Nedarim* 6:1ff and 7:1–2). He also discusses the seasons of the year and their relationship to the ripening of fruits and vegetables (ibid., 9:2–3). Yellow roots of the crocus plant are used by physicians (*Shebi'it* 7:1). The Babylonians ate shewbread raw without baking it because they had strong stomachs (*Menachot* 11:7).

---

1. F. Rosner, *The Medical Aphorisms of Moses Maimonides* (Haifa: Maimonides Research Institute, 1989), pp. 293–312.

2. F. Rosner, "Therapeutic Efficacy of Chicken Soup," *Chest*, 78 (1980): 671–674.

3. F. Rosner, *Maimonides' Treatises on Poisons, Hemorrhoids and Cohabita-*

*tion* (Haifa: Maimonides Research Institute, 1984), pp. 73–76.

4. F. Rosner, *Moses Maimonides' Three Treatises on Health* (Haifa: Maimonides Research Institute, 1990).

5. F. Rosner, "Medicine in Moses Maimonides' Commentary on the Mishnah," *Koroth*, 9 (1988):565–578.

**NUTS**—In his *Treatise on Asthma*,[1] Maimonides describes the virtues and detriments of a variety of foods. He recommends that one avoid gas-producing foods such as beans, peas, rice, lentils, and nuts (Chapter 3:3). An excellent remedy for asthmatic patients, however, is the consumption of pistachio nuts and almonds at the end of a meal since they liquefy phlegm and cleanse the lungs (ibid., 3:10). Also helpful for asthmatics is an opium potion containing numerous ingredients, including completely ripe white, fresh nuts (ibid., 12:4). A variety of nuts are described by Maimonides in his *Glossary of Drug Names*.[2] These include edible nuts, Cypress nuts, metel nuts, elkaya nuts, Sudanese nuts, and the cocoa nut (Section 82). Also discussed are the aromatic nut (nutmeg) (Section 71), the bonduc nut (Section 355), gall-nuts (Section 295), hazelnuts (Section 43), Oriental cashew nuts (Section 62), and areca nuts (Section 311).

In his *Extracts from Galen*,[3] Maimonides recommends the green gallnut as a remedy to heal a wound (p. 44) and to benefit patients who have suffered massive hemorrhage (p. 61). In his *Medical Aphorisms*,[4] he quotes Galen, who describes the King's nut (walnut) and the small nut known as the hazelnut (Chapter 23:102).

1. F. Rosner, *Moses Maimonides' Treatise on Asthma* (Haifa: Maimonides Research Institute, 1994).

2. F. Rosner, *Moses Maimonides' Glossary of Drug Names* (Haifa: Maimonides Research Institute, 1995).

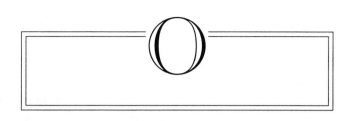

OBESITY—In his *Medical Apho-risms*,[1] Maimonides quotes Galen, who said that obesity is caused by the body flesh drawing most of the blood to it (Chapter 7:18). Obesity is harmful to the body and makes it sluggish, disturbs its functions, and hinders its movements. Therefore, obese people should walk in the sun and bathe in the sea to lose weight, since ocean air causes dissolution of liquids. They should eat foods with little nourishment, such as vegetables, sea fish, and lean meats (ibid., 9:101). Bloodletting should be avoided in people who are extremely obese (ibid., 12:5).

In his *Treatise on Asthma*,[2] Maimonides describes the Sultan as "intermediate between leanness and stoutness," which is helpful because obesity is detrimental to patients with asthma. Maimonides quotes Hippocrates, who said that stoutness or obesity in physical laborers may be dangerous to their health.[3] In his *Extracts from Galen*,[4] Maimonides describes an extensive regimen to treat obesity, including exercise, diet, bathing, and certain medications.

1. F. Rosner, *The Medical Aphorisms of Moses Maimonides* (Haifa: Maimonides Research Institute, 1989).

2. F. Rosner, *Moses Maimonides' Treatise on Asthma* (Haifa: Maimonides Research Institute, 1994), pp. 43–44 and 51.

3. F. Rosner, *Maimonides' Commentary on the Aphorisms of Hippocrates* (Haifa: Maimonides Research Institute, 1987), p. 125.

4. U.S. Barzel, *Maimonides' The Art of Cure. Extracts from Galen* (Haifa: Maimonides Research Institute, 1992), pp. 175–176.

ONIONS—In both his *Mishneh Torah* (*Deot* 4:9) and his *Regimen of Health*[1] (Chapter 1:11), Maimonides includes onions among the detrimental vegetables that one should consume only in small quantities, if at all. The Talmud had already asserted that certain types of onion are bad for the body (*Kiddushin* 62a), whereas others are good (*Nedarim* 66a). In his *Treatise on Asthma*,[2] Maimonides advises that one avoid consuming onions because they produce gas, or flatulence, and also increase heat (Chapter 3:3). However, a good remedy for a patient with a moist body and a phlegmatic constitution is an ounce of oxymel in onion together with an ounce of syrup of roses cooked in honey (ibid., 9:14). One form of onion was used as a rat poison and a skin vesicant, as described in Maimonides' *Glossary of Drug Names*[3] (Section 60), where he also discusses a small species of edible onion imported from Syria into Egypt (Section 61). In his *Medical Aphorisms*,[4] Maimonides quotes the Arabic physician Al Tamimi, who said that the inhalation of the aroma of a cut onion during the drinking of a purgative medication prevents vomiting (Chapter 13:54). Galen is quoted to have said that drinking onion vinegar and onion juice preserves one's health, even if one has unhealthy customs and practices (ibid., 17:24).

---

1. F. Rosner, *Moses Maimonides' Three Treatises on Health* (Haifa: Maimonides Research Institute, 1990).

2. F. Rosner, *Moses Maimonides' Treatise on Asthma* (Haifa: Maimonides Research Institute, 1994).

3. F. Rosner, *Moses Maimonides' Glossary of Drug Names* (Haifa: Maimonides Research Institute, 1995).

4. F. Rosner, *The Medical Aphorisms of Moses Maimonides* (Haifa: Maimonides Research Institute, 1989).

**OPHTHALMOLOGY**—Throughout the twenty-five chapters of his *Medical Aphorisms*,[1] and in his *Extracts from Galen*,[2] Maimonides quotes Galen's pronouncements dealing with the anatomy, physiology, pathology, and diseases of the eye, and remedies for them. Some of Hippocrates' aphorisms on ophthalmology are also cited by Maimonides.[3] Maimonides' own statements about the eyes, eye ailments, and their treatment are found in his *Treatise on Asthma*[4] and *Treatises on Health*.[5] Finally, in his *Mishneh Torah*, he discusses abnormalities of the eyes, eyebrows, eyelids, and eyelashes in humans and animals, and the treatment of serious eye ailments on the Sabbath and Jewish holidays.[6]

---

1. F. Rosner, "Ophthalmology in the Medical Aphorisms of Moses Maimonides," *New York State Journal of Medicine*, 74 (1974):699–703. ·

2. U.S. Barzel, *Maimonides' The Art of Cure. Extracts from Galen* (Haifa: Maimonides Research Institute, 1992).

3. F. Rosner, *Maimonides' Commentary on the Aphorisms of Hippocrates* (Haifa: Maimonides Research Institute, 1987).

4. F. Rosner, *Moses Maimonides' Treatise on Asthma* (Haifa: Maimonides Research Institute, 1994).

5. F. Rosner, *Moses Maimonides' Three Treatises on Health* (Haifa: Maimonides Research Institute, 1990).

6. F. Rosner, *Medicine in the Mishneh Torah of Maimonides* (New York: Ktav, 1984).

ORTHOPEDICS—In his *Medical Aphorisms*, Maimonides discusses fractures of various bones—including the nose, maxilla, clavicle, thigh, and calf bones—the time for healing, and the treatment of fractures.[1] He speaks of splints, bandages, casts, and cushioning. Most of these aphorisms are based on the writings of Galen. Further discussion of broken bones and their healing is found in Maimonides' *Extracts from Galen*.[2]

In his *Mishneh Torah*, Maimonides seems to be describing the healing of a fracture with callus formation when he says that marrow within a bone causes the bone, when injured, to heal on the outside (*Tumat Met* 2:5). He forbids manipulation of the vertebrae of an infant's spine on the Sabbath (*Shabbat* 22:26), perhaps an early reference to chiropractic. Compound fractures in animals render them nonkosher (*Shechitah* 8:12).

---

1. F. Rosner, *The Medical Aphorisms of Moses Maimonides* (Haifa: Maimonides Research Institute, 1989), pp. 255–257.
2. U.S. Barzel, *Maimonides' The Art of Cure. Extracts from Galen* (Haifa: Maimonides Research Institute, 1992), pp. 80–82.

OXYMEL—Oxymel is a medicinal drink made of vinegar and honey that is frequently cited in the Talmud and in Maimonides' medical writings. In his *Treatise on Asthma*,[1] he recommends it for people with moist or phlegmatic constitutions (Chapter 9:14) and for patients with asthma (ibid., 12:1). In his *Medical Aphorisms*,[2] Maimonides quotes Galen, who said that oxymel followed by barley gruel opens the excretory passages (Chapter 8:24 and 8:26). Oxymel is usually prepared with three parts honey to one part vinegar, although a sweeter mixture contains seven parts honey to one part vinegar (ibid., 21:23). It is cooked until well mixed and some of the foam is removed, and is used as either a food or a medication (ibid., 21:24). It is the most appropriate of sweetening things in a simple diet, does not produce harmful humors, and does not harm the stomach (ibid., 21:25). The oxymel beverage, cooked in bitter-vetch soup and imbibed daily on an empty stomach, prevents chest pain and abscesses of internal organs (ibid., 21:26). If used excessively, oxymel produces diarrhea, cough, and nerve damage (ibid., 21:27).

In his *Regimen on Health*,[3] Maimonides reiterates oxymel's value as a good nutritional component of a healthy diet, as well as being good for sick people in general (Chapter 2:7 and 2:9). In his *Causes of Symptoms*, he proposes to purge the Sultan's body by means of medicines and diet including oxymel, hydromel (bees' honey and fine white wine), and the famous ox-tongue concoction. Maimonides emphasizes the importance of drinking wine for better digestion, purer blood, and the inducing of sound sleep. As an alternative to wine, which is forbidden in the Moslem religion, he offers the oxymel drink (Sections 7, 20, 21). Numerous references to oxymel are also found in his *Extracts from Galen*.[4]

1. F. Rosner, *Moses Maimonides' Treatise on Asthma* (Haifa: Maimonides Research Institute, 1994).

2. F. Rosner, *The Medical Aphorisms of Moses Maimonides* (Haifa: Maimonides Research Institute, 1989).

3. F. Rosner, *Moses Maimonides' Three Treatises on Health* (Haifa: Maimonides Research Institute, 1990).

4. U.S. Barzel, *Maimonides' The Art of Cure. Extracts from Galen* (Haifa: Maimonides Research Institute, 1992).

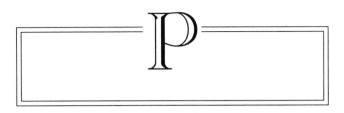

PAIN—In his *Medical Aphorisms*,[1] Maimonides quotes Galen, who said that urinary bladder pains are stronger than uterine pains (Chapter 1:69). An enflamed muscle can be painful (ibid., 3:64). Pain in both temporal muscles may lead to convulsions, fever, stupor, and delirium (ibid., 3:77), seemingly a description of severe temporal arteritis. The pleuritic chest pain of pneumonia (ibid., 6:54), the epigastric pain of diaphragmatic irritation (ibid., 6:53), the right-sided pain of hepatitis (ibid., 6:55), the pain of inflammation of veins or arteries (ibid., 6:62), stomach and intestinal pain (ibid., 7:65), headache (ibid., 6:59 and 9:25), earache (ibid., 9:27), and eye pain (ibid., 12:38) are all described. A variety of medications, including narcotics, to relieve pain are cited (ibid., 8:38–39). The cause of many types of pain was thought to be an excess, or an abnormal combination, of humors (ibid., 7:19).

In his *Commentary on the Aphorisms of Hippocrates* ,[2] Maimonides states that if sleep produces pain in a patient, it is a deadly prognostic sign (Section 2:1). Pain can occur in patients because of an abscess, an ulcer, a fracture, or a contusion (ibid., 2:6). Pain and fever occur more during the development of an abscess than when it is already formed because the abscess forms pus and the pain intensifies (ibid., 2:47). A lengthy discussion of pain is found in Maimonides' *Extracts from Galen*[3] where he states that

The reasons for pain are separation of connections or any quick change which is loathsome to the organ and harmful to it. If the change is introduced gradually it does not hurt. Organs that normally have no sensitivity do not produce any pain. Therefore, if a strong pain appears one must search for its cause whether it is due to a large quantity of humors or to gases that do not find escape or to a bad tumor or to burning moisture or to a dry bad constitution which causes swelling. It may also be due to something which is warming strongly or cooling strongly. One also has to establish whether it is possible to eliminate the cause of the pain itself, which is then not a treatment of the symptom but a treatment of the sickness itself, and which thus alleviates the pain (Chapter 12).

One treats such pains from gases by applying softening foods and drinks, enemas, bandages, ointments, and aromatic baths. If the pain is due to a tumor, the tumor must be cured. If the pain is due to burning moisture (i.e., humors), the damaging substances must be emptied. If that is not possible, one may use analgesic medications (ibid.). For certain pains, cupping glasses and even phlebotomy are recommended.

---

1. F. Rosner, *The Medical Aphorisms of Moses Maimonides* (Haifa: Maimonides Research Institute, 1989).

2. F. Rosner, *Maimonides' Commentary on the Aphorisms of Hippocrates* (Haifa: Maimonides Research Institute, 1987).

3. U.S. Barzel, *Maimonides' The Art of Cure. Extracts from Galen* (Haifa: Maimonides Research Institute, 1992).

*PARALYSIS*—In his *Commentary on the Aphorisms of Hippocrates*,[1] Maimonides comments on a patient with apoplexy, or stroke, as follows: "Every paralysis results from the inability of the spirit of life to pass into the body below the head because of obstruction" from a brain abscess or from white humors filling the brain chambers (Section 2:42). He also states that both epilepsy and paralysis are produced by cold, thick humors (ibid., 2:45). He disputes Galen's assertion that apoplexy and hemiplegia are due to black bile; rather, they occur from white humor and mostly in people over sixty years of age (ibid., 6:57).

In his *Medical Aphorisms*,[2] Maimonides quotes Galen, who said that catarrhs (i.e., humors) that descend from the head may cause hemiplegia (Chapter 3:66). Patients who ingest bad foods may be struck with paralysis until they vomit up that which presses on the stomach (ibid., 9:43), perhaps a form of food poisoning that is due to a neurotoxin. Paralysis and paresis are defined, respectively, as complete cessation or diminution of voluntary activities of the limbs (ibid., 23:22–23). In his *Regimen of Health*,[3] Maimonides states that if the brain retains its superfluities, hemiplegia, facial paralysis, or paralysis agitans (Parkinson's disease?) may develop (Chapter 4:11). [*See also* APOPLEXY, NERVES, and BRAIN]

---

1. F. Rosner, *Maimonides' Commentary on the Aphorisms of Hippocrates* (Haifa: Maimonides Research Institute, 1987).

2. F. Rosner, *The Medical Aphorisms of Moses Maimonides* (Haifa: Maimonides Research Institute, 1989).

3. F. Rosner, *Moses Maimonides' Three Treatises on Health* (Haifa: Maimonides Research Institute, 1990).

*PATHOPHYSIOLOGY*—The twenty-third chapter of Maimonides' *Medical Aphorisms* attempts to elucidate some of the mechanisms or pathophysiology of well-known illnesses, and also to define and explain various technical terms used in medicine.[1] Maimonides first speaks of plethora or hypertonia as representing an excess of blood. Rusty [hyperbilirubinemic] blood is distinguished from watery [anemic] blood. The differences between chyle and chyme, epidemic and pandemic, shaking and trembling, paralysis and paresis, continuous fever and intermittent fever, inflammation and abscess, carbuncle and furuncle, and many others are described. He recognizes that pitting and nonpitting edema represent different signs of illness. Thus he states: "The difference between a swelling [edema] and soft inflammation is that if one presses on a swelling with one's hand, it will not remain depressed. . . . If one presses on the loin of a patient with soft inflammation, it remains depressed and sunken." Further terms, such as varicocele and hydrocele, intestinal hernia and omental hernia, stupor and lethargy, benign ulcer and malignant ulcer, amnesia, melancholia, amentia, and others are discussed. Astonishingly accurate descriptions of conjunctivitis, trachoma, and other ophthalmological diseases are found in this chapter [*see* OPHTHALMOLOGY].

Asthma, a disease concerning which Maimonides wrote a separate essay,[2] is concisely and precisely described: "If someone has rapid breathing . . . without his being febrile, then physicians have long been accustomed to call this occurrence asthma. They also named it upright breathing because the patient with this ailment has an erect chest, during respiration. This illness arises because of constriction that occurs in the chest and abdomen. . . ." Various gastrointestinal and genitourinary illnesses and technical terms are delineated. The chapter ends with a consideration of certain nutriments and drugs and their effects on the human body.

1. F. Rosner, *The Medical Aphorisms of Moses Maimonides* (Haifa: Maimonides Research Institute, 1989), pp. 356–382.
2. F. Rosner, *Moses Maimonides' Treatise on Asthma* (Haifa: Maimonides Research Institute, 1994).

*PATIENT'S OBLIGATION TO SEEK HEALING*—Numerous talmudic citations indicate that patients are allowed, even required, to seek medical attention. Thus, it is said that one who is in pain should go to a physician (*Baba Kamma* 46b); that if one is bitten by a snake, a physician is called even on the Sabbath because all restrictions are set aside in the event of possible danger to human life (*Yoma* 83b). If one's eye is afflicted, one may prepare and apply medication even on the Sabbath (*Abodah Zarah* 28b). Rabbi Judah the Prince, compiler of the *Mishnah*, suffered from an eye ailment and consulted his physician, Mar Samuel, who cured the ailment by placing a vial of chemicals under the rabbi's pillow so that the powerful vapors would penetrate (*Baba Metzia* 85b). In the case of bodily injury, if the offender tells the victim that he will bring a physician who will heal for no fee, the victim can object, saying: "A physician who heals for nothing is worth nothing" (*Baba Kamma* 85a). In Jewish tradition, the patient is obligated to care for his health and life. He is charged with preserving his health. He must eat, drink, and sustain himself, and must seek healing when he is ill in order to be able to serve the Lord in a state of good health. Several biblical precepts are the basis for this mandate (Lev. 18:5; Deut. 4:15).

The strongest evidence in Jewish sources that a patient is mandated to seek healing from a physician is found in Maimonides' *Mishneh Torah*, where he states that "a person should set his heart that his body be healthy and strong in order that his soul be upright to know the Lord. For it is impossible for man to understand and comprehend the wisdoms [of the world] if he is hungry and ailing or if one of his limbs is aching" (*Deot* 3:3).

Maimonides also states (*Deot* 4:23), as does the Talmud (*Sanhedrin* 17b), that no wise person should re-

side in a city that has no physician. Maimonides' position is further expanded and codified in his discussion of preventive medicine (*Deot* 4:1ff). The maintenance of one's health requires Jews to avoid harmful food and activities and to prevent danger wherever possible. Environmental factors such as clean air and sunshine, which affect one's health, are important. One must observe rules of personal hygiene such as hand-washing before eating. Diet, exercise, sex, and bodily functions must all be tended to as outlined by Maimonides.[1]

---

1. F. Rosner, "Moses Maimonides and Preventive Medicine," *Journal of the History of Medicine and Allied Sciences*, 51 (July 1996), pp. 313–324.

**PHTHISIS**—The terms phthisis and consumption, used often in Maimonides' medical writings, refer to a chronic, sometimes fatal, illness of the lungs, perhaps tuberculosis. In his *Medical Aphorisms*,[1] Maimonides quotes Galen, who describes patients dying of phthisis (Chapters 4:100 and 8:58). Clubbing of the fingers, a well-known physical sign in certain pulmonary diseases, including phthisis, is accurately described (ibid., 6:51). Phthisis involving the brain (tuberculous meningitis?) is also discussed (ibid., 10:60). In his *Commentary on the Aphorisms of Hippocrates*,[2] Maimonides characterizes phthisis as a chronic lung disease associated with fever, particularly at night (Section 1:12). Hemoptysis may occur in young patients with phthisis (ibid., 3:29). Patients with phthisis with narrow passages of their lungs should not be given emetics lest they aspirate and asphyxiate (ibid., 4:8). Phthisis occurs mostly in young people (ibid., 5:9). Patients with phthisis who develop diarrhea (tubercular enteritis?) will soon die (ibid., 5:12 and 14). Following hemoptysis, if a patient spits up pus, his phthisis is invariably fatal (ibid., 7:15–16).

In his *Extracts from Galen*,[3] Maimonides writes that hectic fever and consumption may appear in a patient with a hot and dry bad constitution of the lung. Externally applied medicines should wet and cool. Vinegar mixed with water is suitable, as are ointments containing vinegar. A patient with hectic fever and consumption benefits from brief immersion in a hot bath followed by bathing in cold water. The body is then dried with a soft towel and anointed with oil. The patient should be fed wet, cold foods like cold barley groats and spelt wheat boiled in water with leek, aneth, salt, oil, and vinegar. If the fever is prolonged and persistent, one gives the patient fresh milk from a she-ass. Honey must be avoided in patients with hectic fever (pp. 121–126). These measures, which antedated the modern practice of chemotherapy for tuberculo-

sis, were said to be efficacious in some patients. In his *Treatise on Asthma*,[4] Maimonides said that Galen even recommended enemas with linseed sap for patients with consumption because it calms the bad humors (Chapter 9:8).

---

1. F. Rosner, *The Medical Aphorisms of Moses Maimonides* (Haifa: Maimonides Research Institute, 1989).

2. F. Rosner, *Maimonides' Commentary on the Aphorisms of Hippocrates* (Haifa: Maimonides Research Institute, 1987).

3. U.S. Barzel, *Maimonides' The Art of Cure. Extracts from Galen* (Haifa: Maimonides Research Institute, 1992).

4. F. Rosner, *Moses Maimonides' Treatise on Asthma* (Haifa: Maimonides Research Institute, 1994).

---

*PHYSICIAN TREATING HIS PARENTS*—Honoring and revering one's parents is an important biblical commandment described and explained by Maimonides in some detail in his *Mishneh Torah* (*Mamrim* 6:1ff). Cursing or wounding one's father or mother is biblically proscribed, based on Leviticus 20:9 and Exodus 21:15, respectively. Maimonides gives an example of wounding one's father: He who struck his father over the ear so that he became deaf is liable and is put to death because it is impossible to cause deafness without inflicting a wound (*Mamrim* 5:6). Maimonides then cites the mechanism that produced the deafness: A drop of blood got into the ear and led to deafness. However, if a man lets blood from his father, or if he is a physician and cuts off flesh or a limb from his father, he is exempt. But although he is exempt after the fact, he should not do so; nor should he remove a thorn from his father or mother lest he inflict a wound (ibid., 5:7). However, if he is the only one available and his parent is in pain, he may let blood or operate if his parent allows him to do so.

**PHYSICIAN'S LIABILITY**—If a physician intentionally injures a patient, he is obviously liable. If an injury to the patient occurs following an error on the part of the physician, he is held blameless, provided that he is an expert or experienced physician and is licensed to practice by the community authorities. This rule is enunciated by Maimonides in *Mishneh Torah* in relation to the laws of flogging. If a sinner is liable to flogging, his physical strength first must be assessed to estimate how many stripes he is capable of enduring (*Sanhedrin* 17:1). The maximum number is thirty-nine for a robust person, but is reduced in the case of a frail man. If the culprit dies under the hand of the attendant, the attendant is exempt. Similarly, a physician who unintentionally causes physical harm to a patient is placed in the same privileged category as the court official administering corporal punishment; that is to say, the physician is exempt, provided that he is authorized by the court.

**PHYSICIAN'S OBLIGATION TO HEAL**—Maimonides derives the license and obligation for a physician to heal from the scriptural commandment concerning the restoration of lost property (Deut. 22:2). In his *Mishnah Commentary* (*Nedarim* 4:4), he states that this law also includes the restoration of a person's health. His reasoning is based on the Talmud (*Sanhedrin* 73a), which requires a Jew to intervene to save a person's life and health. A physician who refuses to heal the sick with resultant adverse effects on the patient is guilty of transgressing the biblical injunction against "standing idly by the blood of one's neighbor" (Lev. 19:16). This rule is codified by Maimonides in his *Mishneh Torah* (*Rotzeach* 1:14).

In his biblical commentary known as *Torah Temimah*, Rabbi Baruch Halevi Epstein asks why Maimonides fails to invoke the phrase "and heal he shall heal" (Exod. 21:19) as a warrant for the physician to heal. He answers that the phrase in Exodus merely grants permission for a physician to heal, whereas "And thou shalt restore it to him" (Deut. 22:2) makes it obligatory for the physician to heal.

174

**PHYSICIAN'S PRAYER**—The *Physician's Prayer* attributed to Moses Maimonides[1] is a lofty and beautiful prayer that contains moral and ethical standards by which a physician should conduct his professional life. The daily recitation of this prayer serves to remind the physician of these standards, which represent the highest code of medical philanthropy and professional ethics. The prayer was first published anonymously in 1783 in a German periodical called *Deutsches Museum* (vol. 1, pp. 43–45) with the title "Daily Prayer of a Physician Before He Visits His Patients, from the Hebrew Manuscript of a Renowned Jewish Physician in Egypt from the Twelfth Century." The first Hebrew version of the prayer was published in 1790 by Isaac Euchel in *Ha-Me'assef* (vol. 6, pp. 242–244). The title of Euchel's paper indicates that Marcus Herz was the author of the prayer and that Euchel translated it from German into Hebrew at Herz's request. The style, phrasing, and concepts in the 1783 text of the prayer are incompatible with medieval authorship. A phrase such as "Art is great, but the mind of man is ever expanding" is typical and characteristic of eighteenth-century Europe, and is at variance with Maimonidean medieval thinking. Here is the idea of progress, which became even more popular in the nineteenth century. Further evidence for an eighteenth-century author lies in the phrase "Act unceasingly and harmoniously to preserve the whole in all its beauty." This concept of "beauty," or *das Schone*, is characteristic of German literature of the Enlightenment. Moreover, such a phrase as "ten thousand times in ten thousand organs hast Thou combined" presupposed knowledge of the newer sciences of anatomy, biology, and microscopy. The tensions between colleagues discussed in the prayer are also products of a more modern period and are dictated by the new academic hierarchy that arose in the eighteenth century. It is thus evident that the *Physician's Prayer* attributed to Moses Maimonides is a fake, and was probably authored by Marcus Herz in Germany in 1783.[2] A number of other spurious works falsely attributed to Maimonides have recently been published in English.[3,4]

1. H. Friedenwald, "Daily Prayer of a Physician," *Bulletin of the Johns Hopkins Hospital*, 28 (1917):256–261.

2. F. Rosner, "The Physician's Prayer Attributed to Moses Maimonides," *Bulletin of the History of Medicine*, 41 (1967):440–454.

3. F. Rosner, *Six Treatises Attributed to Maimonides* (Northvale, NJ: Jason Aronson, 1991).

4. F. Rosner, *The Existence and Unity of God. Three Treatises Attributed to Moses Maimonides* (Northvale, NJ: Jason Aronson, 1990).

**PHYSIOLOGY**—In Maimonides' *Medical Aphorisms*,[1] the physiology of respiration and the relationship of the diaphragm and accessory muscles of respiration are vividly and accurately described: "The diaphragm alone is responsible for the ease of inhalation and exhalation. However, when exhalation becomes difficult, then intercostal muscles, pectoral muscles, shoulder and neck muscles participate as well." The physiology of sleep is compared to one's state of mentation during intoxication.

Maimonides hints at the lesser (pulmonary) circulation by emphasizing the connection between the right ventricle and the lung when he states: "The right chamber of the two chambers of the heart was created for the benefit of the lung. . . . Should the lung die, the right chamber of the two chambers of the heart also dies." He also subscribes to the three Galenical phases of digestion to explain the physiology of nutrition, and adds a fourth of his own. "The first stage is digestion in the stomach. . . . The second stage is the transition to the intestines where it adds to . . . the liver substance. The third stage . . . the metabolism that occurs in every one of the organs . . . there is an additional metabolic phase, a fourth, which is called assimilation." The development of individual organs, as well as the human organism as a whole, is dependent upon several forces, the procreating force (*vis generationis*), the developmental force (*vis alterationis*), the structure-forming force (*virtus efformatrix*), the growth force (*virtus anctrix*), and the nutritive force (*virtus nutrex*). The nutritive force is composed of four powers: attraction, retention, expulsion, and alteration (digestion or assimilation or metabolism).

The ancient concept of physiology dealing with the four humors—white bile (phlegm), red bile (blood), yellow bile, and black (melancholy) bile—is discussed. The sites of production of these various substances are described, and their various characteristics are outlined. Blood is considered the best, and black bile is the worst. Disease consists of derangements in the normal qualities, quantities, or interrelationships of the body humors. Maimonides, quoting Galen, states that "the illnesses which occur as a result of black bile are: cancer, elephant skin, psoriasis, quartan fever, confusion [depression], and thickness of the spleen." Additional discussions of physiology and pathophysiology are found throughout Maimonides' medical writings, his *Mishnah Commentary*,[2] and his *Mishneh Torah*.[3]

---

1. F. Rosner, *The Medical Aphorisms of Moses Maimonides* (Haifa: Maimonides Research Institute, 1989), pp. 26–33.

2. F. Rosner, "Medicine in Moses Maimonides' Commentary on the Mishnah," *Koroth*, 9 (1988):565–578.

3. F. Rosner, *Medicine in the Mishneh Torah of Maimonides* (New York: Ktav, 1984).

**PNEUMONIA**—In his *Commentary on the Aphorisms of Hippocrates*,[1] Maimonides confirms that pleuritis and pneumonia occur more commonly in the winter months (Section 3:23), affect people of all ages (ibid., 3:30), and are usually associated with fever (ibid., 4:48) and expectoration of pus (ibid., 5:8). He asserts that pleurisy occurs mostly as a result of a thin humor that involves the membrane that covers the rib internally (i.e., the pleura) (ibid., 6:33).

In his *Medical Aphorisms*,[2] Maimonides quotes Galen, who accurately describes the signs and symptoms of pneumonia as follows: acute fever, sticking (i.e., pleuritic) chest pain in the side, short rapid breaths, serrated pulse, and cough mostly associated with sputum (Chapter 6:54). In pleurisy, pain in the scapula is due to stretching of the pleura (ibid., 7:54). Therapy for pneumonia consists of venesection, warm compresses, and soft stools (ibid., 9:81). The compresses should be hot if the patient is expectorating phlegm; otherwise, it should be lukewarm (ibid., 9:83). One should avoid venesection in patients with pneumonia owing to bitter, black, or viscous humors in which the patient spits up blood (ibid., 9:84). Pneumonia usually has an acute onset and a short course (ibid., 11:25). Bathing is beneficial for patients with pleurisy and pneumonia (ibid., 19:25–26). Milk mixed with honey is valuable for pain in the chest and the lung (ibid., 21:17).

---

1. F. Rosner, *Maimonides' Commentary on the Aphorisms of Hippocrates* (Haifa: Maimonides Research Institute, 1987).
2. F. Rosner, *The Medical Aphorisms of Moses Maimonides* (Haifa: Maimonides Research Institute, 1989).

**POISONS**—Maimonides wrote an entire *Treatise on Poisons and Their Antidotes*,[1] which is described elsewhere in this encyclopedia. Discussions of poisons and poisoning are also found in several other Maimonidean works. In his *Medical Aphorisms*,[2] he quotes Galen, who compares patients with acutely occurring and rapidly fatal illnesses to a person who ingests poison or is bitten by a viper (Chapter 3:65). Syncope or collapse may occur if a person ingests a poisonous substance or is bitten by a poisonous snake (ibid., 7:14). The bite of a scorpion produces extremely severe complications because the poison affects nerves, arteries, and veins, and can reach into the depths of the body (ibid., 9:109). Suction cups or direct sucking at the bite site may sometimes remove the poison (ibid., 9:119). Milk, garlic, boiled wine, vinegar, and salt are of value against poisons, depending on the type of poison, plant, or mineral toxin and the particular situation (ibid., 21: 35–36). Other antidotes against poisonings include the Great Theriac (ibid., 21:50–51). Antidotes are of two types: Those that neutralize the poison and render it harmless, and those that expel the poison from the body (ibid., 21:48). In his *Extracts from Galen*,[3] Maimonides states that the aim in treating pain caused by an animal bite or insect sting is to eliminate the poison from the body with cauterizing medications, or cupping glasses, or hollow horns and then treat the pain (p. 156).

The Talmud (*Pesachim* 56a) describes six acts performed by the righteous King Hezekiah of Israel without the prior consent of the sages, three of which they approved and three of which they disapproved. One of the acts that met with the sages' approval was the concealment of the "Book of Remedies." The identity of this book, its authorship, and the possible reasons for its concealment by King Hezekiah are discussed elsewhere.[4] Maimonides gives two reasons. He states that the book contained remedies based on astrological phenomena and magical incantations that might lead people to use them for idolatrous purposes (*Guide for the Perplexed* 3:37), which is why Hezekiah concealed it. Second, Maimonides states that the book contained prescriptions for the preparation of poisons and their antidotes. When corrupt people used this information to kill their enemies by poisoning, Hezekiah concealed the book. [*See*

*also* TREATISE ON POISONS AND THEIR ANTIDOTES]

1. F. Rosner, *Maimonides' Treatises on Poisons, Hemorrhoids and Cohabitation* (Haifa: Maimonides Research Institute, 1984).

2. F. Rosner, *Maimonides' Commentary on the Aphorisms of Hippocrates* (Haifa: Maimonides Research Institute, 1987).

3. U.S. Barzel, *Maimonides' The Art of Cure. Extracts from Galen* (Haifa: Maimonides Research Institute, 1992).

4. F. Rosner, *Medicine in the Bible and the Talmud*, 2nd ed. (Hoboken, NJ: Ktav and Yeshiva University Press, 1995), pp. 60–64.

**PRAYER**—The Talmud discusses the therapeutic efficacy of prayer (*Berachot* 32b). Prayers for healing are answered if the community is in need of the sick person (*Erubim* 29b). One should never be discouraged from praying even under the most difficult circumstances (*Berachot* 10a).

No scientific study has yet satisfactorily proved the efficacy of prayer. The question one might pose is: Does the efficacy of prayer have to be scientifically proved? For what purpose? Will the majority of humankind change its praying habits on the basis of the results, positive or negative, of such a study? The Bible and the Talmud are rich sources of religious and scientific material. Prayer in Judaism is thought to be efficacious if offered by the proper person at the proper time with the proper intent under the proper circumstances.[1]

In his *Guide for the Perplexed* (3:36), Maimonides states that prayer establishes the principle that God watches over us and can make us succeed or fail, that the precept of prayer emanates from a duty to fear and to love Him (3:44 and 3:51). In his *Mishneh Torah*, he states that there are five requisites without which one cannot properly pray: cleansing the hands, covering the body, assurance of the cleanliness of the place where the prayers are to be recited, removal of distractions, and concentration of the mind (*Tefillah* 4:1ff). Thus, a person who had a seminal emission or who suffers from flux (gonorrhea or other venereal disease?; Hebrew, *zav*) should pray only after immersing in a ritual bath (ibid., 4:5). A person with intestinal flatulence should wait until he feels relieved before he prays (ibid., 4:12). A person with urinary incontinence should pause until the dripping ceases and then resume his prayers (ibid., 4:13).

Maimonides points out that Scripture (Num. 10:9) prescribes prayer and the sounding of an alarm with trumpets whenever trouble—such as famine, pestilence, locusts, and the like—befalls the community (*Taanit* 1:1). Fasting is also required on such occasions (ibid., 1:4). Expectant and nursing mothers and minors are not required to fast on fast days observed because of misfortunes (ibid., 1:8).

[*See also* FASTING]

---

1. F. Rosner, "The Efficacy of Prayer: Scientific vs. Religious Evidence," *Journal of Religion and Health*, 14 (1975): 294–298.

**PREGNANCY**—In his *Mishnah Commentary*,[1] Maimonides states that a fetus begins to take form forty days after conception (*Niddah* 3:7). Prior to forty days, it has no form or shape (*Keritot* 1:4). Various types of abortuses and monster births are described (*Niddah* 3:2–6), including those that look like a sandal (i.e., a fish-shaped abortion), an afterbirth (i.e., placenta), or a fully fashioned fetus (*Keritot* 1:3). The afterbirth is "the sac that contains the fetus and that is unfurled" (*Chullin* 4:7). One must do everything necessary, even on the Sabbath, for a parturient woman, including cooking for her and cutting and tying the navel (*Shabbat* 18:3). Maimonides speaks of a woman in labor giving birth to twins, one dead and one alive (*Oholot* 7:6). Elsewhere (*Eduyot* 4:10), he also speaks of multiple births. He also states that a woman pregnant with twins can give birth to one by cesarean section and the second vaginally in the normal manner, and then she dies (*Bechorot* 8:2).

In his *Medical Aphorisms*,[2] Maimonides describes the physiology of procreation (Chapter 1:72–73). He states that the discomforts of pregnancy (e.g., morning sickness) and the cessation of menses are not necessarily clear indications of the existence of a pregnancy (16:1). He describes pica, or abnormal cravings, in pregnancy (16:23). He also states that a fetus is formed in thirty-five to forty-five days, and in twice that many days fetal movement can be detected (16:32). He ridicules the assertion of Galen that male fetuses are conceived by a woman on the right side of the uterus, whereas female fetuses are conceived on the left side.

Maimonides deals extensively with pregnancy, fetal development, and embryology in his legal code, the *Mishneh Torah*.[3] Various forms and shapes of abortuses render a woman ritually unclean. Esophageal atresia, anencephaly, spina bifida, and other congenital abnormalities are clearly described. A woman is considered pregnant from the time that the fetus becomes discernible, that is, at three months. An unborn fetus does not have the status of a person and, therefore, if one transfers ownership through a third party, the transaction is not valid. However, if a man on his deathbed states that a gift be given to his child, which is still an embryo in the womb of its mother, the embryo acquires title to it. An unborn fetus is part of the mother; therefore, if one sells a pregnant female slave, he also sells thereby the unborn fetus.

A one-day-old baby inherits his mother, and need not prove its viability for thirty days. An unborn fetus or embryo does not inherit. A stillbirth is not considered as a firstborn in relation to the laws of inheritance; nor is a child born by cesarean section considered as a firstborn in this regard. If a fetus of a pregnant woman extrudes a limb and then withdraws it, the mother is deemed unclean through childbirth.

---

1. F. Rosner, "Medicine in Moses Maimonides' Commentary on the Mishnah," *Koroth* (Jerusalem), 9 (1988): 565–578.

2. F. Rosner, *The Medical Aphorisms of Moses Maimonides* (Haifa: Maimonides Research Institute, 1989).

3. F. Rosner, *Medicine in the Mishneh Torah of Maimonides* (New York: Ktav, 1984), pp. 165–169.

**PREVENTIVE MEDICINE**—An entire treatise in Maimonides' *Mishneh Torah* (*Deot*) is devoted to moral dispositions or human traits or temperaments. Particularly interesting is the fourth chapter, which deals with a variety of hygienic and medical prescriptions for healthy living and for the prevention of illness.[1] Among the many subjects discussed are normal bodily excretory functions; recommended times for eating; amounts and types of food to be consumed; beverage consumption; exercise; sleep habits; cathartics; climatic and weather effects on eating habits; detrimental and beneficial foods; fruits, meats, vegetables; bathing; bloodletting; sexual intercourse; and domicile. Maimonides repeatedly emphasizes prevention over treatment. Prevention of illness and a healthy lifestyle are obligations upon Jews in order to enable them to serve the Lord. If one is ill, one cannot serve the Lord properly or fulfill the precepts of the Torah. Maimonides concludes Chapter 4 in *Deot* as follows:

> I guarantee anyone who conducts himself according to the directions we have laid down that he will not be afflicted with illness all the days of his life until he ages greatly and expires. He will not require a physician, and his body will be complete and remain healthy all his life. . . .

Maimonides cites exceptions to the goal of preventing rather than treating illness. Genetic diseases and certain epidemics of diseases cannot be prevented. For this reason, the final paragraph in Maimonides' chapter on the regimen of health states that a person should not reside in a city that does not have a physician. A similar pronouncement is found in the Talmud (*Sanhedrin* 17b).

Maimonides' preventive approach to illness and the practice of medicine is also evident throughout his medical writings.[2] The maintenance of one's health requires Jews to avoid harmful foods and activities and to prevent danger wherever possible. This principle is exemplified by the precept of building a parapet on one's roof. One must be concerned about ecological and environmental factors, such as clean air and sunshine, that may affect one's health. One must observe rules of personal hygiene, such as hand-washing, before eating. Diet, exercise, sex, and bodily functions must all be tended to as described by Maimonides. [ *See also* HYGIENE]

1. F. Rosner, "The Hygienic Principles of Moses Maimonides," *Journal of the American Medical Association*, 194 (1965):1352–1354.
2. F. Rosner, *The Medical Legacy of Moses Maimonides* (Hoboken, NJ: Ktav, 1998).

**PROCREATION**—Marriage in Judaism is a basic commandment (Deut. 22:13) and is so codified by Maimonides in his *Mishneh Torah* (*Eeshut* 1:1). Its purposes include procreation and the attainment of a holy state that comes with the avoidance of sin, i.e., illicit sex outside the sanctioned relationship. Deferral of marriage must be justified (ibid., 15:2).

Maimonides discusses the biblical commandment of "Be fruitful and multiply" (Gen. 1:28; 9:1 and 9:7; and 35:11), and defines the obligation of how one fulfills it. How many children must a man have before he can be regarded as having fulfilled this commandment? One male child and one female (*Eeshut* 15:4), as it is written, "Male and female He created them" (Gen. 5:2). Maimonides cautions against marrying a sterile woman, an old woman, a barren woman, or a girl who is still a minor who is incapable of giving birth unless the man has already fulfilled the commandment to be fruitful and multiply (*Eeshut* 15:7).

Maimonides recognized that in order for the wife to become impregnated by her husband, his semen during intercourse must be ejected with "the force of an arrow" (ibid., 15:8). A man should not compel his wife to have intercourse with him against her will. Rather, he should do it only with her consent, accompanied by pleasant discourse and enjoyment (ibid., 15:17). The mutual love and admiration of husband and wife are beautifully described by Maimonides (ibid., 15:19–20). The relationship of husband and wife during her menstrual period is such that physical contact and sexual intercourse are forbidden (ibid., 21:8). Further discussion of Maimonides' laws pertaining to marriage and the duty of procreation can be found elsewhere.[1]

---

1. F. Rosner, *Medicine in the Mishneh Torah of Maimonides* (New York: Ktav, 1984), pp. 177–180.

**PROGNOSIS**—At the beginning of his *Commentary on the Aphorisms of*

*Hippocrates*,[1] Maimonides states that it is very difficult to accurately prognosticate the outcome of illness. Often the prognosis seems grave and the signs and symptoms are extremely malignant, yet the patient recovers. Just as often, the signs may indicate that the prognosis is good, yet that which seems indicated does not materialize.

In his *Medical Aphorisms*,[2] Maimonides quotes Galen, who said that one can prognosticate regarding a stroke called apoplexy: If it is severe, the patient will die, but if it is minor, cure is possible, although difficult (Chapter 6:1). Maimonides then devotes a long aphorism to many aspects of prognosis and describes a schema by which one can predict whether or not an illness will be fatal. He cites mentally retarded and psychotic people who may live a long life because their physical bodies are strong and their illness is limited to the brain, rather than being caused by the weakening of the "sovereign force" or "overall reigning force" such as occurs to patients in the agonal stages of their illness. Blind and deaf people may also live long lives. Facial appearance is also an important prognostic sign: "If it is normal, it signifies that nature is strong; if it is far from normal, it is a sign of weakening of the overall reigning force" (ibid., 6:94).

---

1. F. Rosner, *Maimonides' Commentary on the Aphorisms of Hippocrates*

(Haifa: Maimonides Research Institute, 1987).

2. F. Rosner, *The Medical Aphorisms of Moses Maimonides* (Haifa: Maimonides Research Institute, 1989).

*PSYCHOSOMATIC MEDICINE—* The third chapter of Maimonides' medical treatise *Regimen of Health*[1] contains his concept of "a healthy mind in a healthy body," one of the earliest descriptions of psychosomatic medicine. He indicates that the physical well-being of a person is dependent on his mental well-being, and vice versa. Maimonides here teaches public and private hygiene for the preservation of the health of body and soul. He emphasizes preventive medicine and mental hygiene as factors of fundamental importance in the maintenance of health. For this reason, he expounds on the religious and philosophical aspects of this subject in his *Commentary on the Mishnah* and *Mishneh Torah* (*Deot* 1:11ff). He prescribes exercise for the body and soul. Maimonides demands total treatment of the patient, including his physical body and also his soul. He stresses the treatment of the patient, not the illness. Maimonides' theory on mental and physical therapy is holistic rather than dualistic, requiring parallel treatment of body and soul, which form a single psychosomatic unit.

The *Regimen of Health* shows Maimonides not only as scholar and physician, but also as a healer of the mind,

comforting and encouraging those who turn to him for help. It is a mark of his greatness that, while treating the Sultan for whom this treatise was written with all the honor and respect due to him and expressing fervent prayers and hope for his speedy recovery, he does not hesitate to condemn, in an indirect manner, the Sultan's overindulgences in wine and women, his gluttony and his lusts. Physical and mental well-being are interdependent, teaches Maimonides. A healthy person is cheerful and content, while a sick one is always depressed and dissatisfied. Complete recovery therefore can be furthered by strengthening the patient's moral convictions through study of the moral exhortations of the prophets and philosophers, leading the patient to regulate his life accordingly. Peace of mind, even in adverse circumstances, is an essential requisite for the well-being of the soul. Acceptance with humility and gratitude of the good fortunes and favors of life, as well as its miseries and tribulations, is part of the teachings of all great religions.

This theme—the paramount importance of the preservation of body health and the maintenance of psychological peace of mind—appears in Chapter 8 of Maimonides' *Treatise on Asthma*,[2] where he asserts that if a person is emotionally upset or mentally agitated, his physical well-being suffers, and eventually he becomes physically ill. This early description of psychosomatic medicine indicates that a deranged psyche can profoundly affect a person's somatic or physical well-being. Conversely, continues Maimonides, gaiety and joy gladden the heart and stimulate the blood and mental activity. Excessive indulgence in the pursuit of pleasure, however, is injurious to one's health. The avoidance of illnesses induced by such excesses is accomplished by conducting oneself according to ethical and moral principles.

---

1. F. Rosner, *Moses Maimonides' Three Treatises on Health* (Haifa: Maimonides Research Institute, 1990), pp. 1–116.

2. F. Rosner, *Moses Maimonides' Treatise on Asthma* (Haifa: Maimonides Research Institute, 1994).

**PUBERTY**—In a lengthy chapter in his *Mishneh Torah* (*Eeshut* 2:1ff), Maimonides details the anatomical and physiological signs of puberty in both boys and girls, and enumerates the signs and symptoms of barrenness in women and eunuchism in men. Such signs of puberty include two pubic hairs and, in girls, breast development.

Maimonides' rulings on the signs that determine the legal boundary between minority and majority[1] are based on several talmudic discussions. To come to maturity in Jewish law requires not only the signs of sexual maturity, but also the attainment of a certain age—in girls and boys, twelve and thirteen complete years, respectively. Naturally, a physical examination is necessary to determine majority.

In his *Mishnah Commentary*,[2] Maimonides describes sexual development in both boys and girls. An adolescent girl (*bogeret*) is one who is six months past the time when she developed signs of puberty (*Yebamot* 6:4). The tokens of puberty are that she have two pubic hairs after she is a full twelve years of age; the presence of two hairs before that time does not represent a token, but a mole (*Niddah* 5:7–8 and *Ketubot* 3:7). Similarly, if she does not develop the two hairs after twelve years of age, she is considered a minor until she is twenty years old.

Scattered references to puberty and sexual development can also be found in Maimonides' medical writings, including his *Medical Aphorisms*,[3] *Commentary on the Aphorisms of Hippocrates*,[4] and *Extracts from Galen*.[5]

---

1. F. Rosner, *Medicine in the Mishneh Torah of Maimonides* (New York: Ktav, 1984), pp. 143–153.

2. F. Rosner, "Medicine in Moses Maimonides' Commentary on the Mishnah," *Koroth* (Jerusalem), 9 (1988): 565–578.

3. F. Rosner, *The Medical Aphorisms of Moses Maimonides* (Haifa: Maimonides Research Institute, 1989).

4. F. Rosner, *Maimonides' Commen-*

*tary on the Aphorisms of Hippocrates* (Haifa: Maimonides Research Institute, 1987).

5. U.S. Barzel, *Maimonides' The Art of Cure. Extracts from Galen* (Haifa: Maimonides Research Institute, 1992).

*PULMONOLOGY*—Maimonides' *Treatise on Asthma* provides medieval and modern concepts of lung disease causation, symptomatology, and therapy.[1] His *Medical Aphorisms* is replete with references to the anatomy, physiology, and pathology of the lungs, heart, and other parts of the chest.[2] He describes the process of respiration as follows: "When the diaphragm stretches . . . the inhalation [of air] is facilitated . . . the diaphragm alone is responsible for the ease of inhalation and exhalation. However, when exhalation becomes difficult [as in asthma], intercostal muscles, pectoral muscles, shoulder and neck muscles participate as well." He recognizes that respiration continues during sleep. He describes the lesser pulmonary circulation. Coughing and the production of sound and speech are also clearly described.

Maimonides discusses many diseases of the lungs and pleura including pneumonia and pleurisy. Cyanosis and clubbing of the fingers associated with pulmonary disease are beautifully depicted, as are illnesses involving the larynx and bronchi. Hemoptysis—perhaps owing to tuberculosis—and related pulmonary disorders, together with certain therapeutic approaches, are mentioned in a series of aphorisms.[3]

_____

1. F. Rosner, *Moses Maimonides' Treatise on Asthma* (Haifa: Maimonides Research Institute, 1994).

2. F. Rosner, *The Medical Aphorisms of Moses Maimonides* (Haifa: Maimonides Research Institute, 1989).

3. F. Rosner, "Moses Maimonides and Diseases of the Chest," *Chest*, 60 (1971):68–72.

*PULSE*—An entire chapter in Maimonides' *Medical Aphorisms*[1] is devoted to the pulse and its interpretation. Quoting Galen, Maimonides says that the pulse is normal if body strength is at equilibrium. A bad body or organ constitution leads to a low pulse. The pulse exists to maintain natural body warmth and to distribute pneuma for respiration. Pneuma was thought to be "pumped" by the heart to the lungs and throughout the body in arteries (perhaps derived from "air-tery," meaning an air-containing vessel). A normal pulse is totally regular. The pulse of a newborn is very rapid and full. The pulse of old people is very slow and weak. All irregular types of pulses in more than one beat are due to an abnormal constitution of the heart. The weakening of one's strength rarely causes pulse irregularities. However, if the body is strong but an excess of humors burden it, the pulse becomes irregular in its beat. A hard pulse, as in an excited person, strikes a forceful beat. Heartburn, nausea, emesis, and excitation can cause the pulse to become accelerated and small. Maimonides also describes fluttering, vermiculate, thready, and other types of pulses.

In one of his *Treatises on Health*,[2] Maimonides tells the Sultan that emotional experiences or excitement produce numerous changes in the body: The facial expression falls and loses its glow, the posture drops, the voice becomes hoarse and weak, the eyelids become heavy, and the pulse becomes small and weak.

---

1. F. Rosner, *The Medical Aphorisms of Moses Maimonides* (Haifa: Maimonides Research Institute, 1989), pp. 61–77.

2. F. Rosner, *Moses Maimonides' Three Treatises on Health* (Haifa: Maimonides Research Institute, 1990), p. 59.

---

**PUS**—In his *Medical Aphorisms*,[1] Maimonides quotes Galen, who said that bad blood leads to decay and pus formation (Chapter 3:31). Inflammation may also lead to pus or abscess formation (ibid., 3:48). Medications to draw out pus from a mastoid and other abscesses are recommended (ibid., 3:85). Pus is formed when natural body warmth dominates and alters the humors, producing pain and fever. When the pus is expelled, the organ returns to complete health (ibid., 6:10). When an abscess ripens and reaches a sharp head, it is on the verge of expelling the pus (ibid., 6:68). Specific salves or ointments to apply on pustules are described (ibid., 9:105–106). Cauterization can also be used to expel pus from the site of infection (ibid., 15:8). Care must be taken when incising an abscess to empty the pus therefrom (ibid., 15:35). It should be incised at its highest point to let the pus flow out (ibid., 15:48). Fig compresses should then be applied (ibid., 15:52).

In his *Commentary on the Aphorisms of Hippocrates*,[2] Maimonides states that the evacuation of pus from putrefied boils by incision and drainage is beneficial and cleanses the affected organ (Section 4:47). Pus in the urine indicates that there is an ulceration in the kidneys or urinary bladder (ibid., 4:75). Empyema is clearly depicted as "pleurisy with pus" (ibid., 5:15 and 6:27). Empyema in those days was treated by cauterization (ibid., 7:44). The formation of pus in wounds is said to be a favorable prognostic sign (ibid., 5:22). Sinusitis and otitis media are relieved by the drainage of pus or mucus (ibid., 6:10). Hepatic or subphrenic abscesses are also described, and are not always fatal, depending on the type, amount, and location of the pus (ibid., 7:45). Additional references to pus, pustules, carbuncles, furuncles, and abscesses are found in Maimonides' *Extracts from Galen*,[3] where incision and drainage followed by the application of various medications are recommended. [*See also* ABSCESS]

---

1. F. Rosner, *The Medical Aphorisms of Moses Maimonides* (Haifa: Maimonides Research Institute, 1989).

2. F. Rosner, *Maimonides' Commentary on the Aphorisms of Hippocrates* (Haifa: Maimonides Research Institute, 1987).

3. U.S. Barzel, *Maimonides' The Art of Cure. Extracts from Galen* (Haifa: Maimonides Research Institute, 1992).

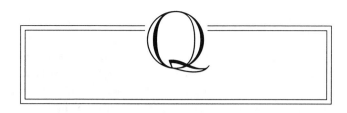

QUAIL—The biblical story of the consumption of quails by Israelites in the desert (Num. 11:30ff and Exod. 16:11ff) and their subsequent sudden death is explained by various writers as some type of food poisoning.[1] Extensive discussions of this biblical incident are found in Psalms (78:26–31 and 106:13–15) and in the Talmud (*Yoma* 75b, *Sanhedrin* 17a; *Avot* 5:4; *Chullin* 27b; *Arachin* 15a). In his *Medical Aphorisms*,[2] Maimonides quotes Galen, who said that many people who indulge greatly in quail develop cramps in the muscle because of the hellebore (a veratrum alkaloid) upon which the quail feeds (Chapter 12:32). Maimonides may be describing rhabdomyolysis and myoglobinuria secondary to the hellebore contained in quail meat. This suggestion was made by a recent Greek writer.[3] Later in *Medical Aphorisms*, Maimonides describes the benefit of quail and other fowl meat for both healthy people and those convalescing from illness, and its efficacy in dissolving kidney stones and promoting urine flow (ibid., 20:69). In one of his treatises on health, he warns against quail consumption because it constipates.[4] [*See also* CHICKEN SOUP and MEAT]

1. F. Rosner, "The Biblical Quail Incident," in *Medicine in the Bible and the Talmud*, 2nd augmented ed. (Hoboken, NJ, and New York: Ktav and Yeshiva University Press, 1975), pp. 292–294.
2. F. Rosner, *The Medical Aphorisms of Moses Maimonides* (Haifa: Maimonides Research Institute, 1989).
3. T. Ouzounellis, "Some Notes on Quail Poisoning," *Journal of the American Medical Association*, 211 (1970): 1186–1187.
4. F. Rosner, *Moses Maimonides' Three Treatises on Health* (Haifa: Maimonides Research Institute, 1990), p. 144.

QUINCES—In his *Treatise on Asthma*,[1] Maimonides states that the sucking of quinces (Cydonia vulgaris) after the meal is good, but that one should not use them excessively because they may be harmful to asthmatics (Chapter 2:10). Consuming a lot of quince juice helps to regulate the stools by virtue of the astringent property of quinces (ibid., 9:5). Oxymel in quinces, or lemon juice in quinces, improves the digestion and cleanses the stomach of phlegm (ibid., 9:15). Quince oil rubbed in the middle of the head helps to strengthen the brain in patients with asthma (ibid., 12:6). The constipating or binding properties of quinces are reiterated by Maimonides in his *Mishneh Torah* (*Deot* 4:6) and in his *Extracts from Galen*,[2] where he also cites the stomach-cleansing actions of quinces. Aromatic baths with quince oil are helpful for patients with liver tumors. Finally, a quince confection is mentioned by Maimonides in his *Glossary of Drug Names* (drug no. 119).[3]

---

1. F. Rosner, *Moses Maimonides' Treatise on Asthma* (Haifa: Maimonides Research Institute, 1994).

2. U.S. Barzel, *Maimonides' The Art of Cure. Extracts from Galen* (Haifa: Maimonides Research Institute, 1992).

3. F. Rosner, *Moses Maimonides' Glossary of Drug Names* (Haifa: Maimonides Research Institute, 1996).

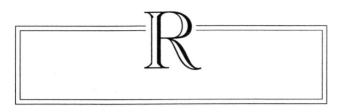

## RABBINOWICZ, ISRAEL MICHEL

—Lithuanian-born Israel Rabbinowicz (1818–1883) lived most of his life in France, and is best known for his translations into French of parts of the Talmud and works on talmudic medicine. He also translated Maimonides' *Treatise on Poisons* into French.[1]

---

1. I.M. Rabbinowicz, *Maïmonide Traité des Poisons* (Paris: A. Delahaye, 1865). Reprinted by Lipschutz (Paris) in 1935.

## RABIES

—In his *Treatise on Poisons and Their Antidotes*,[1] Maimonides not only details the signs and symptoms of rabies, but also notes that anyone bitten by a mad dog should immediately be treated with "ligature, incision, sucking, and copious bloodletting from the affected site." Additional treatments are suggested, but he warns that the treatment is "only efficacious if used prior to the onset of hydrophobia. If applied after . . . I have never seen anyone survive." Most

remarkable is his recognition of the varying incubation periods. The "serious symptoms . . . do not begin to appear until eight days have passed . . . one should not continue treatment of the bite victim . . . for a minimum of forty days." He closes the chapter with the case of a weaver's boy who was bitten by a dog. As there was no indication that it was a mad dog, the wound was closed at the end of a month. "The child recovered, much time elapsed, and he performed activities like healthy people. Later symptoms became apparent, he developed fear of water and died."

The remedy suggested by the Talmud (*Yoma* 84a) for the bite of a mad dog is derived from folk medicine. On the other hand, the treatment advocated by Maimonides—bandaging, incision, sucking out, and copious bloodletting from the affected site— is very modern in its approach. [*See also* TREATISE ON POISONS]

---

1. F. Rosner, *Maimonides' Treatises on Poisons, Hemorrhoids and Cohabita-*

*tion* (Haifa: Maimonides Research Institute, 1984), pp. 19–115.

**RADISHES**—In both *Mishneh Torah* (*Deot* 4:9) and *Regimen of Health* (Chapter 1:11),[1] Maimonides writes that radishes are among the vegetables that are bad for people. Yet in his *Treatise on Asthma*,[2] he recommends radish juice to soften the stools without harm and to cleanse the internal organs, including the lungs (Chapter 9:2). Later in the same treatise, he again lists the radish among the detrimental sharp foods (ibid., 9:12) but allows its use as an emetic (ibid., 12:10). In his *Extracts from Galen*,[3] he reiterates the stomach-cleansing properties of radish, which "dissolves the phlegm," (p. 67) and the use of radish as an emetic (p. 97). The long radish is listed in Maimonides' *Glossary of Drug Names* (drug no. 273).[4]

1. F. Rosner, *Moses Maimonides' Three Treatises on Health* (Haifa: Maimonides Research Institute, 1990).

2. F. Rosner, *Moses Maimonides' Treatise on Asthma* (Haifa: Maimonides Research Institute, 1994).

3. U.S. Barzel, *Maimonides' The Art of Cure. Extracts from Galen* (Haifa: Maimonides Research Institute, 1992).

4. F. Rosner, *Moses Maimonides' Glossary of Drug Names* (Haifa: Maimonides Research Institute, 1996).

**RAISINS**—In his *Regimen of Health*,[1] Maimonides states that dried fruits such as raisins, dried figs, and pistachio kernels are healthful foods and are especially beneficial for the liver (Chapter 1:13). Raisins are good for the liver; they fatten and nourish it, color the blood, and increase the humors (ibid., 3:6). In his *Medical Aphorisms*,[2] he quotes Galen, who said that raisins neutralize bad humors and improve the liver (Chapter 20:57 and 20:73).

In his *Treatise on Asthma*,[3] Maimonides recommends a concoction made from seeded raisins soaked in vinegar, crushed with peeled almonds, and filtered into a roasted meat soup. He attests to its benefit for asthmatics in that it "liquefies and digests foods and warms to an intermediate degree" (Chapter 4:2). The raisins in this preparation also fatten the liver and greatly benefit it, eliminate epigastric burning, and cleanse the lungs (ibid., 4:3). He further writes that he personally ate peanuts and fresh raisins without their pips, or dried raisins and almonds (ibid., 6:4). A mild remedy for asthma consists of equal parts of seeded raisins and fenugreek cooked in clear water, sifted, and left standing for a prolonged period. More potent remedies are also described (ibid., 12:1).

1. F. Rosner, *Moses Maimonides' Three Treatises on Health* (Haifa: Maimonides Research Institute, 1990).

2. F. Rosner, *The Medical Aphorisms of Moses Maimonides* (Haifa: Maimonides Research Institute, 1989).

3. F. Rosner, *Moses Maimonides' Treatise on Asthma* (Haifa: Maimonides Research Institute, 1994).

### RECOVERY FROM ILLNESS—

Maimonides' *Mishneh Torah* states that four categories of individuals are required to recite a thanksgiving blessing (*birchat hagomel*); one of the four is one who was sick and who has recovered (*Tefillah* 10:8). This blessing is also to be recited by persons who have been in peril of their lives, during journeys by sea or on land, or who are delivered from captivity (ibid.). To this day, a dangerously ill Jewish patient—irrespective of the nature of the illness, whether medical, surgical, or otherwise—upon recovery from the illness, comes to the synagogue and recites the blessing of thanksgiving.

When Rabbi Judah recovered from an illness, Rabbi Channa of Baghdad and other sages visited him, and said: "Blessed is God, Who gave you back to us." Rabbi Judah answered Amen, and was absolved of reciting the prayer of thanksgiving (*Berachot* 54b). Rabbi Abbahu made a feast to celebrate the recovery of Rabbi Zera from a serious illness (ibid., 46a).

Men or women recovering from illness or women after childbirth brought offerings of thanks to the Lord, often in the form of shekels or other coins that were used for the upkeep of the Temple or the purchase of sacrifices (*Shekalim* 2:2).

### REMEDIES—

The twenty-second chapter of Maimonides' *Medical Aphorisms* discusses specific remedies for a variety of conditions.[1] The first half of the chapter consists of quotations from Galen; the second half, citations from Ibn Zuhr and Al Tamimi. They are mostly of historical interest, although an occasional modern therapeutic regimen is described, such as the treatment of gout with colchicine. The following are a few excerpts: ". . . mouse excrement, if pulverized in vinegar, is beneficial for alopecia. The brain of a camel, if dried, prepared in vinegar and imbibed, is of value against epilepsy. If one rubs the gums of children with brains of an ewe lamb, it will facilitate growth of the teeth without pain. Earthworms, if pulverized, [dissolved] and imbibed by a patient with icterus, immediately cleanse his body. Cattle's milk is of aid against intestinal ulcers. . . . The spleen of wild donkey or the spleen of a wild horse should be dried and pulverized and given to drink to a patient with illness of the spleen. . . . The consumption of rabbit heads, as much as one is able to eat, helps against tremors. A lotion made of the liquid of roses and sugar strengthens vision . . . the gilly flower [eugenia caryophyllata carnefolium], pulverized and filtered [and placed] on the forehead during the winter is a reliable remedy for preventing catarrhal colds. The ingestion of radish or cabbage eliminates hoarseness.

Hedgehog meat, if dried and some of it imbibed in oxymel, is beneficial for pain in the kidneys . . . if one takes pulverized, dried snakeroot and three parts of wheat flour and places all this in sesame oil and kneads it with leavening and salt and bakes it and dries this bread and pulverizes it and snuffs about ten drachmas of its dust every morning in a spiced honey drink, the hemorrhoids will be obliterated in three days." Numerous other remedies for many different ailments are discussed by Maimonides in all his medical writings.

---

1. F. Rosner, *The Medical Aphorisms of Moses Maimonides* (Haifa: Maimonides Research Institute, 1989), pp. 342–355.

*RESPIRATION*—In his *Treatise on Asthma*,[1] Maimonides discusses a variety of therapeutic suggestions for asthmatics relating to climate and domicile. He endorses a remedy of Rhazes to clear the lungs of moisture, ease respiration, and eliminate the cough. In his *Regimen of Health*,[2] Maimonides states that vigorous exercise produces an increase in the depth and rate of breathing. He describes shortness of breath as being due to an abundance of humors in the chest that suffocate the patient. In his *Commentary on the Aphorisms of Hippocrates*,[3] Maimonides asserts that paralysis from a stroke may inhibit movement of the chest and,

hence, respiration. Weakness of respiration occurs because of dryness and hardness of the respiratory organ so that there is insufficient strength to exhale. In his *Extracts from Galen*,[4] he speaks of the benefits of breathing and of shivering in aeration of the body and the dissolution of its wastes.

In his *Medical Aphorisms*,[5] Maimonides quotes Galen, who said that respiratory impairment owing to weakness of the chest muscles occurs because of generalized body weakness, narrowing of the respiratory passages, or heat prevailing in the heart and lungs (Chapters 6:42 and 7:47). Flaring at the nostrils indicates body weakness. Narrowing of the respiratory passages produces expansion of the chest (ibid.), an obvious description of obstructive emphysema. Short, rapid breaths occur in patients with pneumonia (ibid., 6:54). The lung is the organ of both respiration and voice (ibid., 1:53). Accelerated respiration may also occur owing to a loss of mentation (ibid., 7:48). Inspiration was recognized as the entrance of air into the larynx and trachea (ibid., 23:12). The expulsion of air during respiration is mediated by the chest muscles (ibid., 3:43). Respiration was thought to be of two types, one being movements of the chest and the other movements of the pulse (ibid., 3:80). In medieval times, the blood was thought to pump air or pneuma into the lungs. Cessation of respiration as a sign of death is discussed by Maimonides in *Mishneh Torah*.[6]

1. F. Rosner, *Moses Maimonides' Treatise on Asthma* (Haifa: Maimonides Research Institute, 1994).

2. F. Rosner, *Moses Maimonides' Three Treatises on Health* (Haifa: Maimonides Research Institute, 1990), pp. 24 and 84.

3. F. Rosner, *Maimonides' Commentary on the Aphorisms of Hippocrates* (Haifa: Maimonides Research Institute, 1987), pp. 62 and 183.

4. U.S. Barzel, *Maimonides' The Art of Cure. Extracts from Galen* (Haifa: Maimonides Research Institute, 1992), p. 127.

5. F. Rosner, *The Medical Aphorisms of Moses Maimonides* (Haifa: Maimonides Research Institute, 1989).

6. F. Rosner, *Medicine in the Mishneh Torah of Maimonides* (New York: Ktav, 1984), pp. 215–220.

**RESURRECTION**—Maimonides' *Treatise on Resurrection*, written in 1991, is an extended discussion of God's unity, the messianic age, the resurrection of the dead, and the world-to-come.[1] He had already briefly mentioned the resurrection of the dead in his *Mishnah Commentary* (*Sanhedrin* 10:1), which he wrote in 1168 and in which he lists resurrection as one of the thirteen fundamental principles, or articles, of the Jewish faith.[2] Brief statements on resurrection also appear in his *Mishneh Torah* (e.g., *Teshuvah*). Because of the brevity of his comments on resurrection in the *Mishnah Commentary* and *Mishneh Torah*, Maimonides was asked to expand and amplify his view on the subject. Controversy regarding his views arose because he espoused a view contrary to the prevailing one, which held that the resurrection of the dead and the world-to-come are a single continuum of spiritual existence. Maimonides' view is that the resurrection of the dead includes not only spiritual resurrection but also physical resurrection, and that the world-to-come that is separate from and will follow the resurrection will be wholly a spiritual world—with spiritual beings without corporeality. Thus, the bodies of the righteous will be resurrected at the beginning of the messianic era, but upon its termination will die again to enjoy everlasting existence in spirit only. Similar theories were propounded by Abraham bar Chiya and Abraham Ibn Ezra.[3]

1. F. Rosner, *Moses Maimonides' Treatise on Resurrection* (New York: Ktav, 1982).

2. F. Rosner, *Maimonides' Commentary on the Mishnah, Tractate Sanhedrin* (New York: Sepher Hermon, 1981), pp. 134–158.

3. J. Finkel, *Maimonides' Treatise on Resurrection* (New York: American Academy for Jewish Research, 1939).

**RHUBARB**—In his *Treatise on Asthma*,[1] Maimonides describes rhubarb as a powerful purgative when combined with cassia fistula, agaricon, and myrobalan (Chapter 13:41). Rhubarb may also be used in a concoction to serve as a mild stool softener (ibid., 9:1–2). Rhubarb has no efficacy, however, in cleansing the head or lungs of asthmatic patients (ibid., 12:8). In his *Regimen of Health*,[2] Maimonides reiterates the laxative properties of rhubarb (Chapter 3: 2–3) and gives a detailed description of the preparation of the cassia fistula, agaricon, myrobalan, and rhubarb purgative concoction (ibid., 3:9). In his *Medical Aphorisms*,[3] Maimonides quotes Galen, who said that rhubarb benefits the liver in an overt manner (Chapter 21:30).

3. F. Rosner, *The Medical Aphorisms of Moses Maimonides* (Haifa: Maimonides Research Institute, 1989).

*RICE*—In his *Treatise on Asthma*,[1] Maimonides advises people to avoid seeds that produce flatulence, such as beans and peas; those that fatten, such as rice and lentils; those that produce gases in the head, such as nuts; and foods that increase heat, such as leek, onions, and garlic (Chapter 3:3). In his *Regimen of Health*,[2] he states that if a person constantly ate rice—as do some peoples and cultures—he would certainly become ill (Chapter 1:13).

1. F. Rosner, *Moses Maimonides' Treatise on Asthma* (Haifa: Maimonides Research Institute, 1994).

2. F. Rosner, *Moses Maimonides' Three Treatises on Health* (Haifa: Maimonides Research Institute, 1990).

1. F. Rosner, *Moses Maimonides' Treatise on Asthma* (Haifa: Maimonides Research Institute, 1994).

2. F. Rosner, *Moses Maimonides' Three Treatises on Health* (Haifa: Maimonides Research Institute, 1990).

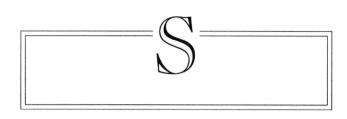

SACHS, SCHNEYER—A Hebraic literature scholar and author, Schneyer Sachs (1815–1892) edited various literary and scholarly journals. He also edited a fragment of the Hebrew translation by Nathan Ha-Meati of Maimonides' *Medical Aphorisms* (*Pirkei Moshe*) missing in the Lemberg edition of 1834–1835 (*Hatechiyah*, folio 1 (1850), pp. 35–38).[1]

_____

1. J.I. Dienstag, "Translators and Editors of Maimonides' Medical Works: A Bio-bibliographical Survey," in J.O. Leibowitz, ed., *Memorial Volume in Honor of Prof. S. Muntner* (Jerusalem: Israel Institute of the History of Medicine, 1983), pp. 95–135.

SAPHIR, JACOB—A scholar and traveler, Jacob Saphir (1822–1885) is best known for his work *Eben Saphir* (Lyck, 1866; Mayence, 1974), in which he vividly describes the history and conditions of Jews in Yemen, India, Egypt, and Australia. He also published *Iggeret Teman* (Vilna, 1868), not to be confused with Maimonides' *Iggeret Teman* (Epistle to Yemen). Saphir edited Moshe Ibn Tibbon's Hebrew translation of Maimonides' *Regimen of Health*, the manuscript of which was in his possession (Jerusalem: A.M. Luntz, 5645–1885).[1]

_____

1. J.I. Dienstag, "Translators and Editors of Maimonides' Medical Works: A Bio-bibliographical survey," in J.O. Leibowitz, ed., *Memorial Volume in Honor of Prof. S. Muntner* (Jerusalem: Israel Institute of the History of Medicine, 1983), pp. 95–135.

SAVITZ, HARRY AUSTRYN—A U.S. physician and writer, Harry A. Savitz translated into English Chapter 3 of Maimonides' *Regimen of Health*, which deals with psychosomatic medicine. Savitz called his translation Maimonides' "Hygiene of the Soul" (*Annals of Medical History*, new series, 4 (1932):80–86) and reprinted it in his *Profiles of Erudite Jewish Physicians and Scholars* (Chicago: Spertus

College of Judaica Press), 1955, p. 664.[1]

---

1. J.I. Dienstag, "Translators and Editors of Maimonides' Medical Works: A Bio-bibliographical Survey," in J.O. Leibowitz, ed., *Memorial Volume in Honor of Prof. S. Muntner* (Jerusalem: Israel Institute of the History of Medicine, 1983), pp. 95–135.

*SCHWARZ, MICHAEL*—An Orientalist and Arabist at Tel Aviv University, Michael Schwarz translated into Hebrew Maimonides' *Responsum on Longevity*. Based upon G. Weil's Arabic and German edition, Schwarz' translation also includes Weil's introduction to this work (Tel Aviv University Student Press, 1979).[1]

---

1. J.I. Dienstag, "Translators and Editors of Maimonides' Medical Works: A Bio-bibliographical Survey," in J.O. Leibowitz, ed., *Memorial Volume in Honor of Prof. S. Muntner* (Jerusalem: Israel Institute of the History of Medicine, 1983), pp. 95–135.

*SEX ETHICS*—In addition to his *Treatise on Sexual Intercourse*,[1] numerous statements on sex, sexual intercourse, and forbidden sexual relations are found in the other medical writings of Maimonides, as well as in his philosophical and theological works.[2] In his *Treatise on Hemor-* rhoids, his *Regimen of Health*, and elsewhere, he states that sexual intercourse immediately after a meal interferes with digestion. In his *Treatise on Asthma* and *Mishneh Torah* (*Deot* 4:19), he warns against excessive indulgence in sexual intercourse, stating that a person who "immerses himself therein will be assailed by premature aging, his strength will wane, his eyes will weaken . . . the hair of his head, eyebrows, and eyelashes will fall out. . . ."

Maimonides' *Medical Aphorisms* is replete with references to sexual intercourse. He again describes the consequences of excessive indulgence in sexual intercourse, since "a sudden strong and strenuous pleasure may lead to death." He recognizes, however, that sexual intercourse is one of the requirements for the maintenance of health, provided that there are adequate periods of abstinence between episodes so that "no noticeable enfeeblement or weakness should ensue." He states that the consumption of fowl "aids the libido in a strongly perceptible manner" and that eggs are good aphrodisiacs, especially if cooked with onion or turnip.

The subject of forbidden sexual relations such as incest and idolatry is discussed at length by Maimonides in *Mishneh Torah* (*Issurei Biyah*). Briefly, all unions between the sexes that are repellent to the moral inner feelings of humans, or would taint the natural affection between close relatives, are strictly prohibited. Such prohibited marriages and illicit sexual intercourse comprise two major categories: first, blood relations such as mother, sister, daughter, granddaughter, father's sister, and mother's sister; and second, cases of affinity such as the wives of blood relations and of the wife's blood relations. All sexual unions, whether temporary or permanent, between persons belonging to these groups are called incestuous, and are prohibited and abhorrent. They have no binding force whatsoever in Jewish law; such unions are not deemed to be a marriage, no bill of divorce is required for their dissolution, and the children that issue from them are illegitimate.

Maimonides also discusses sodomy, homosexuality, lesbianism, masturbation, orgasm, rape, bestiality, incest, and adultery. He also prescribes the time, place, and quantity of sexual intercourse considered desirable according to the Torah. In his *Mishnah Commentary* (*Sanhedrin* 7:4), he also provides a lengthy discussion of forbidden unions, bestiality, lesbianism, homosexuality, and other matters pertaining to sex ethics.

Finally, in his *Guide for the Perplexed* (3:33 and 3:49), Maimonides provides the philosophical basis for the laws concerning forbidden intercourse. To be holy, humans must forgo sensual excess. Maimonides stresses the disciplinary intent of the laws, which counteract the worldly tendency to regard pleasure as the purpose of human existence. Chastity and temperance are seen as higher disciplines. The path to holy living, shown by the Law, lies in self-disciplined abstention from that which is characteristically bestial, and wholehearted practice of that which is characteristically divine. [*See also* TREATISE ON SEXUAL INTERCOURSE]

---

1. F. Rosner, *Maimonides' Treatises on Poisons, Hemorrhoids and Cohabitation* (Haifa: Maimonides Research Institute, 1984), pp. 153–182.

2. F. Rosner, *Sex Ethics in the Writings of Moses Maimonides* (New York: Bloch, 1974).

*SEX, LEGITIMATE*—In his *Mishneh Torah*, Maimonides rules that a man is obligated to provide his wife with food, clothing, and sexual pleasure (*Eeshut* 6:10). In a Jewish marriage, over and above the question of procreation, exists the conjugal rights of the wife, technically termed *onah*. Thus, nonprocreative intercourse, such as occurs if the wife is too young to bear children, barren, pregnant, postmenopausal is not only allowed, but required. Improper emission of seed is not involved or is canceled out so long as the intercourse is in the manner of procreation. Not only are such sexual activities permitted, but they are, in fact, required by biblical law.

According to Jewish law, when a man marries a woman, he obligates himself to her for ten things (*Eeshut* 12:1). Of the ten, three are biblical in origin: "her food, her raiment, and her conjugal rights" (Exod. 21:10). "Her food" refers to her maintenance; "her raiment" is self-explanatory; and "her conjugal rights" means sexual intercourse with her according to the way of the world (*Eeshut* 12:2). Although some of the other obligations can be waived, her conjugal rights are not subject to stipulation either by a husband who wishes to exempt himself or by a wife who wishes him to forfeit that privilege. If the husband stipulates that his wife is to have no conjugal rights from him, the condition is null and void, and he remains obligated for her conjugal rights (ibid., 12:7). Conjugal rights are obligatory upon each man according to his physical powers and his occupation (ibid., 14:1). Elsewhere in *Mishneh Torah*, Maimonides describes the proper manner of sexual intercourse and intimacy between husband and wife (*Issurei Biyah* 21:9–14).

In his *Medical Aphorisms*,[1] Maimonides describes the physiology of sexual intercourse, mentions aphrodisiacs and antiaphrodisiacs, and discusses a variety of other matters relating to coitus. For example, he asserts that the penis, genitalia, and cervix possess an abundance of nerves necessary for sensation and feeling during coitus (Chapter 3:62). He who has an excess of black bile in his body is very fond of sexual intercourse (ibid., 7:17). The case of sudden death during or following sexual intercourse is reported by Maimonides (ibid., 7:61).

He also affirms that indulgence in sexual intercourse is one of the requirements for the maintenance of health, providing that there are adequate intervals of abstinence between periods of indulgence, so that no noticeable enfeeblement or weakness ensues; rather, one's body should feel lighter than before the act. During the time that one performs coitus, a person should be neither filled with food, nor completely empty thereof; neither very cold, nor very warm. The same applies to dryness and moisture (ibid., 17:8). For the preservation of health, a person should first perform physical exercise, then strive for food and drink, and then strive for sleep (ibid., 17:10). Thereafter, he can indulge in sexual intercourse if he so desires (ibid., 17:12). No one is harmed by coitus, except one whose body is warm and moist, or one whose nature is to produce warm semen (ibid., 17:13).

Maimonides advises righteous people not to conduct themselves in the manner of many people who behave in animallike custom, meaning the seeking of the most pleasurable in life, and nothing else (i.e., hedonism) (ibid., 17:20). Healthy sexual practices, including moderation in sexual intercourse and the use of aphrodisiacs, are described in some detail in his other medical writings, particularly the *Treatise on Cohabitation*[2] and the *Treatises on Health*[3] and his *Mishneh Torah* (*Deot* 4:19). [*See also* SEX ETHICS and TREATISE ON SEXUAL INTERCOURSE]

---

1. F. Rosner, *The Medical Aphorisms of Moses Maimonides* (Haifa: Maimonides Research Institute, 1989).
2. F. Rosner, *Maimonides' Treatises on Poisons, Hemorrhoids and Cohabitation* (Haifa: Maimonides Research Institute, 1984), pp. 153–182.
3. F. Rosner, *Moses Maimonides' Three Treatises on Health* (Haifa: Maimonides Research Institute, 1990).

**SEXUAL INTERCOURSE**—Maimonides wrote an entire *Treatise on Sexual Intercourse* described elsewhere in this encyclopedia. This subject is also dealt with from a medical viewpoint in several of his other writings. In his *Medical Aphorisms*,[1] he quotes Galen, who said that a person whose body is dominated by black bile is very fond of sexual intercourse (Chapter 7:17). One who indulges excessively in sexual intercourse becomes weak because the entire body becomes devoid of pneuma and humors. Many people have a sudden strong and strenuous pleasure and then die (ibid., 7:16). One can only speculate on the cause of death. Epileptic convulsions may also occur in people who indulge excessively (ibid., 9:43). Cessation of sexual activity in a person who is accustomed thereto may result in the body becoming cold and movements burdensome because of the putrefaction of the retained semen (ibid., 9:110). Indulgence in sexual intercourse is one of the requirements for the maintenance of health, provided that there are adequate intervals of abstinence so that no weakness or enfeeblement occurs. At the time of coitus, one should be neither filled with food, nor completely empty thereof; neither very cold, nor very warm (ibid., 17:8).

In his *Mishneh Torah* (*Deot* 4:19), Maimonides codifies some important rules about sexual intercourse. His words speak for themselves.

> Effusion of semen represents the strength of the body and its life, and the light of the eyes. Whenever semen is emitted to excess, the body becomes consumed, its strength terminates, and its life perishes. This is what Solomon in his wisdom stated: "Give not thy strength unto women" (Prov. 31:3). He who immerses himself in sexual intercourse will be assailed by premature aging. His strength will wane, his eyes will weaken, and a bad odor will emit from his mouth and his armpits. The hair of his head, his eyebrows, and his eyelashes will fall out, and the hair of his beard and armpits and the hair of his legs will increase excessively. His teeth will fall out, and many maladies other than these will afflict him. The wise physicians have

stated that one in a thousand dies from other illnesses and the remaining 999 in a thousand from excessive sexual intercourse. Therefore, a man must be cautious in this matter if he wishes to live wholesomely. He should not cohabit unless his body is healthy and very strong and he experiences many involuntary erections, and when he diverts his thoughts to another thing, the erection persists, and when he senses a heaviness from his loins down, as if the testicular cords were being tightened, and his flesh is warm. Such a person requires coitus, and it is therapeutic for him to have sexual intercourse. A person should not cohabit when he is satiated nor when he is hungry but after the food is digested in his intestines. He should examine whether need for excretion [of urine or feces] exists before coitus and after coitus. One should not have sexual intercourse standing or sitting, and not in a bathhouse, nor on the day when he takes a bath, nor on the day of phlebotomy, nor on the day when setting out on a journey or returning from a journey, nor on the previous or following days of such occurrences.

Some of these rules are based on talmudic statements—for example, the occurrence of premature aging in people who indulge excessively in sexual intercourse (*Shabbat* 152a). Furthermore, one should cohabit after food is digested, but not when one is hungry or satiated (*Nedarim* 20b). Finally, the last paragraph in this citation from Maimonides is derived

from a talmudic discussion (*Gittin* 70a).

---

1. F. Rosner, *The Medical Aphorisms of Moses Maimonides* (Haifa: Maimonides Research Institute, 1989).

**SHATIBI, JOSHUA**—Fourteenth-century Joshua Shatibi was probably born in Xativa; hence his name. Shatibi's unpublished Hebrew translation of Maimonides' *Treatise on Asthma* is manuscript 280 of the Munich State Library. The manuscript closes with a poem by Shatibi in praise of Maimonides.[1]

---

1. J.I. Dienstag, "Translators and Editors of Maimonides' Medical Works: A Bio-bibliographical Survey," in J.O. Leibowitz, ed., *Memorial Volume in Honor of Prof. S. Muntner* (Jerusalem: Israel Institute of the History of Medicine, 1983), pp. 95–135.

**SHMUKLER, I.K.**— Shmukler translated Maimonides' *Regimen of Health* into Russian.[1] His work was published in *Vrachebnae Delo* (no. 14–16), 1930.[2]

---

1. I.K. Shmukler, *Pismo Moiseh Maimonida K Egupefskomu Sultanu.* Gugienicheskie Sovietia Perevod S Drevneevreiskogo Doctora I.K. Shmuklera (Kiev). Otdelnii Ottisk Iz, "Vrach Delo" (no. 14–15 and 16). Charkov. "Nuachnaja Misl." Uchr. NKZ. USSR (1930).

2. J.I. Dienstag, "Translators and Editors of Maimonides' Medical Works: A Bio-bibliographical Survey," in J.O. Leibowitz, ed., *Memorial Volume in Honor of Prof. S. Muntner* (Jerusalem: Israel Institute of the History of Medicine, 1983), pp. 95–135.

*SIMON, ISIDOR*—Born in Romania in 1906, the French physician and historian of Hebrew medicine Isidor Simon founded and edited the *Revue d'Historie de la Médecine Hebraique* from 1948 until his death more than four decades later. Among his many articles in numerous professional journals is his French translation of Muntner's Hebrew edition of Maimonides' *Treatise on Asthma.*[1]

---

1. S. Muntner and I. Simon, "Le Traité de l'Asthme de Maïmonide (1135–1204) Traduit Pour la Première Fois en Français d'Après le Texte Hebreu," *Rev. d'Hist. Méd. Héb.*, 16 (1963):171–186; 17 (1964):5–13, 83–97, 127–139, 187–196; 18 (1965): 5–15.

*SKIN*—In his *Medical Aphorisms,*[1] Maimonides quotes Galen, who describes the space between skin and underlying flesh (Chapter 3:48) and the nerves that connect the skin to underlying organs (ibid., 3:52). Loss of sensation in the skin does not affect the movement of muscles (ibid., 3:54). Maimonides describes pores or vessels in the skin (ibid., 7:13). Ill-

nesses of the skin owing to black bile are eczema and psoriasis (ibid., 9:98). Psoriasis is treated with purgation (ibid., 13:30). Psoriatic skin lesions may be caused by thick chymes or humors (ibid., 3:25). Erysipelas is said to be a redness or inflammation of the skin (ibid., 3:110) that may produce an abscess (ibid., 23:42). This erysipelas-like inflammation is also described by Maimonides in his *Commentary on the Aphorisms of Hippocrates*[2] (Section 6:25), as is eczema (ibid., 6:9). In his *Extracts from Galen,*[3] Maimonides discusses skin grafting and the healing of the skin over wounds (Chapter 3). When bathing, the skin loosens and the pores open (Chapter 10). Desquamation of the outer skin layer is also described (Chapter 14). [*See also* LEPROSY]

---

1. F. Rosner, *The Medical Aphorisms of Moses Maimonides* (Haifa: Maimonides Research Institute, 1989).
2. F. Rosner, *Maimonides' Commentary on the Aphorisms of Hippocrates* (Haifa: Maimonides Research Institute, 1987).
3. U.S. Barzel, *Maimonides' The Art of Cure. Extracts from Galen* (Haifa: Maimonides Research Institute, 1992).

*SKOSS, SOLOMON LEON*—Born in Russia, educator and Semitic scholar Solomon Skoss (1884–1953) pursued his studies at Dropsie College in the United States, where he became a leading Judeo-Arabic philologist.[1] He translated the first two chapters of Maimonides' *Regimen of Health* into English from the Arabic.[2]

---

1. J.I. Dienstag, "Translators and Editors of Maimonides' Medical Works: A Bio-bibliographical Survey," in J.O. Leibowitz, ed., *Memorial Volume in Honor of Prof. S. Muntner* (Jerusalem: Israel Institute of the History of Medicine, 1983), pp. 95–135.
2. S.L. Skoss, *Portrait of a Jewish Scholar; Essays and Addresses* (New York: Bloch, 1957), pp. 99–116.

---

**SLEEP**—In his *Mishneh Torah* (*Deot* 4:4–5), Maimonides recommends that people sleep eight hours per night, preferably lying on one's side, not on one's face or back. One should not go to sleep shortly after eating, or sleep during the day—although a brief nap is acceptable. In his *Medical Aphorisms*,[1] Maimonides quotes Galen, who said that during sleep muscles are idle and completely at rest (Chapter 1:27). Only the chest muscles continue to be active during sleep (ibid., 1:32). During sleep, some people talk, cry out, turn from side to side, or even walk (ibid., 1:33), although the cause for such activities is unclear. Galen himself once admitted to walking sixty *mils* (about 20 kilometers) while asleep (ibid., 24:21). Excessive sleep is detrimental to health (ibid., 3:69), although it is helpful for patients recovering from illness (ibid., 6:95). Sleep moistens the body by increasing humors, whereas insomnia dries the body (ibid., 7:58). Sleep is harmful in patients with cold humors or abscesses (ibid., 8:29). A very deep sleep or coma following poisoning in which the patient appears to be dead is also described (ibid., 24:51).

In his *Treatises on Health*,[2] Maimonides recommends that one exercise an hour after arising from sleep or a bath. Some wine mixed with oxtongue at bedtime is very helpful to induce deep sleep. Chapter 10 of his *Treatise on Asthma*[3] deals with the effects of sleeping, waking, massage, and coitus on this disease. Sleeping immediately after a meal is said to be harmful, but sleeping after bathing is efficacious. In some illnesses, sleep is harmful; in others, it is helpful. If natural body heat prevails over abnormal humors, sleep will produce tranquility and subsidence of delirium.[4]

---

1. F. Rosner, *The Medical Aphorisms of Moses Maimonides* (Haifa: Maimonides Research Institute, 1989).
2. F. Rosner, *Moses Maimonides' Three Treatises on Health* (Haifa: Maimonides Research Institute, 1990).
3. F. Rosner, *Moses Maimonides' Treatise on Asthma* (Haifa: Maimonides Research Institute, 1994), pp. 84–90.
4. F. Rosner, *Maimonides' Commentary on the Aphorisms of Hippocrates* (Haifa: Maimonides Research Institute, 1987), pp. 43–44.

**SMELL**—In his *Guide for the Perplexed*, Maimonides describes the senses of hearing, sight, and smell—but not those of taste and touch—as being attributed to God (Part 1:47). He also finds fault with the senses since they cannot perceive some objects (e.g., we cannot smell at a distance) or may misapprehend an object (e.g., abnormal smell sensations) (Part 1:73).

In his *Medical Aphorisms*,[1] Maimonides quotes Galen, who said that a pleasant smell is beneficial to the body, equilibrates its faulty temperament, and strengthens the natural warmth (Chapter 3:75). Maimonides distinguishes living beings from plants in that the former have the five senses of touch, taste, smell, hearing, and sight (ibid., 7:73). Aromatic foods and medications are described throughout his medical writings. For example, malodorous spices and foods cause anorexia and produce body weakness, whereas fragrant-smelling ones strengthen the stomach (ibid., 9:51). Good odors, which strengthen the psychic power (appetite?) of a person, include hot aromatics like musk, amber, basilicon leaves, and others.[2]

[*See also* HEARING and TASTE]

---

1. F. Rosner, *The Medical Aphorisms of Moses Maimonides* (Haifa: Maimonides Research Institute, 1989).

2. F. Rosner, *Moses Maimonides' Three Treatises on Health* (Haifa: Maimonides Research Institute, 1990), p. 47.

**SNEEZING**—Quoting Galen, Maimonides writes that sneezing, in pleuritis, pneumonia, and other illnesses, is a favorable sign. Sneezing may abort hiccoughs that accompany abscesses of the liver. Sneezing sometimes indicates healing and recuperation, particularly if fluids had gathered in the lungs or stomach. However, patients with coryza are adversely affected by sneezing because the humors are still raw and withheld. Sneezing is beneficial for watery humors, but detrimental for bitter humors since it incites and increases them. Sneezing may be induced by instilling finely pulverized caraway mixed in oil into the nose, with the patient's head tilted as far back as possible.[1]

Elsewhere, Maimonides asserts that sneezing alleviates illnesses of the uterus because sneezing indicates the awakening of nature and its functional activities in evacuating harmful humors. Sneezing heals hiccoughs in a similar manner by eliminating excessive fluids. He also says that sneezing sometimes occurs when the brain is heated and the empty space within it becomes filled with humors and converts the humors to vapor. Sometimes air rises from below during coughing. When these vapors pass through the nasal passageways, they are the cause of sneezing.[2]

---

1. F. Rosner, *The Medical Aphorisms of Moses Maimonides* (Haifa: Maimonides Research Institute, 1989).

2. F. Rosner, *Maimonides' Commentary on the Aphorisms of Hippocrates* (Haifa: Maimonides Research Institute, 1987).

**SOTAH**—An entire treatise in Maimonides' *Mishneh Torah* (*Sotah*) deals with the procedures to be followed in the case of a suspected adulteress, or *sotah*. At the time of the Temple, if a man seriously suspected his wife of infidelity, he could subject her to the biblically described ordeal of jealousy. Following the destruction of the Temple, this procedure was abrogated.

The scriptural passage dealing with the ordeal of jealousy (Num. 5:11–31), including the drinking of the water of bitterness by a wayward woman or suspected adulteress, is the subject of lengthy discussion by the talmudic sages and biblical commentators. An entire tractate of the Talmud (*Sotah*) is devoted thereto. Briefly, the husband brings his wife to the priest (*kohen*), who places her before God. He then places holy water in an earthen vessel and adds to it some dust from the floor of the Temple. Then the priest uncovers the woman's head and charges her by an oath. The priest writes these curses on a scroll and blots them out in the water of bitterness, and then makes the woman drink the water. Then follows the offering. If the woman was defiled and had committed a trespass against her husband, the water of bitterness enters her and becomes bitter, her belly swells, her thighs fall, and she becomes a curse among her people. But if the woman is innocent, she remains unhurt and conceives seed from her husband.

Maimonides describes in detail the entire procedure for administering the bitter water to the wayward wife (*Sotah* 3:1ff), as well as the consequences if she was guilty of infidelity. Her face immediately turned pale, her eyes bulged, and her veins filled up. Then her belly became swollen, her thighs fell away, and finally she died (ibid., 3:16). The bitter water is compared to a dry drug that is placed upon living flesh: If there is a wound thereon the drug enters, but if there is no wound, the drug does nothing (ibid., 4:5).

Is it possible to rationally explain these signs and symptoms from a medical or scientific viewpoint? Maimonides, in *Mishneh Torah* (*Sotah* 4:3), and *Guide for the Perplexed* (3:46), refers to the fear and dread of the bitter water that might cause the *sotah* to refuse to drink at first. Most biblical and talmudic commentators consider the pallor of the face, the eye protrusion, the prominence of veins, the falling thighs, and the abdominal swelling to be miraculous occurrences by divine intervention.

**SOUL**—Maimonides' *Guide for the Perplexed* is replete with discussions of the soul. He states that the Hebrew word *nefesh* (soul) is a homonymous noun signifying the vitality that is common to all living sentient beings (Section 1:41). The word also denotes blood; reason; the part of human beings that remains after death; and, lastly, will (ibid.). The soul that remains after a person's death is not the soul that lives in him when he is born; the latter type is a mere faculty, whereas the former is a reality (ibid., 1:70). He further states that the Mutakallemim disagree about the soul, but that in the most predominant view, the soul is an accident existing in one of the atoms of which humans are composed. The aggregate is called a being endowed with a soul, insofar as it includes that atom (ibid., 1:73). The soul is immortal (ibid., 1:74). The souls of the pious are immortal in that the bodies of the pious enjoy everlasting happiness. Maimonides takes issue with this last part of the statement (ibid., 2:27). Later, he discusses evil-disposed persons and their evil souls (ibid., 3:12). The soul is that part of man over which the adversary (Satan, or Angel of Death?) has no power (ibid., 3:22). The object of the Torah is twofold: the well-being of the soul, and the well-being of the body (ibid., 3:26). The soul derives no benefit from the perfection of a person's possessions or the perfection of his body. It does benefit, however, from moral perfection—the highest degree of excellence in one's character—and from the true perfection of humans, which is the possession of the highest intellectual faculties leading to true metaphysical opinions regarding God (ibid., 3:54).

*SPASMS*—In his *Commentary on the Aphorisms of Hippocrates*,[1] Maimonides describes three types of spasms: extensor and flexor muscle spasms, and tetany, in which no cramps are visible because the extensors and flexors pull with equal force (Section 4:57). Spasms occur because of the overfilling or emptying of nerve organs (ibid.) or because of high fever that dries the nerves (ibid., 2:26 and 4:66). Spasms or convulsions from the ingestion of hellebore (veratrum alkaloid) may result in death (ibid., 5:1). Tetanus is probably the illness referred to in the fatal spasms resulting from wounds (ibid., 5:6). Spasms or cramps in the uterus may occur during menstruation (ibid., 5:56–57). Spasms may also occur in patients with quartan fever, and is due to overfilling with a bad humor (ibid., 5:70).

In his *Medical Aphorisms*,[2] Maimonides quotes Galen, who said that patients who develop convulsions or spasms following the ingestion of a potent laxative medication will die (Chapter 6:70). Certain illnesses are associated with cramps called spasms (ibid., 7:30). Spasms also result from overfilling or from emptying. If they are due to insomnia, physical exertion, anxiety, or a dry, burning fever, the cause is drying and emptying (ibid., 7:37). Maimonides points out the relationship between spasms and epileptic seizures, which he calls "neighbors" (ibid., 9:24). He defines spasm as the detrimental tightening of limbs (ibid., 23:22). It is not always clear from Maimonides' writings whether the word "spasms" refers to muscle cramps, tetany, or epileptic seizures. All three are obviously interrelated.

---

1. F. Rosner, *Maimonides' Commentary on the Aphorisms of Hippocrates* (Haifa: Maimonides Research Institute, 1987).

2. F. Rosner, *The Medical Aphorisms of Moses Maimonides* (Haifa: Maimonides Research Institute, 1989).

**SPLEEN**—Numerous references to the spleen occur in many of Maimonides' medical writings. The anatomical location of the spleen on the left side of the upper abdomen was known to Maimonides.[1] "Its parenchyma is loose, permeated and soft and resembles a sponge. It contains many large arteries. . . ." (Chapter 1:61) The spleen is said to purify the blood (ibid., 2:9). The red and black biles are attracted to the spleen (ibid., 2:34). The spleen becomes hard (abscess?) if a person neglects the red and black biles by ingesting viscous foods (ibid., 3:91). The best therapy for a hardened spleen consists of compresses prepared from caper roots, wormwood, vinegar, and honey (ibid., 9:77). Melancholy may develop because of an illness of the spleen (ibid., 9:79). Milk mixed with honey is harmful for the spleen (ibid., 21:17).

In his *Extracts from Galen*,[2] Maimonides says that if the spleen is ill, the patient should be phlebotomized from the veins of the left hand. Here he recommends vinegar-containing medicines to treat a hard tumor in the spleen. Quoting Galen in his *Treatise on Asthma*,[3] Maimonides asserts that wheat products cause hardening and enlargement of the spleen. In his *Commentary on the Aphorisms of Hippocrates*,[4] he states that if a patient with an enlarged spleen develops bloody diarrhea, he is expelling thick humors from the black bile that caused the disease of the spleen.

In his *Mishneh Torah* (*Maachalot Assurot* 6:9), he rules that it is permitted to cook the spleen even with meat, since it does not consist of forbidden blood, but is merely flesh that resembles blood. Absence of the spleen, compatible with life, does not render a priest unfit to serve in the Temple (*Biyat Mikdash* 6:7). The anatomy, functions, and illnesses of the spleen are discussed at length in the post-talmudic literature,[5] including the writings of Maimonides. Both surgical and medical splenectomy are described.

1. F. Rosner, *The Medical Aphorisms of Moses Maimonides* (Haifa: Maimonides Research Institute, 1989).

2. U.S. Barzel, *Maimonides' The Art of Cure. Extracts from Galen* (Haifa: Maimonides Research Institute, 1992).

3. F. Rosner, *Moses Maimonides' Treatise on Asthma* (Haifa: Maimonides Research Institute, 1994).

4. F. Rosner, *Maimonides' Commentary on the Aphorisms of Hippocrates* (Haifa: Maimonides Research Institute, 1987).

5. F. Rosner, "The Spleen," in *Medicine in the Bible and the Talmud,* augmented ed. (Hoboken, NJ, and New York: Ktav and Yeshiva University Press, 1995), pp. 102–106.

**SPONTANEOUS GENERATION** —Chapter 24 of Maimonides' *Medical Aphorisms,*[1] which is based mainly on the writings of Galen, deals with medical curiosities, strange occurrences, and unusual and rare happenings. One example is the statement that, following a complete solar eclipse in Sicily, women gave birth to bicephalic monsters. Another is the remarkable description of teratomas: "Abscesses that are called 'tumors' are found to be of varying types when cut open. Sometimes, objects resembling mud, urine, feces, honey, excrement, stone, teeth, and flesh are found therein. Sometimes one even finds living creatures therein that arise from putrefaction." The last sentence seems to indicate the belief in spontaneous generation, an accepted fact until Spallanzani disproved it in the eighteenth century. In his *Mishneh Torah* (*Shabbat* 11:3), Maimonides asserts that "lice originate in perspiration," another allusion to spontaneous generation.

In his *Mishnah Commentary* (*Chullin* 9:6), Maimonides comments as follows about a mouse thought to be generated from earth itself: "This mouse is said to be half flesh and half earth because it is generated [spontaneously] from the earth . . . many people told me they saw such a creature . . . it seems nearly impossible and there is no explanation for it."

The Talmud (*Betzah* 7a) speaks of chickens who lay eggs from the heat of the ground without copulating with male chickens. Based on another talmudic passage (*Shabbat* 107b), Rabbi Meir Simchah Hakohen of Dvinsk, in his biblical commentary known as *Meshech Chochmah* (Gen. 9:9–10), speaks of "creatures born from garbage and putrefaction." This statement is reminiscent of Maimonides' allusions to spontaneous generation.

1. F. Rosner, *The Medical Aphorisms of Moses Maimonides* (Haifa: Maimonides Research Institute, 1989), p. 385.

**SPURIOUS WORKS**—It is not surprising that many writers in medieval and modern times tried not only to emulate Maimonides, but even to attach his name to their own writings. Such is the case with several famous works, including the well-known and widely quoted "Prayer of Maimonides" for physicians, which was actually written by Marcus Herz in Germany in 1783. Other treatises also have been falsely attributed to Maimonides for a variety of reasons. These works are now available to the English-speaking world[1] and, although spurious, are important for those interested in medieval Judaism in general and Moses Maimonides in particular. It is also important to emphasize and demonstrate, once and for all, that works commonly spoken of as Maimonidean, such as the *Treatise on Eternal Bliss* (*Pirkei Hahatzlachah*), the *Book of Remedies* (*Sefer Refu'ot*), the *Gates of Moral Instruction* (*Sha'are Hamusar*), the *Scroll of the Unrevealed* (*Megillat Setarim*), and the *Letter to the Jews of Fez about the Messiah in Isfahan* are all medieval fabrications and were not written by Maimonides.

In addition to these, the *Treatise on the One Who Exists* (*Sefer Hanimtzah*), a small and somewhat obscure medial and moral work, provides telltale clues, such as flowery language, that set it apart from the plain, precise prose of Maimonides.[2] Finally, the *Nine Chapters on the Unity of God* (*Tisha Perakin Miyichud*) includes passages from the kabbalistic *Book of Creation*, which is never mentioned or alluded to in any Maimonidean work.

Particularly, certain letter combinations of the Divine Name and *gematria* concepts completely clash with ideas expressed by Maimonides in his *Guide for the Perplexed*. The *Nine Chapters* obviously was not written by Maimonides because the text is similar in style, content, and purpose to many other Jewish medieval writings that attempt to harmonize Greco-Arabic philosophy and *Kabbalah*. [*See also* PHYSICIAN'S PRAYER]

---

1. F. Rosner, *Six Treatises Attributed to Maimonides* (Northvale, NJ: Jason Aronson, 1991).

2. F. Rosner, *The Existence and Unity of God. Three Treatises Attributed to Moses Maimonides* (Northvale, NJ: Jason Aronson, 1990).

**SPUTUM**—In medieval times, cold, moist humors were called phlegm. White phlegm usually refers to sputum. In the introduction to his *Treatise on Asthma*,[1] Maimonides describes the symptoms of the Sultan, for whom the treatise was written, and his difficulty in expelling phlegm from his lungs. Maimonides prescribes a variety of remedies to loosen and liquefy the phlegm (Chapter 4:4 and 11:12), including certain potions composed of many ingredients (ibid., 12:3–5). Chicken soup is also recommended to assist in the expectoration of phlegm from the lungs (ibid., 12:6). In his *Regimen of Health*,[2] Maimonides suggests a vinegar-based concoction to liquefy sputum or white phlegm (Chapter 3:6).

In his *Medical Aphorisms*,[3] Maimonides quotes Galen, who said that in pleuritis one should first examine the sputum and then the urine (Chapter 5:1). Black (bloody?) sputum indicates a life-threatening condition (ibid., 6:23). Viscous sputum that collects in the chest may produce a serious cough (ibid., 65:41). Sputum is a cardinal sign of pleurisy and pneumonia (ibid., 6:44). Inability to expectorate sputum is due to its viscosity and its spread throughout the bronchial tree (ibid., 6:50). If one's sputum tastes salty like sea water, it indicates the presence of sores in the lung (ibid., 9:39). In his *Commentary on the Aphorisms of Hippocrates*,[4] Maimonides states that foul-smelling sputum is evidence of the putrefaction of the humors and is a poor prognostic sign (Section 5:11). [*See also* PLEURISY and PULMONOLOGY]

---

1. F. Rosner, *Moses Maimonides' Treatise on Asthma* (Haifa: Maimonides Research Institute, 1994).

2. F. Rosner, *Moses Maimonides' Three Treatises on Health* (Haifa: Maimonides Research Institute, 1990).

3. F. Rosner, *The Medical Aphorisms of Moses Maimonides* (Haifa: Maimonides Research Institute, 1989).

4. F. Rosner, *Maimonides' Commentary on the Aphorisms of Hippocrates* (Haifa: Maimonides Research Institute, 1987).

**STEINSCHNEIDER, MORITZ—** An Orientalist and bibliographer, Moritz Steinschneider (1816–1907) unearthed a wealth of data on the history of Jewish research in the sciences, including medicine. He compiled a complete bibliography of Hebrew literature in Latin at Oxford in his masterly *Catalogus Librorum Hebraeorum in Bibliotheca Bodleiana* (Berolini, 1852–1860). In Berlin, his literary output was unmatched and encyclopedic. A list of his writings in the *Steinschneider Festschrift* on his eightieth birthday (1896) occupies thirty-nine large pages of small print. He also edited twenty-one volumes of the *Hebraeische Bibliographe* (1858–1882). His articles in Hebrew, Italian, Dutch, French, English, and Latin appeared in all the scholarly journals of his day.[1] His important contributions to Maimonidean scholarship are listed by Dienstag.[2]

Among Steinschneider's translations and editions of Maimonides' medical writings are "The Introduction of Maimonides to His *Commentary on the Aphorisms of Hippocrates*" (*Zeitschrift der Deutschen Morgenlandischen Gesellschaft* 48 (1894): 218–234), "Maimonides' *Treatise on Poisons and their Antidotes*" (*Archiv fur Pathologische Anatomie und Physiologie*, 57 (1873):62–120) and "Maimonides Concerning Galen According to Zerachiah's Translation of Maimonides' Aphorisms" (M. Steinschneider,

*Al-Farabi, des Arabischen Philosophen, Leben, und Schriften* (St. Petersburg: 1869), pp. 230–238.

———————

1. J.I. Dienstag, "Translators and Editors of Maimonides' Medical Works: A Bio-bibliographical Survey," in J.O. Leibowitz, ed., *Memorial Volume in Honor of Prof. S. Muntner* (Jerusalem: Israel Institute of the History of Medicine, 1983), pp. 95–135.
2. J.I. Dienstag, "M. Steinschneider as Maimonidean Scholar," *Sinai*, 66 (1970):347–366 (Heb.).

rabbis in Provence (*Tzion*, 16 (5711–1951):18–29); and Maimonides' *Mishnah Commentary* (*Tarbitz* year 23, 2 (Tevet 5712–1952):72–88; ibid. year 27 (5718–1958):536–546; ibid. year 29, 2 (Nisan 5720–1960):261–267).

———————

1. J.I. Dienstag, "Translators and Editors of Maimonides' Medical Works: A Bio-bibliographical Survey," in J.O. Leibowitz, ed., *Memorial Volume in Honor of Prof. S. Muntner* (Jerusalem: Israel Institute of the History of Medicine, 1983), pp. 95–135.

*STERN, SAMUEL MIKLOS*—Born in Hungary and educated at the Hebrew University and Oxford, Orientalist Samuel M. Stern (1920–1969) served as secretary-general of the new edition of the *Encyclopedia of Islam*. A prolific writer, he published a variety of studies on Maimonides,[1] including several medical items in *Maimonides Commentarius in Mischnam* (vol. 3, Hafniae: Munksgaard, 1966, pp. 12–15, 15–17, 17–21, and 27–28); autographs of Maimonides in the Bodleian library (*Bodleian Library Record*, 5 (1954–1956):180–202); a review of G. Weil's edition of Maimonides' *Responsum on Longevity* (*Bulletin of the School of Oriental and African Studies*, 16 (1954):397–398); comments on Maimonides' attitude to music (*Hispano-Arabic Strophic Poetry*, Oxford: Clarendon Press, 1974, pp. 79–80); the exchange of letters between Maimonides and the

*STOMACH*—Extensive discussions are found about the stomach, its anatomy, physiology, disorders and remedies for them throughout Maimonides' medical writings. In his *Medical Aphorisms*,[1] where he extensively quotes Galen, Maimonides asserts that the stomach attracts nutrients from the liver by way of blood vessels (Chapter 1:51). When the stomach fills with food, its layers of skin extract the best therein and eliminate the rest (ibid., 1:57). He describes in detail the several stages of digestion and food assimilation (ibid., 1:58). White bile produced in the stomach becomes blood that ascends to the liver (ibid., 3:50). Bad humors at the mouth of the stomach may produce nausea (ibid., 9:55) or an irregular pulse (ibid., 4:19). An abscess of the stomach (ibid., 3:90) can be treated with wax plaster prepared with asparagus oil (ibid., 9:57). Maimonides states that one should constantly strengthen the stomach and avoid foods that are difficult to digest (ibid., 7:15). If food remains undigested in the stomach, pyrosis—and even a bloody abscess—may develop (ibid., 7:53). Epilepsy was erroneously thought to be due to stomach ailments (ibid., 9:43). Such ailments can be treated with light foods, emesis, laxatives and a variety of therapeutic concoctions such as hiera picra juice (ibid., 9:45–46). The stomach's expulsion of damaging substances or poorly digested food may eliminate dyspepsia and other symptoms (ibid., 23:80 and 23:95).

In his *Treatise on Asthma*,[2] Maimonides recommends that people eat only when the stomach is empty (Chapter 6:3). One should not drink much water during meals, but may do so two hours later (ibid., 7:3). Regular vomiting is recommended to maintain health and to eliminate stomach superfluities (ibid., 9:10). Weakness of the stomach is one of the results of excessive indulgence in coitus (ibid., 10:8). In his *Regimen on Health*, Maimonides again warns against overeating, and against eating at all unless the stomach is empty and one is hungry (Chapter 1:1ff). He describes remedies to strengthen the stomach (ibid., 3:8). One should not engage in sexual intercourse before the food is digested in the stomach, or when one is hungry, thirsty, or intoxicated (ibid., 4:9). He repeats the fact that stomach irritation (gastritis?) may develop from catarrhs descending into it (ibid., 4:12) and prescribes remedies to combat this ailment (ibid., 4:14). In another of his *Treatises on Health*,[3] Maimonides states that when the stomach is moist and weak, all three digestions suffer. He prescribes oxymel with quince juice and other concoctions to improve digestion. Additional references to the stomach are found in Maimonides' *Extracts from Galen*[4] and *Commentary on the Aphorisms of Hippocrates*.[5]

---

1. F. Rosner, *The Medical Aphorisms of Moses Maimonides* (Haifa: Maimonides Research Institute, 1989).

2. F. Rosner, *Moses Maimonides' Treatise on Asthma* (Haifa: Maimonides Research Institute, 1994).

3. F. Rosner, *Moses Maimonides' Three Treatises on Health* (Haifa: Maimonides Research Institute, 1990).

4. U.S. Barzel, *Maimonides' The Art of Cure. Extracts from Galen* (Haifa: Maimonides Research Institute, 1992).

5. F. Rosner, *Maimonides' Commentary on the Aphorisms of Hippocrates* (Haifa: Maimonides Research Institute, 1987).

**STOOLS**—In his *Medical Aphorisms*,[1] Maimonides quotes Galen, who says that normal digestion results in the excretion of normal solid stool in an amount commensurate with food intake (Chapter 6:73). He then describes numerous abnormalities of the stools, including dry, soft, or bulky stools (ibid., 6:74–76). Bloody stool is a sign of weakness of the liver (ibid., 6:78). Melena, or black stool, is dangerous to life (ibid., 6:23). Stools of various colors and odors and their significance are also described (ibid., 6:80–84). Fatty or foamy stools are indicative of certain pathophysiological conditions (ibid., 6:85–86). For colitis associated with watery stools, the treatment is an enema of dust water or of water and honey (ibid., 15:45). To remain healthy, one should strive for slightly soft stools and no constipation (ibid., 17–19). Elderly people should soften their stools with a confection of prunes cooked in honey prior to meals (ibid., 17:32).

In his *Mishneh Torah* (*Deot* 4:113), Maimonides also recommends that "man should always strive to have his intestines relaxed all the days of his life [based on the Talmud, *Ketubot* 10b] and his stools should be soft. A fundamental principle in medicine is that whenever the stool is withheld or is extruded with difficulty, grave illnesses result." The recommendation to regulate one's stools is again made by Maimonides in his *Treatise on Asthma*,[2] where he devotes the entire twelfth chapter to regimens for retention and evacuation of body wastes. Various clues to illness from an examination of the color, consistency, odor, and other characteristics of the stools are discussed in Maimonides' *Commentary on the*

*Aphorisms of Hippocrates.*[3] [*See also* CONSTIPATION and DIARRHEA]

1. F. Rosner, *The Medical Aphorisms of Moses Maimonides* (Haifa: Maimonides Research Institute, 1989).
2. F. Rosner, *Moses Maimonides' Treatise on Asthma* (Haifa: Maimonides Research Institute, 1992).
3. F. Rosner, *Maimonides' Commentary on the Aphorisms of Hippocrates* (Haifa: Maimonides Research Institute, 1987).

**STRANGURY**—Strangury refers to slow and painful urination that is due to spasm of the urethra and bladder, often because of prostatic enlargement. In his *Commentary on the Aphorisms of Hippocrates*,[1] Maimonides criticizes Hippocrates for stating that certain illnesses, including strangury, occur in association with a paucity of rain (Section 3:16). Although there may be a relationship between meteorology and medicine (the talmudic tractate *Yebamot* 62b relates that Rabbi Akiba's disciples died of *askara* only during the summer), strangury is not affected by the climate. Rather, claims Maimonides, strangury occurs because of weakness of the bladder or because of a stinging urine. Inflammation in the rectum or uterus may also produce strangury (Section 5:58). Drinking wine or alcohol is beneficial for strangury, but venesection is contraindicated (ibid., 7:48). [*See also* UROLOGY]

1. F. Rosner, *Maimonides' Commentary on the Aphorisms of Hippocrates* (Haifa: Maimonides Research Institute, 1987).

*SUCTION CUPS*—Suction cups to draw out pus or blood were used throughout antiquity and the Middle Ages. In his *Medical Aphorisms*,[1] Maimonides quotes Galen, who said that suction cups should be applied for discharges from the roots of the ears if medications fail (Chapter 3:85). Suction cups are one of the most powerful therapeutic measures to extract that which is in the depths of the body and to uproot chronic abscesses (ibid., 3:106). Applying a suction cup over the orbit prevents bad humors from pouring into the eye (ibid., 3:107 and 12:43). The idea that rapid alleviation of rheumatic pains by the application of large suction cups is a type of magical therapy was rejected by reputable physicians who used them frequently (ibid., 8:37). Suction cups without heat scarification of the skin are beneficial because they allow the "pneuma" to exit through the skin without obstructing the pores (ibid., 8:54). To treat severe epistaxis, suction cups were applied below the loins and resulted in cessation of bleeding (ibid., 9:2). If not, the cups were applied to the nape of the neck together with cold compresses to the head (ibid., 9:5). Suction cups were also applied at the site of a poisonous animal bite to suck out the poison (ibid., 9:119).

In his *Regimen of Health*,[2] Maimonides lists the removal of blood by cupping among the mild remedies for such people in general when a physician is not available (Chapter 2:7).

1. F. Rosner, *The Medical Aphorisms of Moses Maimonides* (Haifa: Maimonides Research Institute, 1989).
2. F. Rosner, *Moses Maimonides' Three Treatises on Health* (Haifa: Maimonides Research Institute, 1990).

*SUICIDE*—Judaism regards suicide as a criminal act that is strictly forbidden by Jewish law. The cases of suicide in the Bible, as well as those in the Apocrypha, Talmud, and *Midrash*, took place under unusual and extenuating conditions.[1]

In general, a suicide is not accorded full burial honors. The Talmud and codes of Jewish law decree that rending one's garments, delivering memorial addresses, and other rites of mourning, which are an honor for the dead, are not to be performed for a suicide victim. The strict definition of a suicide to which these laws apply is one who had previously announced his intentions and then killed himself immediately thereafter by the method he announced. Children are never regarded as deliberate suicides, and are afforded all burial rites. Similarly, those who commit suicide under extreme physical or mental strain, or while not in full possession of their faculties, or in order to atone for past sins are not considered as willful suicides, and none of the burial and mourning rites are withheld.

In his *Mishneh Torah*, Maimonides states:

> For one who has committed suicide intentionally we do not occupy ourselves at all with the funeral rites, and we do not mourn for him nor eulogize him. However, we do stand in a row for him, and we recite the mourner's benediction, and we do all that is intended as a matter of honor for the living (*Avel* 1:11).

Maimonides then defines an intentional suicide exactly as defined in the Talmud (*Semachot* 2:2). The commentators on Maimonides' code—Rabbi David ben Zimra, known as Radvaz; Rabbi Joseph Karo, known as Keseph Mishneh; and Rabbi Abraham Boton, known as Lechem Mishneh—all point out that Maimonides considers mourning an honor for the dead and therefore prohibited for intentional suicides.

The aforementioned considerations may condone the numerous acts of suicide and martyrdom committed by Jews throughout the centuries, from the priests who leaped into the flames of the burning Temple to the martyred Jews in the time of the Crusades; from the Jewish suicides during the medieval persecutions to the martyred Jews in more recent pogroms. Only for the sanctification of the name of the Lord should a Jew ever intentionally take his own life or allow it to be taken as a symbol of his extreme faith in God. Otherwise, intentional suicide is strictly forbidden because it constitutes a denial of the divine creation of the human being, the immortality of the soul, and the atonement of death.

---

1. F. Rosner, "Suicide in Jewish Law," *Journal of Psychology and Judaism*, 18 (1994):283–297.

**SUNSTROKE**—In his *Medical Aphorisms*,[1] Maimonides quotes Galen, who said that fever and shivering are classic signs of sunstroke (Chapter 7:45). The treatment of choice is bathing followed by the pouring of cooled oil of roses on the patient's head (ibid., 19:35). The same recommendation is found in Maimonides' *Extracts from Galen*,[2] where he says that the head of a patient afflicted with fever because of sunburn should be made to sweat with cooling oils after the bath (p. 101). Several cases of sunstroke are also described in the Bible and the Talmud.[3]

---

1. F. Rosner, *Moses Maimonides' Treatise on Asthma* (Haifa: Maimonides Research Institute, 1994).

2. U.S. Barzel, *Maimonides' The Art of Cure. Extracts from Galen* (Haifa: Maimonides Research Institute, 1992).
3. F. Rosner, *Medicine in the Bible and the Talmud*, 2nd ed. (Hoboken, NJ: Ktav and Yeshiva University Press, 1995), pp. 65–68.

*SURGERY*—Chapter 15 of Maimonides' *Medical Aphorisms* deals with surgery[1] and contains many modern concepts. The principles of sterilization and cauterization are outlined when Maimonides cautions against infecting open wounds. The recognition of gangrene and the necessity for surgical intervention are pointed out. Early cure of cancer by wide excision is advocated. The surgical approach to varicose veins, nasal polyps, peritonsillar abscess, various tumors, and a variety of other conditions is described. For effective hemostasis, Maimonides advocates the application of ligatures to bleeding vessels. Incision and drainage of abscesses is described. The final several aphorisms are devoted exclusively to orthopedics. Splinting of fractures, cast application, positioning of limbs, and healing time are all described.

Maimonides disapproves of surgery for hemorrhoids.[2] He mentions the surgical reconstruction of the prepuce by some Jews during times of persecution.[3] He also describes the surgical procedures for closure of abdominal wounds and the treatment of bone fractures.[4]

1. F. Rosner and S. Muntner, "The Surgical Aphorisms of Moses Maimonides," *American Journal of Surgery*, 119 (1970):718–725.
2. F. Rosner, *Maimonides' Treatises on Poisons, Hemorrhoids and Cohabitation* (Haifa: Maimonides Research Institute, 1984), pp. 117–152.
3. F. Rosner, *Medicine in the Mishneh Torah of Maimonides* (New York: Ktav, 1984), p. 264.
4. U.S. Barzel, *Maimonides' The Art of Cure. Extracts from Galen* (Haifa: Maimonides Research Institute, 1992), pp. 75ff.

*SYNCOPE*—In his *Medical Aphorisms*,[1] Maimonides is strongly critical of Galen's description of the causes of syncope, saying that it is disorganized and incomplete. Since syncope is a very serious occurrence that may herald death or a prefatal condition, Maimonides asserts that it is important for the physician to know all its causes, how to prevent it, and how to treat it (Chapter 7:8). Syncope represents the loss of the essential powers of the body as well as the spirit of life, owing to abnormalities in one or more major organs (heart, brain, liver) or an alteration of humors or the spirits of life (respiration?) (ibid., 7:10). The causes of syncope constitute six groups and twenty-one types (ibid., 7:14). The term "syncope" includes not only fainting, but shock and collapse from acute or chronic illnesses; high fever; ingestion of a poison or bite of a poisonous snake; severe pain;

insomnia; lack of food; excessive diarrhea; and other conditions (ibid.). To prevent syncope, one must maintain the health of the major organs and their function and equilibrate the spiritual, physical, and natural pneumas (ibid., 7:15). One must avoid eating detrimental foods and ensure proper digestion and bowel function (ibid.).

The treatment of syncope depends on its cause. If it is due to "red bile that pours into the stomach," the patient should be given cold, spiced dilute wine to drink (ibid., 9:49) or an emetic oil (ibid., 14:4). If it is due to a respiratory disorder, the patient should be nourished with foods such as barley bread, pureed groats, and egg yolks (ibid., 9:116). Syncope from excess sweating in a bath is very detrimental to one's health (ibid., 19:4). In his *Treatise on Asthma*,[2] Maimonides states that constant eructation and heartburn may lead to syncope (Chapter 5:3). Excessive bloodletting may also produce fainting (ibid., 13:10 and 13:33). In his *Regimen of Health*,[3] Maimonides warns against sleeping in a bath lest the person faint (p. 83). In his *Causes of Symptoms,* he asserts that people with hot temperaments may suffer from heart palpitations and fainting (p. 141). In the twelfth chapter of his *Extracts from Galen*,[4] Maimonides confirms the treatment for fainting to be the administration of aromatic wine to the patient to drink. He also discusses strong pain, sleeplessness, excessive voiding, and strenuous exercise as reasons for fainting.

1. F. Rosner, *The Medical Aphorisms of Moses Maimonides* (Haifa: Maimonides Research Institute, 1989).

2. F. Rosner, *Moses Maimonides' Treatise on Asthma* (Haifa: Maimonides Research Institute, 1994).

3. F. Rosner, *Moses Maimonides' Three Treatises on Health* (Haifa: Maimonides Research Institute, 1990).

4. U.S. Barzel, *Maimonides' The Art of Cure. Extracts from Galen* (Haifa: Maimonides Research Institute, 1992).

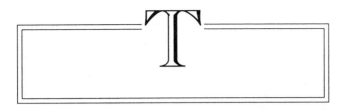

**TASTE**—In his *Treatise on Poisons,*[1] Maimonides describes the senses of taste, smell, and sight. Regarding taste, he states that an item may be considered extremely sweet by one person and extremely bitter by another. To one person, it is pleasant and sweet; another person cannot taste it without suffering extreme discomfort because to him it tastes bitter or acrid. All people know that colocynth tastes bitter, but it is tasty to swine, who eat it with avidity. The same situation pertains to different types of odors; an object can emit an odor that is pleasant to one person or animal, but offensive to another. The pleasantness of taste and the goodness of an odor depend upon the constitution of the species of living creature. When something is appropriate for a particular constitution, it tastes sweet and has a pleasant odor. Maimonides warns against consuming bitter, acrid, or sharp-tasting foods, and certainly those with altered or abnormal tastes, lest these foods contain harmful substances or ingredients.

In his philosophical work *Guide for the Perplexed,* Maimonides asserts that the senses of hearing, sight, and smell are attributed to God, but not those of taste and touch, which "act only when in close contact with the object" (Section 1:47). He further posits that "the senses are not always to be trusted" (ibid., 1:73).

In his *Medical Aphorisms,*[2] he quotes Galen, who said that the sensation of taste and the sense of touch in the tongue come from the same cranial nerve. In spite of this, taste may be lost without loss of the tongue's touch sensation because taste has more widespread and sensitive functions (Chapter 1:45). The tongue transfers the taste of a food from that food to the humors concealed in the tongue (ibid., 7:70). Bad-tasting foods prevent proper digestion (ibid., 20:5). Sweet-tasting food is especially nourishing, although tasteless foods may also be nourishing (ibid., 20:64). Finally, the following citation from Galen concerning therapeutic foods and medications speaks for itself:

Four tastes indicate [that a therapy is] warming in its effect and they are: sweetness which is the least warming, after which is saltiness, and then bitterness and finally sharpness which is the strongest. The tastes which indicate [that a remedy is] cooling are also four and these are: tastelessness which is the least cooling, after which is sourness, followed by astringency, and finally ponticity. An oily taste signifies an intermediate quality between warming and cooling (ibid., 21:56).

[*See also* SMELL and HEARING]

1. F. Rosner, *Maimonides' Treatises on Poisons, Hemorrhoids and Cohabitation* (Haifa: Maimonides Research Institute, 1984), pp. 77–81.
2. F. Rosner, *The Medical Aphorisms of Moses Maimonides* (Haifa: Maimonides Research Institute, 1989).

**TESTICLES**—In his *Medical Aphorisms*,[1] Maimonides quotes Galen, who said that the blood vessels that supply the testicles and the breasts come from distant sites to prolong the mixing of blood until the semen and milk are thoroughly ripe (Chapter 1:4). Testicles have only small nerves (ibid., 3:62). The right testicle and the right womb are said by Galen to have more warmth than the left, and that therefore male fetuses develop on the right side and females on the left (ibid., 3:39). Maimonides ridicules this assertion by saying that a man has to be a prophet or a logical

deducer to make such an unusual assertion. Testicles of fat chickens are said to be very tasty and to provide good nourishment (ibid., 20:22a). The therapeutic efficacy of chicken soup is discussed elsewhere in this encyclopedia. Hydrocele, or water in the scrotum surrounding the testicles, is clearly discussed in this work (ibid., 23:57) and in Maimonides' *Extracts from Galen*.[2]

1. F. Rosner, *The Medical Aphorisms of Moses Maimonides* (Haifa: Maimonides Research Institute, 1989).
2. U.S. Barzel, *Maimonides' The Art of Cure. Extracts from Galen* (Haifa: Maimonides Research Institute, 1992), p. 174.

**THIRST**—In his *Regimen of Health*,[1] Maimonides advises a person to drink water only when truly thirsty. The drinking of water immediately after a meal is harmful to digestion, except for someone accustomed thereto (Chapter 1:4). In his *Mishneh Torah* (*Deot* 4:2), he rules that when the food begins to be digested in the intestines, one may drink as much water as necessary. However, even after the food has been digested, one should not imbibe water excessively. The Talmud (*Niddah* 24b) states that he who takes in more drink than food undermines his health. On the other hand, the Talmud also states that he who eats without drinking—his food is like blood and causes intestinal ailments (*Shabbat* 41a), and that he who softens his food with water does not develop intestinal ailments (*Berachot* 40a). In his *Regimen of Health*, Maimonides also recommends that one be careful not to drink cold water immediately after leaving the bath. Rather, one should tolerate thirst until the body cools off and then drink water. If he cannot wait, because of severe thirst, he should mix the water with lemon peel, mastic, or rose syrup (Chapter 4:11).

In his *Medical Aphorisms*,[2] Maimonides quotes Galen, who seems to be describing diabetes mellitus and the extreme thirst that may occur in such patients (Chapter 6:9). [*See* DIABETES.] Severe thirst may be an indication of other serious illnesses (ibid., 6:71), often in association with shivering (ibid., 7:46) and abnormal bad temperaments (humors) in the stomach or pylorus, or in the esophagus, the lung, or even the kidney, which are then transferred to the stomach, thus strengthening the thirst (ibid., 7:57).

tongue (Chapter 1:15) and its arteries, veins, and nerves (ibid., 1:22). The tongue is an unpaired organ, like the brain and the womb (ibid., 1:21). The tongue is the organ of taste (ibid., 1:45 and 7:70). A coated or colored tongue may be a sign of illness of the stomach or lungs (ibid., 6:19). Movement of the tongue is mediated by the seventh pair of cranial nerves (ibid., 6:36). Below the root of the tongue are the larynx, the vocal cords, and the esophagus (ibid., 23:76). The tongue was lacerated as punishment for people who spoke crookedly and excessively, thereby inflicting harm (ibid., 24:57). A growth on the tongue resembling a black ricinus plant kernel may signify a fatal disease (ibid., 6:24). Tumors of the tongue are also discussed in Maimonides' *Extracts from Galen*.[2] Also described is a man with a markedly swollen tongue who was cured by drinking a concoction prepared with aloe, scammony, and colocynth and by holding lettuce in his mouth (p. 171).

1. F. Rosner, *Moses Maimonides' Three Treatises on Health* (Haifa: Maimonides Research Institute, 1990).

2. F. Rosner, *The Medical Aphorisms of Moses Maimonides* (Haifa: Maimonides Research Institute, 1989).

1. F. Rosner, *The Medical Aphorisms of Moses Maimonides* (Haifa: Maimonides Research Institute, 1989).

2. U.S. Barzel, *Maimonides' The Art of Cure. Extracts from Galen* (Haifa: Maimonides Research Institute, 1992).

**TONGUE**—In his *Medical Aphorisms*,[1] Maimonides quotes Galen, who describes the muscles of the

**TREATISE ON ASTHMA**—Maimonides' *Treatise on Asthma*[1] was written for a member of the Sultan's family who suffered from violent headaches that prevented him from wearing a turban. The patient's symptoms began with a common cold, especially in the rainy season, forcing him to gasp for air until phlegm was expelled. The patient asked whether a change of climate would be beneficial. Maimonides, in thirteen chapters, explains the rules of diet and climate in general and those rules specifically suited for asthmatics. He outlines the recipes of food and drugs and describes the various climates of the Middle East. He states that the dry Egyptian climate is efficacious for sufferers from this disease, and he warns against the use of very powerful remedies.

In the introduction of this book, Maimonides praises his benefactor for having asked him to write the book. Maimonides points out that asthma should be treated according to the various causes that bring it about. He further states that one can manage the disease properly only with thorough knowledge of the patient's constitution and his individual organs, the age and habits of the patient, the season, and the climate. Maimonides asserts that in this book he intends to include general principles that may be useful to all people to preserve their health and to prevent disease. He discusses hygienic principles relating to clean air; correct eating and drinking; regulation of the emotions; exercise and rest; sleep and wakefulness; excretion or retention of wastes; bathing and massage; and appropriate indulgence in sexual intercourse.

Maimonides' logical and systematic approach to the prevention, diagnosis, and treatment of illness is typical of all his medical and other writings. One should note his allusions to psychosomatic medicine and his discussion of iatrogenic disease, seemingly modern concepts. His teachings that a bad physician is worse than none, that one should treat patients and not diseases, and that *primum non nocere* (first do no harm), among others, should be taken to heart by all students of medicine and medical practitioners.

---

1. F. Rosner, *Moses Maimonides' Treatise on Asthma* (Haifa: Maimonides Research Institute, 1994).

### TREATISE ON HEMORRHOIDS

—Maimonides wrote a short *Treatise on Hemorrhoids*[1] in which he provides an insight into the etiology of disease in general, in that he regards operative excision of hemorrhoids with skepticism because surgery may not remove the underlying cause that produced the hemorrhoids. He first describes the three phases of digestion (cephalic, gastric, and intestinal), which the science of physiology has clarified only in the last century. Maimonides' systematic approach to a healthy dietary regimen, including the quantity and quality of ingested food, the sequence and timing of its consumption, water consumption, and physical exercise, is reminiscent of his preventive-medicine recommendations in *Mishneh Torah* (*Deot*) and his *Treatise on Health*.[2]

He then describes the pathology, pathogenesis, and types of hemorrhoids. The medieval concept of the four humors (black bile, yellow bile, blood, and phlegm) is apparent. Black bile is considered to be the cause of hemorrhoids in most instances. The theory is geared to eliminate the excess black bile by bloodletting, various foods, or specific remedies such as oral decoctions, cataplasms, syrups, pills, oils, ointments, suppositories, and fumigation.

The *Supplement* concludes the *Treatise on Hemorrhoids* and puts the entire treatise into perspective regarding its purpose and significance. Maimonides concludes, as he began, with a short prayer to Almighty God, a feature noted throughout his medical works and indicative of his deep religious convictions. This concern perhaps contributed to his enormous success as a physician.

1. F. Rosner, *Maimonides' Treatises on Poisons, Hemorrhoids and Cohabitation* (Haifa: Maimonides Research Institute, 1984), pp. 117–152.

2. F. Rosner, *Moses Maimonides' Three Treatises on Health* (Haifa: Maimonides Research Institute, 1990).

**TREATISE ON POISONS AND THEIR ANTIDOTES**—One of Maimonides' ten authentic medical essays and books[1] is his *Treatise on Poisons and Their Antidotes*,[2] which was written at the request of the Vizier al-Fadhil, who asked Maimonides to import costly remedies lacking in Egypt for the preparation of the two famous poisoning antidotes, the Great Theriac and the Electuary of Mithridates. The Vizier also asked Maimonides to write a short treatise on the treatment of poisoning by venomous animals before the arrival of a physician. The first section of the treatise deals with the bites of snakes and mad dogs and the stings of scorpions, bees, wasps, and spiders. The description of the emergency care for a victim of a snakebite is as up-to-date as any modern textbook on toxicology or poisoning. He prescribes a variety of local measures and medications for treating venomous bites or stings.

The *Treatise on Poisons* show Maimonides to be a scientist who did not abide by medical dogma, but experimented for himself or accepted valid investigations of others. His originality, conciseness, and lucidity are reflected in every chapter.[3] His recommendations in the twelfth century concerning first aid for poisonings still have much validity. For this reason, Maimonides' *Tractatus De Venemis* was considered to be one of the foremost textbooks of toxicology and therapeutics throughout Europe and the Near East in the Middle Ages. The age-old adage, "An ounce of prevention is worth a pound of cure," is evident from Maimonides' emphasis on preventive or prophylactic measures. Perhaps most interesting of all in this work is the distinction he makes between "hot" and "cold" poisons, which may be equivalent to the modern hemolysins and neurotoxins. Neurotoxins, or "cold poisons," are exemplified by the scorpion's poison, which "cools" and paralyzes the victim's respiratory center with fatal outcome. Hemolysins, or "hot" poisons, are found in adder's poison; they produce hemorrhage, intravascular hemolysis, hypertension, fever, and death.

---

1. F. Rosner, "The Medical Writings of Moses Maimonides," *New York State Journal of Medicine*, 87 (1987):656–661.
2. F. Rosner, "Moses Maimonides' Treatise on Poisons," *New York State Journal of Medicine*, 80 (1980):1627–1630.
3. F. Rosner, *Maimonides' Treatises on Poisons, Hemorrhoids and Cohabitation* (Haifa: Maimonides Research Institute, 1984), pp. 19–115.

### TREATISE ON SEXUAL INTERCOURSE—Maimonides' short *Treatise on Sexual Intercourse* was written at the request of the nephew of Saladin the Great, the Sultan al-Muzaffar Omar Ibn Nur ad-Din. The Sultan,

who indulged heavily in sexual activities, asked Maimonides, his physician, to help him to increase his sexual potential. The work consists mainly of recipes of foods and drugs that are either aphrodisiac or antiaphrodisiac in their actions. Maimonides advises moderation in sexual intercourse, and describes the physiology of sexual temperaments. As in several of his other medical works, Maimonides begins by showering praises upon the Sultan, and ends the treatise with another flowery expression of praise.

There exists an additional longer work with an identical title—*Treatise on Sexual Intercourse*—that was erroneously attributed to Maimonides by such renowned scholars as Steinschneider and Kroner. Kroner considered this longer work as the unabridged version of the smaller authentic work. This error was perpetuated until Muntner proved the spurious nature of the longer work.[1]
[*See also* SEX ETHICS]

---

1. F. Rosner, *Maimonides' Treatises on Poisons, Hemorrhoids and Cohabitation* (Haifa: Maimonides Research Institute, 1984), pp. 153–182.

### TREATISES ON HEALTH—Maimonides wrote the *Regimen of Health* (*Regimen Sanitatis*) in 1198, during the first year of the reign of Sultan al-Malik al-Afdal, eldest son of Saladin

the Great. The Sultan was a frivolous and pleasure-seeking man of thirty, subject to fits of melancholy or depression owing to his excessive indulgences in wine and women and to his warlike adventures against his own relatives and in the Crusades. He complained to his physician of constipation, dejection, bad thoughts, and indigestion. Maimonides answered his royal patient in four chapters. The first chapter is a brief abstract on diet taken mostly from Hippocrates and Galen. The second chapter deals with advice on hygiene, diet, and drugs in the absence of a physician. The third, and extremely important, chapter contains Maimonides' concept of "a healthy mind in a healthy body," one of the earliest descriptions of psychosomatic medicine. He indicates that the physical well-being of a person is dependent on his mental well-being, and vice versa. The final chapter summarizes his prescriptions relating to crime, domicile, occupation, bathing, sex, wine-drinking, diet, and respiratory infections.

The whole treatise on the *Regimen of Health* is short and concise, but to the point. This is the whole reason for its great success and popularity throughout the years. The scientific value of the treatise is supported by many quotations in medieval Hebrew literature and in the frequent Latin editions beginning with the Florence incunabulum of 1481. During the Middle Ages, the *Regimen of Health* served as a textbook in academies and universities.

The *Regimen of Health* shows Maimonides not only as a scholar and physician, but also as a healer of the mind, comforting and encouraging those who turn to him for help. It is a mark of his greatness that, while treating his sovereign with all the honor and respect due to him and expressing fervent prayers and hope for his speedy recovery, he does not hesitate to condemn, in an indirect manner, the Sultan's overindulgences in wine and women, his gluttony, and his lusts. Physical and mental well-being are interdependent, teaches Maimonides. A healthy person is cheerful and content, while a sick one is always depressed and dissatisfied. Complete recovery can be furthered, therefore, by strengthening the patient's moral convictions through study of the moral exhortations of the prophets and philosophers leading the patient to regulate his life accordingly. Peace of mind, even in adverse circumstances, is an essential requisite for the well-being of the soul. The acceptance with humility and gratitude of the good fortunes and favors of life, as well as its miseries and tribulations, is part of the teachings of all great religions.

Another treatise on health written by Maimonides is his *Causes of Symptoms*.[1] This work has been called Maimonides' swan song; it was thought to be the last of his medical works, having been written in the year 1200, four years before his death. It was also written for the Sultan al-Malik al-Afdal, and is sometimes considered to represent Chapter 5 of the *Regimen of Health*. The Sultan persisted in his overindulgences and wrote to Maimonides, who was himself ill, asking advice about his health. Maimonides confirms most of the prescriptions of the Sultan's other physicians regarding wine, laxatives, bathing, exercise, and the like, and, near the end, gives a very detailed hour-by-hour regimen for the daily life of the Sultan.

In this treatise, Maimonides assumes the role of the medical arbiter, pronouncing judgment on the views of his fellow physicians. He does it in all humility toward the Sultan who asked his advice, and toward God, the King of Kings, the Lord of his conscience. Viewed in the light of contemporary medical art, Maimonides' judgment is generally sound. He stresses the medical approach in his desire to serve his Sultan wholeheartedly; for many years, he knew what ailed the Sultan better than anybody else.

A third treatise on health composed by Maimonides appears as Chapter 4 of *Hilchot Deot* in his *Mishneh Torah*.[2] This chapter deals with a variety of hygienic and medical prescriptions for healthy living and for the prevention of illness. Among the many subjects discussed are normal bodily excretory functions; recommended times for eating; amounts and types of food to be consumed; beverage consumption; exercise; sleep habits; cathartics; climatic and weather effects on eating habits; detrimental and beneficial foods; fruits, meats, vegetables; bathing; bloodletting; sexual intercourse; and domicile. The other chapters of this treatise are just as interesting, and deal with recommended moral traits and ethical standards of practice for which a person should strive. All three of these treatises on health have been published in a single volume.[3]

1. J.O. Leibowitz and S. Marcus, *Moses Maimonides on the Causes of Symptoms* (Berkeley: University of California, 1974).

2. F. Rosner, *Medicine in the Mishnah Torah of Maimonides* (New York: Ktav, 1984), pp. 69–107.

3. F. Rosner, *Moses Maimonides' Three Treatises on Health* (Haifa: Maimonides Research Institute, 1990).

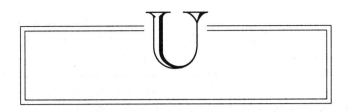

ULCERS—In his *Commentary on the Aphorisms of Hippocrates*,[1] Maimonides writes that suckling babes may develop mouth ulcers (stomatitis or aphthous ulcers) because of the softness of their limbs and mouth dryness related to the milk they drink (Section 3:24). Foul-smelling urine indicates an ulcer in the urinary bladder (ibid., 4:81). Aggressive, spreading ulcers cause loss of adjacent hair and skin (ibid., 6:4). A chronic skin ulcer that suppurates may affect the underlying bone, causing osteomyelitis and bone sequestration (ibid., 6:45). In his *Medical Aphorisms*,[2] Maimonides provides a lengthy list of remedies helpful for all ulcers that arise anywhere in the body (Chapter 9:88). Intestinal ulcerations are not always fatal, especially if only one of the two intestinal membranes is affected (ibid., 9:90). Malignant ulcers that become infected require medications with sharpness, like that of fire, that should be placed in the central crater (literally "fireplace") of the ulcer (ibid., 15:9). If the border of an ulcer

changes its appearance or becomes indurated, the ulcer should be totally excised up to healthy flesh (ibid., 15:43). Finally, Maimonides quotes Galen, who describes the differences between benign, malignant, and phagadenic ulcers (ibid., 23:44).

---

1. F. Rosner, *Maimonides' Commentary on the Aphorisms of Hippocrates* (Haifa: Maimonides Research Institute, 1987).
2. F. Rosner, *The Medical Aphorisms of Moses Maimonides* (Haifa: Maimonides Research Institute, 1989).

UROLOGY—Maimonides was knowledgeable about the anatomy and pathophysiology of the urinary tract.[1] In his medical works, he describes two kidneys from which urine passes through the "two vessels" (ureters) into the "reservoir" (urinary bladder), where it is kept until the sphincter relaxes and the urine is excreted through the urethra. He also describes the testicles, the scrotum, the penis, and the uterus. In his *Mishneh Torah* (*Shechitah*

8:26), he describes diseases and defects in animals, including very small kidneys, which are possibly due to end-stage renal disease or chronic nephritis.

Maimonides accurately describes the symptoms of lower-urinary-tract obstruction, including hesitancy, a narrow stream, dripping, and urinary retention. He distinguishes between urinary retention in the elderly (which is due perhaps to prostatic hypertrophy) and anuria, a condition in which "no urine reaches the reservoir because the kidneys cease to function." He also speaks of patients who discharge copious amounts of thick white urine (pus or pyuria?) or who urinate blood. Fat in the urine, he asserts, is evidence of dissolution of the kidneys. Strangury occurs because of weakness of the bladder or sharpness of the urine. A tear in the bladder or kidneys is not always fatal. Maimonides speaks of bladder stones and describes renal colic, calculi, and abscesses. Kidney disease is present if the patient micturates rusty, thin urine.

Maimonides usually advocates conservative management of genitourinary ailments, with the exception of renal abscesses, for which he advises early surgery to evacuate the pus. He states that radish juice cleanses the kidneys and bladder and that diuresis should be induced not in healthy people, but only in patients with certain illnesses. Catheters or tubes to collect urine from the bladder are described. Some kidney sicknesses are treated by bloodletting.

In Maimonides' major medical work, his *Medical Aphorisms*,[2] the entire fifth chapter is devoted to the examination of the urine in health and in disease. He seems to allude to hemoglobinuria when he writes that ". . . every urine which is black in extremely dangerous. I have never seen anyone who urinated black urine who survived. . . ." The final aphorism in this chapter is a concise outline by Maimonides of Galen's views on the four basic types of urine.

---

1. F. Rosner, "Nephrology and Urinalysis in the Writings of Moses Maimonides," *American Journal of Kidney Diseases*, 24 (1994):222–227.

2. F. Rosner, *The Medical Aphorisms of Moses Maimonides* (Haifa: Maimonides Research Institute, 1989), pp. 72–77.

**UTERUS**—In his *Medical Aphorisms*,[1] Maimonides quotes Galen, who says that the womb is an unpaired but double organ (Chapter 1:21). It has a neck—the uterine cervix—and is located adjacent to the urinary bladder (ibid., 1:65). It is attached to the spine on both sides with ligaments, which prevents it from prolapsing (ibid., 3:33). The breasts and the uterus share common arteries and veins in order to perform their unique function in human reproduction (ibid., 3:40). Sores or abscesses in the uterus were treated with intravaginal clysters (ibid., 13: 39) or by phlebotomy (ibid., 16:13). Spasms of the uterus occur if menses are withheld and the uterus becomes filled with blood and its ligaments stretched (ibid., 16:16). Intravaginal suppositories may alleviate the situation (ibid., 16:19). During pregnancy, the uterus protrudes through the abdomen (ibid., 16:21). If a woman is pregnant with twins and one of her breasts shrivels, she will abort one of her fetuses (ibid., 16:26). The cervix uteri is closed during pregnancy until a woman is ready to give birth (ibid., 16:29). Extra "flesh that sometimes arises within the womb" may refer to fibroid tumors or to a hydatid mole (ibid., 23:97). Eclampsia also seems to be described (ibid., 24:58).

In his *Commentary on the Aphorisms of Hippocrates*,[2] Maimonides repeats the assertion that a pregnant woman whose breasts suddenly shrink in size will abort her fetus because of the known partnership between the breasts and the uterus (Section 5:37). Infection in the uterus (endometritis) in a pregnant woman can be fatal to both mother and fetus (ibid., 5:43). Maimonides describes the anatomy of the uterus with its long neck and the opening or cervical os at the end of the neck (ibid., 5:46). He also discusses various abnormalities of the uterus that may affect a woman's ability to become pregnant (ibid., 5:62). In his *Extracts from Galen*,[3] Maimonides discusses instruments for the treatment of various uterine diseases (p. 60) by inserting medications directly into the uterus (p. 63). Hectic fever can occur in association with uterine disease (p. 120). Some uterine sicknesses are treated by bloodletting (p. 157). Uterine tumors are also mentioned (p. 155).

---

1. F. Rosner, *The Medical Aphorisms of Moses Maimonides* (Haifa: Maimonides Research Institute, 1989).

2. F. Rosner, *Maimonides' Commentary on the Aphorisms of Hippocrates* (Haifa: Maimonides Research Institute, 1987).

3. U.S. Barzel, *Maimonides' The Art of Cure. Extracts from Galen* (Haifa: Maimonides Research Institute, 1992).

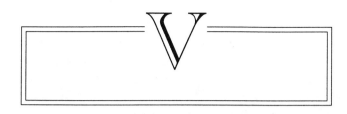

VEGETABLES—The preparation, storage, and nutritive value of certain vegetables is discussed by Maimonides in his *Mishneh Torah*.[1] In his *Medical Aphorisms*,[2] he quotes Galen, who said that most vegetables are of little nutritional value and usually weaken the body (Chapter 20:46). Horseradish is a vegetable that cools without damaging the body. Rhubarb is between bad and good; after it is corchorus, and then wormwood, bliton, and portulaca (ibid., 20:47). Among the chyme-thinning vegetables are garlic; onion; watercress; leek; mustard; mountain celery; fennel; mints; inula; satureia; caraway; seseli; garden rocket; celery; lettuce; basilicon; radish; cabbage; and senna (ibid., 20:49).

In his *Treatise on Asthma*,[3] Maimonides describes the virtues and detriments of a variety of vegetables for this disease. Efficacious for asthmatics are fennel, parsley, mint, pennyroyal, origanum, watercress, and radish, whereas lettuce, pumpkin, cauliflower, and turnip are harmful.

[*See also* specific vegetables and NUTRITION and FOODS AND BEVERAGES]

1. F. Rosner, *Medicine in the Mishneh Torah of Maimonides* (New York: Ktav, 1984), pp. 251–253.
2. F. Rosner, *The Medical Aphorisms of Moses Maimonides* (Haifa: Maimonides Research Institute, 1989).
3. F. Rosner, *Moses Maimonides' Treatise on Asthma* (Haifa: Maimonides Research Institute, 1994), pp. 52–57.

VEINS—In his *Medical Aphorisms*,[1] Maimonides quotes Galen, who describes veins as nonpulsating vessels (Chapter 1:3). Whereas arterial movements can be sensed, those of veins cannot (ibid., 1:49). Phlebitis or inflammation in veins causes a unique stretching-type pain (ibid., 6:62). The vena cava connects to the liver (ibid., 7:54). Venesection is performed from the popliteal or saphenous veins (ibid., 12:28), the basilic vein (ibid., 12:29), or the median antecubital veins (ibid., 12:33). The jugular vein should be used only as a last resort (ibid.). In his *Extracts from Galen*,[2] Maimonides discusses phlebotomy for the treatment of liver tumors and recommends "the basilic vein, the inside vein of the right arm, which is connected with the vena cava. . . . If you do not find this vein, bleed the median vein . . . [or] the cephalic vein" (Chapter 13). To ensure hemostatis following bleeding that is due to a severed vein, in addition to local pressure, olibanum and aloe mixture is applied and serves as a glue (ibid., 5). [*See also* ARTERIES]

1. F. Rosner, *The Medical Aphorisms of Moses Maimonides* (Haifa: Maimonides Research Institute, 1989).

2. U.S. Barzel, *Maimonides' The Art of Cure. Extracts from Galen* (Haifa: Maimonides Research Institute, 1992).

**VERTIGO**—Maimonides quotes Hippocrates,[1] who said that vertigo, headache, and apoplexy are illnesses that occur during the winter (Chapter 3: 23) and mostly in old people (ibid., 3:31). Maimonides defines vertigo as a condition in which the patient feels as if everything is spinning around and he suddenly loses his sense of vision (ibid., 4:17). In his *Medical Aphorisms*,[2] he quotes Galen, who said that a patient with vertigo may vomit from the slightest stimulus and that vertigo may be due to a stomach ailment (Chapter 5:34) or cessation of the excretion of superfluities from the brain

(ibid., 9:3). Vertigo is also known as scotodinia (ibid., 9:25). Pressure in the pit of the stomach may result in vertigo (ibid., 9:44). Patients with vertigo are sometimes benefited by bloodletting from the pulsating arteries behind the ears (ibid., 15:14). Dizziness is produced when the head becomes filled with gases (ibid., 20:26).

1. F. Rosner, *Maimonides' Commentary on the Aphorisms of Hippocrates* (Haifa: Maimonides Research Institute, 1987).

2. F. Rosner, *The Medical Aphorisms of Moses Maimonides* (Haifa: Maimonides Research Institute, 1989).

**VETERINARY MEDICINE**—In his *Mishneh Torah*, Maimonides reviews animal anatomy, physiology, and pathology; lists seventy physical defects in animals that render them *terefah*, or nonviable; and discusses other animal and bird disorders, diseases, and defects.[1] For example, he discusses compound fractures, removal of the liver, very small kidneys, plethora, and a variety of other topics related to veterinary medicine. He also describes a variety of routine practices related to animals, such as the tying of a leather pouch to the male organ of rams to prevent their copulating with ewes (*Shabbat* 20:12), and the leather shields tied over rams' hearts to protect them against attacks by wolves. He also cites the prohibition of intentionally mating two different species of animals (*Kilayim* 9:1).

In his *Mishnah Commentary*, Maimonides also writes about the anatomy and pathology of animals.[2] He states that fractured ribs in an animal may not kill it, but a ruptured spleen is incompatible with life (*Chullin* 3:1). He describes the carotid arteries as "the pulsating vessels in the neck on the two sides of the windpipe" (ibid., 2:1). He describes simple and compound fractures of birds' legs and broken wings.

---

1. F. Rosner, *Medicine in the Mishneh Torah of Maimonides* (New York: Ktav, 1984), pp. 229–238.
2. F. Rosner, "Medicine in Moses Maimonides' Commentary on the Mishnah," *Koroth*, 9 (1988):565–578.

*VINEGAR*—In his *Treatises on Health*,[1] Maimonides repeatedly describes vinegar as an important ingredient in a variety of therapeutic concoctions. A mixture of honey and vinegar is known as oxymel syrup. If raisins are added, it is a very efficacious remedy and protects and preserves the liver, since vinegar alone may damage the liver. He recommends that the Sultan eat dishes sweet to the taste or that have only a little sourness, such as foods prepared with a little vinegar. Oxymel is very effective in fortifying the stomach and the heart, in improving digestion, and in widening the spirit. It also helps to evacuate wastes.

He says that he and others have tested it many times. In his *Mishneh Torah* (*Deot* 4:8), Maimonides asserts that in the warm summer months one should eat cooling foods, refrain from using seasoning to excess, and consume vinegar. The Talmud (*Shabbat* 111b) also states that vinegar is good on a hot day.

In his *Treatise on Asthma*,[2] Maimonides reiterates the harmful effects of vinegar on the liver. He recommends vinegar, however, in a variety of therapies for asthma. He personally used one of these therapies to cleanse his stomach of phlegm. In his *Medical Aphorisms*,[3] he quotes Galen, who said that a liquid mixture of vinegar and honey is effective therapy for a child with epilepsy (Chapter 9:13) and for patients with hardened spleens (ibid., 9:77–78). Vinegar is also useful with oil of roses for cerebral illnesses (ibid., 21:19). Vinegar damages the womb and other organs richly endowed with nerves (ibid., 21:20). Oxymel has a variety of medicinal uses (ibid., 21:21–27). When wine putrefies, it turns into vinegar (ibid., 23:109). Further references to vinegar and its therapeutic uses are found in Maimonides' *Extracts from Galen*.[4]

---

1. F. Rosner, *Moses Maimonides' Three Treatises on Health* (Haifa: Maimonides Research Institute, 1990).
2. F. Rosner, *Moses Maimonides' Treatise on Asthma* (Haifa: Maimonides Research Institute, 1994), pp. 59–61 and 83.

3. F. Rosner, *The Medical Aphorisms of Moses Maimonides* (Haifa: Maimonides Research Institute, 1989).

4. U.S. Barzel, *Maimonides' The Art of Cure. Extracts from Galen* (Haifa: Maimonides Research Institute, 1992).

**VIRGINITY**—In his *Mishneh Torah*, Maimonides defines a virgin as one who has never had a menstrual flow, even if she had a discharge of blood because of marital intercourse or childbirth (*Issurei Biyah* 9:5). An old woman is one who has had no flow for ninety days at a time adjacent to her old age. When does her old age set in? When she no longer resents being called an old woman (ibid.).

A minor girl three years old or less who has had sexual intercourse with an adult male eventually recovers her virginity and becomes like other virgins (*Eeshut* 11:3). The intercourse of a minor boy who is nine years old or less is not regarded as effective intercourse, whereas if he is nine years and one day old or over, it is (ibid.). A minor boy should not be given in marriage until he is examined and is found to exhibit the tokens of puberty (ibid., 11:6). Although a minor girl may eventually contract full marriage for herself, the sages instituted marriage for her to prevent her from being used wantonly (ibid.).

The case of disputed virginity is discussed by Maimonides in some detail (ibid., 11:12). Maimonides recognized that starvation or certain illnesses may produce amenorrhea, and that there may be genetic or anatomical causes for failure to bleed—i.e., absent hymen.

Defamation of a virgin girl by falsely accusing her of unchastity is punishable by a fine and lashes (*Naarah Betulah* 3:1). If the girl is found guilty as charged, she is liable to be put to death (ibid., 3:2). Defamation is defined in detail (ibid., 3:6). The proof of a woman's virginity should consist of testimony in court, not an actual display of the garment (Deut. 22:17) to prove the tokens of virginity. The scriptural statement is a euphemism, because these matters are of an intimate nature (*Naarah Betulah* 3:12).

**VISITING THE SICK**—Every Jew is required to visit the sick, for God visits the sick and we must emulate Him. This general rule is based on: "You shall walk after the Lord your God" (Deut. 13:5). Since this command is clearly impossible to fulfill literally, the reference is to our obligation to try to emulate His attributes. Just as He visited the sick (Gen. 18:1), so, too, should we (*Sotah* 14a). Some well-known cases of visiting the sick are recorded in the Bible.[1]

In his *Mishneh Torah* (*Avel* 14:1ff) Maimonides deals with duties characterized as deeds of lovingkindness, such as visiting the sick, comforting mourners, joining a funeral procession, dowering a bride, escorting departing guests, and the like. Maimonides asserts that it is a commandment upon everyone to visit the sick. Even a prominent person should visit a less important person. One should visit the sick many times each day; the more often, the more praiseworthy, provided that the patient is not bothered thereby. He who visits the sick is as if he would take away part of his sickness and make it lighter for him (ibid., 14:4).

Judaism views visiting the sick as more than just a social obligation—it is a commandment. The visit itself also entails more than paying a social call. Since there were no hospitals in biblical and talmudic times, a person who visited a sick friend or relative was expected to provide for the physical and emotional needs of the patient. In addition to cheering up the patient and giving him the courage to recover, the visitor would cook, clean, and perform other needed tasks. Furthermore, Jewish law requires that the visitor pray for the recovery of the patient, as codified by Maimonides (ibid., 14:6). These activities are all essential components of visiting the sick and are applicable to this day.

---

1. F. Rosner, "Visiting the Sick (*Bikkur Cholim*)," in *Medicine in the Bible and the Talmud*, augmented ed. (Hoboken, NJ: Ktav and Yeshiva University Press, 1995), pp. 176–181.

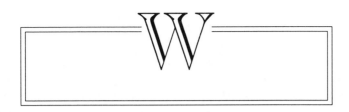

**WATER**—Chapter 7 of Maimonides' *Treatise on Asthma*[1] is devoted to beverages. He recommends that water be sweet, clear, and pure, boiled a little, and drunk from a clean vessel after it cools off. The best time to drink water is about two hours after eating. If imbibed with food, it counteracts it and impedes digestion. A water-and-honey mixture is described as an emetic (Chapter 12:10). In his *Regimen of Health*,[2] Maimonides repeats the danger of drinking a lot of water during a meal (Chapter 1:1). One should not drink water unless one is truly thirsty (ibid., 1:4). He discusses the temperature of bathwater, from cold to tepid to hot (ibid., 4:11). For some people, drinking a lot of water is harmful, but for others, it is a remedy to loosen the bowels and combat a fever (ibid., 4:8).

A similar statement is found in Maimonides' *Medical Aphorisms*,[3] where the drinking of cold water is recommended for febrile patients (Chapter 8:22 and 8:24). Drinking cold water before meals is said to be harmful to the food and the liver (ibid., 20:32). The best drinking water is pure, clear rainwater that has no perceptible taste or odor (ibid., 20:35 and 20:38). Drinking water on an empty stomach stimulates thirst, weakens the body, produces gurgitation, and has other detrimental effects, all of which can be avoided if the water is mixed with oxymel (ibid., 21:7). Maimonides erroneously suggests that diabetes is caused by drinking the suave waters of the River Nile (ibid., 8:69). Numerous references to water are also found in Maimonides' *Extracts from Galen*.[4] In his legal code, the *Mishneh Torah*, he rules that one may not bathe in purgative water on the Sabbath (*Shabbat* 21:29); one may not drink from a water pipe or drink at night from rivers, ponds, or water left uncovered overnight (*Rotzeach* 11:6–7), because of possible danger. He also describes the drinking of the water of bitterness in the case of a suspected adulteress (*Sotah* 3:1ff), as prescribed in the Bible (Num. 5:11–

31). Finally, his medical advice about drinking only water when one is thirsty and not during meals, except a little mixed with wine, is codified in his *Mishneh Torah* (*Deot* 4:1–2) in a lengthy chapter dealing exclusively with a regimen of life that all people should follow to remain healthy.

1. F. Rosner, *Moses Maimonides' Treatise on Asthma* (Haifa: Maimonides Research Institute, 1994).

2. F. Rosner, *Moses Maimonides' Three Treatises on Health* (Haifa: Maimonides Research Institute, 1990).

3. F. Rosner, *The Medical Aphorisms of Moses Maimonides* (Haifa: Maimonides Research Institute, 1989).

4. U.S. Barzel, *Maimonides' The Art of Cure. Extracts from Galen* (Haifa: Maimonides Research Institute, 1992).

**WEIL, GOTTHOLD**—An Orientalist and Semitic philologue, Gotthold Weil (1882–1960) was the chief librarian at the National and Hebrew University Library in Jerusalem. He edited and published Maimonides' *Responsum on Longevity* in its original Arabic, accompanied by an introduction and German translation.[1] It has since been translated into English by Fred Rosner.[2]

1. G. Weil, *Maimonides. Uber die Lebensdauer* (Basel and New York: S. Karger, 1953), pp. 1–59.

2. F. Rosner, "Moses Maimonides' Responsum on Longevity," *Geriatrics,* 23 (1968):170–178.

**WHEAT**—In his *Treatise on Asthma,*[1] Maimonides points out that food prepared from well-sifted wheat flour is very nourishing, but may be difficult to digest (Chapter 3:1). For the maintenance of normal stools, wheat bran soaked in water, cooked and strained with a little oil, is an effective enema (ibid., 9:7). An effective oral remedy for asthmatics is almonds and licorice soaked with wheat bran and cooked (ibid., 12:2). This and other remedies cleanse the lungs and facilitate breathing. In his *Extracts from Galen,*[2] Maimonides describes a hemostatic medication prepared from cooked resins, crushed wheat flour, and gypsum (Chapter 5). To treat hectic fever in a patient with a hot constitution, one should use barley groats or spelt wheat to which a little vinegar is added (Chapters 8, 10, and 12). In his *Glossary of Drug Names,*[3] Maimonides describes "edible lichen" (drug no. 69), which signifies wheat kernel, and may be identical to the biblical manna. He also lists *sawiq,* which is "wheat, barley, and other similar roasted cereals, agitated with butter and then ground" (drug no. 284). Another drug called *handarus* refers to grains of wheat or spelt, coarsely ground or crushed, and also to the wheat flower itself (drug no. 389). In his *Regimen of Health,*[4] Maimonides says that bread made from fully ripened wheat whose moisture is dried out is very nutritious (Chapter 1:6). Finally, in his *Mishneh Torah* (*Berachot* 2:1ff), he cites wheat, barley, spelt, oats, and rye as the five types of grain, products of which require the recitation of certain blessings.

_____

1. F. Rosner, *Moses Maimonides' Treatise on Asthma* (Haifa: Maimonides Research Institute, 1994).
2. U.S. Barzel, *Maimonides' The Art of Cure. Extracts from Galen* (Haifa: Maimonides Research Institute, 1992).
3. F. Rosner, *Moses Maimonides' Glossary of Drug Names* (Haifa: Maimonides Research Institute, 1995).
4. F. Rosner, *Moses Maimonides' Three Treatises on Health* (Haifa: Maimonides Research Institute, 1990).

**WINE**—In the Talmud, the rabbis considered that wine taken in moderation induces appetite and is beneficial to health (*Berachot* 35b) and "gladdens the heart" (Psalms 104:15). Wine is the greatest of all medicines; where wine is lacking, drugs are necessary (*Baba Batra* 58b). Old wine benefits the intestines, whereas ordinary wine may do harm (*Berachot* 51a). Rabbi Eleazar suggested that old wine was among the good things that Joseph sent to his aging father (*Megillah* 16b).

In his *Medical Aphorisms*, Maimonides also speaks of the value and beneficial effects of wine.[1]

Wine mixed with cold water sometimes tranquilizes a fainting spell which occurs following a strong evacuation (*Aphorisms* 8:34). People suffering from a strong midline headache or the like, secondary to thick blood or internal coldness, are overtly benefited by drinking undiluted wine . . . by the warming effect of the wine and its thinning [of the blood] . . . (ibid., 9:4). Wine diluted with an equivalent amount of water is beneficial . . . since it neutralizes bad liquids and warms the stomach, aids digestion, dissolves cold gases, and helps to combat shivering . . . (ibid., 9:42). It is appropriate to give anyone who develops syncope a drink of spiced wine (ibid., 9:49). Wine to which an equal quantity of water has been added warms the entire body and stimulates all limbs to more rapid movement. It also improves or moistens the liquids of the body and eliminates the bad thereof (ibid., 20:24). . . .

Most of Maimonides' statements in his medical aphorisms concerning wine are based upon statements made by Greek medical writers, including Galen and Hippocrates. Other assertions about the benefits of wine are found throughout Maimonides' other medical writings, including his *Treatise on Asthma*,[2] his *Treatise on Poisons and Their Antidotes*,[3] his *Extracts from Galen*,[4] and his *Treatises on Health*.[5] Since these treatises were written for one or more members of the royal family of Sultan Saladin the Great of Egypt, who were Moslems to whom wine was religiously proscribed, Maimonides offered a substitute of a nonalcoholic honey drink.

In his *Mishneh Torah*, Maimonides also extols the virtue of wine in his treatise on human temperaments (*Deot* 4:1ff). He also mentions wine in other parts of his *Code*. For example, he points out that fasting and funeral eulogies are forbidden on festivals (*Yom Tov* 6:17). One must rejoice and, together with one's family, be of cheerful heart. Children are given roasted seeds, nuts, and other dainties. Women should have pretty clothes and trinkets, and men should eat meat and drink wine (ibid., 6:18). However, one should not overindulge in wine, merriment, and frivolity, for drunkenness, excessive merrymaking, and frivolity are not rejoicing, but madness and folly (ibid., 6:20). Feasting on Purim (*Megillah* 2:14) and rejoicing on Chanukah (*Chanukah* 3:3) are religious duties. Purim is the only occasion in Judaism when one is told to drink wine until it overcomes him and makes him sleep (*Megillah* 2:15). A special headnet was used to amuse drinkers of strong drink (*Kelim* 27:151). For some people, new wine is bad for the stomach, whereas aged wine is good for the stomach (*Nedarim* 8:7).

Based on a talmudic discussion (*Sanhedrin* 43a) describing the value of alcohol as an analgesic, Maimonides codifies the rule that, prior to being led out to execution, a condemned person is given a cup of wine containing a grain of frankincense to benumb his senses or to induce a state of stupor, and only then he is executed by the mode of death prescribed for the offense of which he is guilty (*Sanhedrin* 13:2). The commentaries explain that benumbing of the senses is an act of compassion to minimize or eliminate the anxiety of the accused during the execution. The Talmud has a similar pronouncement (*Semachot* 2:9).

In his *Guide for the Perplexed* (3:48), Maimonides writes that the object of Naziritism (Num. 6:1ff) is to keep a person away from wine, which has ruined people in ancient and modern times. Many strong men have been slain by it, and priests and prophets have erred through wine (Isaiah 28:7).

1. F. Rosner, *The Medical Aphorisms of Moses Maimonides* (Haifa: Maimonides Research Institute, 1989).

2. F. Rosner, *Moses Maimonides' Treatise on Asthma* (Haifa: Maimonides Research Institute, 1994).

3. F. Rosner, *Maimonides' Treatises on Poisons, Hemorrhoids and Cohabitation* (Haifa: Maimonides Research Institute, 1984), pp. 19–115.

4. U.S. Barzel, *Maimonides' The Art of Cure. Extracts from Galen* (Haifa: Maimonides Research Institute, 1992).

5. F. Rosner, *Moses Maimonides' Three Treatises on Health* (Haifa: Maimonides Research Institute, 1990).

**WINTERNITZ, DAVID**—David Winternitz was a nineteenth-century physician in Prague.[1] He translated Maimonides' *Regimen of Health* into German (Vienna: Braumüller and Seidel, 1843, 64 pp.).

1. J.I. Dienstag, "Translators and Editors of Maimonides' Medical Works: A Bio-bibliographical Survey," in J.O. Leibowitz, ed., *Memorial Volume in Honor of Prof. S. Muntner* (Jerusalem: Israel Institute of the History of Medicine, 1983), pp. 95–135.

**WORMS**—In his *Medical Aphorisms*,[1] Maimonides quotes Galen, who describes three types of abdominal worms—one found in the small intestine, the second in the large intestine, and the third in the perianal region (Chapter 9:93). Worms that resemble gourd grains or cucumbers (ascaris?) consume all that an individual has eaten, thus making the body slender (ibid., 7:31). Intestinal worms can be eliminated by killing them with bitter medicines; if they die, they come out with the excrement.[2] Small worms (oxyuris?) and large worms (trematodes, ascaris, taenia?) are also cited.[3]

In his *Mishneh Torah* (*Maachalot Assurot* 2:17), Maimonides speaks of worms found in the entrails of fish or in animal brains or flesh. It is not clear which types of worms are meant—ascaris, fish tapeworm, or other worms. [*See also* ABDOMEN]

1. F. Rosner, *The Medical Aphorisms of Moses Maimonides* (Haifa: Maimonides Research Institute, 1989).

2. U.S. Barzel, *Maimonides' The Art of Cure. Extracts from Galen* (Haifa: Maimonides Research Institute, 1992), p. 29.

3. F. Rosner, *Maimonides' Commentary on the Aphorisms of Hippocrates* (Haifa: Maimonides Research Institute, 1987), p. 85.

**WOUNDS**—An entire treatise of Maimonides' legal code, the *Mishneh Torah* is devoted to wounds and damages and deals with cases of assault and damages. The treatise begins with the assertion that if one wounds another, he must pay compensation to him for five effects of injury: damages, pain, medical treatment, enforced idleness (i.e., loss of employment), and humiliation (*Chovel Umazik* 1:1). Maimonides explains that the scriptural passage "an eye for an eye" (Exod. 21:24 and Lev. 24:20) represents payments of monetary compensation, and is not to be interpreted literally (*Chovel Umazik* 1:2). The assessments or estimations of pain (ibid., 2:9–10), enforced idleness (ibid., 2:11), medical treatment (ibid., 2:14), and humiliation (ibid., 3:1ff) are precisely defined. For example, the assessment of humiliation depends in part on the relative status of the one who caused the humiliation and the one who was humiliated (ibid., 3:1). The prohibition of assault includes self-wounding (ibid., 5:1) and wife-beating (ibid., 4:16). One is also forbidden to wound one's father or mother (ibid., 4:7). An interesting difference between personal injury and property damage is the following: If one damages another's property, atonement is effected for him as soon as he pays what is required. But if one wounds another person, atonement is not effected for him even if he has paid for all five effects of the injury, until he begs forgiveness of the injured person and is pardoned (ibid., 5:9). Forgiveness is a virtue in that whoever forgives quickly is praiseworthy, and his behavior meets with the approval of the sages (ibid., 5:10).

Elsewhere in his *Mishneh Torah*, Maimonides rules that any internal wound is regarded as dangerous to life, and that the Sabbath may be violated for the patient without hesitation (*Shabbat* 2:5). In his *Medical Aphorisms*,[1] Maimonides quotes Galen, who said that internal wounds not associated with abscess formation heal rapidly with constricting medications (Chapter 9:89). Some wounds

should be left open to heal (ibid., 15:17), whereas others should be sutured and bandaged (ibid., 15:37) with the application of binding medications (ibid., 15:56). The treatment of wounds is discussed in some detail in Maimonides' *Extracts from Galen*.[2] For example, he states that in an abdominal wound, the intestine can be returned to the cavity and the peritoneum closed before the skin is sutured. The remainder of his description of wound care and healing and the treatment of simple fractures, hemorrhage, and injuries enhances his stature as a teacher and observant and careful practitioner of medicine.

---

1. F. Rosner, *The Medical Aphorisms of Moses Maimonides* (Haifa: Maimonides Research Institute, 1989).

2. U.S. Barzel, *Maimonides' The Art of Cure. Extracts from Galen* (Haifa: Maimonides Research Institute, 1992).

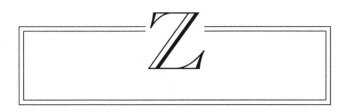

**ZERACHIAH, BEN ISAAC BEN
SHEALTIEL**—A philosopher, physician, and translator, thirteenth-century Zerachiah was a native of Spain, but lived most of his life in Italy. He wrote important philosophical and theological commentaries on the Book of Job and the Book of Proverbs in the spirit of Maimonides' *Guide for the Perplexed*. He also wrote commentaries on the Pentateuch and the *Guide*, which remain unpublished.[1] Zerachiah translated from the original Arabic into Hebrew Maimonides' *Medical Aphorisms*, Maimonides' *Treatise on Sexual Intercourse*, and Maimonides' *Treatise on Poisons*, all of which were edited, annotated, and published by Suessman Muntner.

---

1. J.I. Dienstag, "Translators and Editors of Maimonides' Medical Works: A Bio-bibliographical Survey," in J.O. Leibowitz, ed., *Memorial Volume in Honor of Prof. S. Muntner* (Jerusalem: Israel Institute of the History of Medicine, 1983), pp. 95–135.

# INDEX

# ABOUT THE AUTHOR

Dr. Fred Rosner is Director of the Department of Medicine of the Mount Sinai Services at the Queens Hospital Center and Professor of Medicine at New York's Mount Sinai School of Medicine. Dr. Rosner is an internationally known authority on medical ethics and has lectured widely on Jewish medical ethics. He is the author of five widely acclaimed books on Jewish medical ethics, including *Modern Medicine and Jewish Ethics* and *Medicine and Jewish Law*. These books are up-to-date examinations of the Jewish view on many important bioethical issues in medical practice. Dr. Rosner is also a noted Maimonidean scholar and has translated and published in English most of Maimonides' medical writings.